Cambridge History of Medicine
Editors: CHARLES WEBSTER and CHARLES ROSENBERG

The colonial disease

T0283699

The Belgians commonly referred to their colonisation of the Congo as a 'civilising mission', and many regarded the introduction of Western biomedicine as a central feature of their 'gift' to Africans. By 1930, however, it was clear that some features of their 'civilising mission' were in fact closely connected to the poor health of many of the Congolese. The Europeans had indeed brought scientific enquiry and Western biomedicine; but they had also introduced a harsh, repressive political system which, coupled with a ruthlessly exploitative economic system, led to the introduction of new diseases, while already existing diseases were exacerbated and spread.

Tropical, or 'colonial', medicine was a new field at the turn of the century, linked closely both to European expansionism and human trypanosomiasis, or sleeping sickness. In 1901 a devastating epidemic had erupted in Uganda, killing well over 250,000 people by 1905. Over the next decades other African colonies, including the Belgian Congo, experienced epidemic sleeping sickness. By the 1960s and independence, many Africans had come to regard sleeping sickness as the 'colonial disease' because of the truly draconian measures taken by some colonial administrations in their attempts to check the spread of the disease. Sleeping sickness captured the colonial imagination to such an extent that it continued to dominate medical attention for many years. As a consequence, other glaring public health needs of the Congolese were ignored over decades.

Cambridge History of Medicine

Editors

CHARLES WEBSTER, *All Souls College, Oxford*

CHARLES ROSENBERG, *Professor of History and the Sociology of Science, University of Pennsylvania*

The colonial disease

A social history of sleeping sickness in
northern Zaire, 1900–1940

Maryinez Lyons
Institute of Commonwealth Studies, University of London

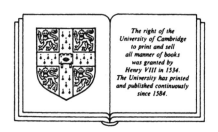

The right of the
University of Cambridge
to print and sell
all manner of books
was granted by
Henry VIII in 1534.
The University has printed
and published continuously
since 1584.

Cambridge University Press
Cambridge
New York   Port Chester   Melbourne   Sydney

PUBLISHED BY THE PRESS SYNDICATE OF THE UNIVERSITY OF CAMBRIDGE
The Pitt Building, Trumpington Street, Cambridge, United Kingdom

CAMBRIDGE UNIVERSITY PRESS
The Edinburgh Building, Cambridge CB2 2RU, UK
40 West 20th Street, New York NY 10011–4211, USA
477 Williamstown Road, Port Melbourne, VIC 3207, Australia
Ruiz de Alarcón 13, 28014 Madrid, Spain
Dock House, The Waterfront, Cape Town 8001, South Africa

http://www.cambridge.org

© Cambridge University Press 1992

First published 1992
First paperback edition 2002

A catalogue record for this book is available from the British Library

Library of Congress Cataloguing in Publication data
Lyons, Maryinez.
The colonial disease: a social history of sleeping sickness in
northern Zaire, 1900–1940 / Maryinez Lyons.
        p.   cm. – (Cambridge history of medicine)
Revision of the author's thesis.
Includes bibliographical references.
Includes index.
ISBN 0 521 40350 2 (hardback)
1. African trypanosomiasis – Zaire – History.   2. Social medicine –
Zaire – History.   I. Series.
[DNLM: 1. Trypanosomiasis, African – epidemiology – Zaire.
2. Trypanosomiasis, African – history. WC 705 L991c]
RA644.T69L96   1992
614.5'33'0096751–dc20   91-192   CIP
DNLM/DLC
for Library of Congress

ISBN 0 521 40350 2 hardback
ISBN 0 521 52452 0 paperback

Contents

Maps

Plates

Tables

Preface

In revising my Ph.D. thesis for publication, I have tried to draw out the relevance of the study to public health issues in Africa today. While I do not concur with the view that history is prescriptive, I do believe there is much that can be learned from the past which can be of help with present-day issues. The history of medicine and public health in Africa, particularly during this century, can assist greatly in understanding some of the issues and problems confronting health workers today. The histories of epidemics, such as those of sleeping sickness, are especially helpful, highlighting as they do a broad spectrum of issues ranging from purely medical ones to political and economic considerations. In this way, the history of sleeping sickness in a region of colonial Belgian Congo, now known as Zaire, has an importance reaching far beyond the confines of African history but is of relevance also to the wider history of health in the developing world. The present epidemic of AIDS has once again reminded us of the complexities involved in monitoring health on a global scale as well as those involved when attempting to intervene in the highly sensitive and deeply entrenched cultural realm of human responses to disease. As I discuss in this volume, the declaration of an epidemic is very much a political act, but not as widely recognised are the political aspects of public health programmes. This topic has been much discussed in the media in connection with AIDS in Africa and I hope that my study of sleeping sickness in early colonial Zaire will contribute to a broader understanding of the issues involved in public health programmes in the developing world.

A large number of individuals and institutions were of enormous assistance in the preparation of this study, too many to name each one. First and foremost, I want to thank Professor Jan Vansina of the University of Wisconsin for his excellent advice and guidance. My warmest thanks go to my Ph.D. supervisor, Dr Christopher Ehret of the University of California, Los Angeles; thanks also to Professor T. O.

Ranger of the University of Oxford; to Dr William Bynum, Head of the Academic Unit of the Wellcome Institute for the History of Medicine, London – I owe special thanks for his support. I would also like to thank the Trustees of the Wellcome Trust for their financial support of my work over three years. Professor David J. Bradley of the London School of Hygiene and Tropical Medicine has been most helpful and I thank him. Also in that institution, I would like to extend my thanks to Mary Gibson and John Eyers of the library. Dr Jean-Luc Vellut of the Catholic University of Louvain has been a good friend throughout and has made helpful comments on my work.

Many institutions assisted with this study. In addition to the Wellcome Institute for the History of Medicine, I would like to acknowledge the Musée de l'Afrique Centrale in Tervuren, Belgium; the African Archives in the Ministry of Foreign Affairs, Brussels; the Royal Palace Archives, Brussels; the Prémontré Abbey at Tongerloo, Belgium; and the Liverpool School of Tropical Medicine.

Grateful acknowledgement is made to the following for permission to reproduce maps and photographs: Longman Academic, Scientific and Technical for map 4 (from A. M. Jordan, *Trypanosomiasis Control and African Rural Development*, 1986); Musée Royal de l'Afrique Centrale, Tervuren, Belgium for plates 1, 2 and 8–17; Mr W. B. Petana for plate 3; Wellcome Institute for the History of Medicine, London, for plates 4–7.

Abbreviations

AE	Affaires Etrangères
AGR	Archives Général Royaume
AIMO	Affaires Indigènes Main d'Oeuvre
APR	Archives Palais Royal
ARSC	Académie Royale des Sciences Coloniales
ARSOM	Académie Royale des Sciences d'Outre-mer
CO	Colonial Office
DC	District Commissioner
FO	Foreign Office
GC	General Commissioner
GG	Governor-General
IRCB	Institut Royal Colonial Belge
LSHTM	London School of Hygiene and Tropical Medicine
LSTM	Liverpool School of Tropical Medicine
MAEAA	Ministère des Affaires Etrangères, Archives Africaines
Min.	Minister
MMSU	Mission Maladie du Sommeil Uele
MRAC	Musée Royal de l'Afrique Centrale
PC	Post Chief
PRO	Public Record Office
RCS	Royal Commonwealth Society
RGS	Royal Geographical Society
SC	Sector Chief
SS	Secretary of State
TA	Territorial Administrator
VGG	Vice Governor-General
WIHM	Wellcome Institute for the History of Medicine
WTI	Wellcome Tropical Institute
ZC	Zone Chief

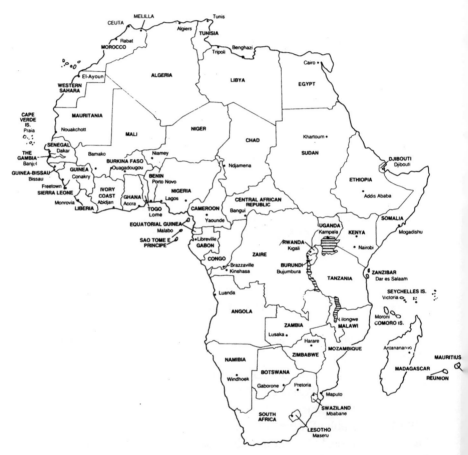

Map 1. Africa: political.

1

Disease and medicine in the history of Africa

The historian can approach the subjects of disease and medicine in a number of ways. More traditional historians of medicine concentrate on the impressive scientific achievements in Western medicine, beginning their story with medical knowledge and practices of the ancient Greeks and Romans. Other medical historians are concerned with the social history of medicine although their focus remains on technical and scientific achievements. They discuss societal relations in connection with the development of medical science and they tend to be more critical and analytical than their more traditional colleagues. Both of these groups of historians are generally of the opinion that Western biomedicine is the correct path to pursue in the effort to salve and solve the ills of mankind. A number of twentieth-century works have dealt with the history of medicine in the African context. Most have been written by former colonial or missionary medics who often follow the more traditional approach and take the form of a celebration of man's intellectual advance as demonstrated by his increasing ability not only to comprehend his environment but to shape it to suit himself. Titles such as Gelfand's *Tropical Victory* and Ransford's *Bid the Sickness Cease* espouse this notion.[1]

What is needed now is for historians to begin to put such work back into its historical context. The study of medicine *in* history can result in a much richer view of man's past by pulling into the analysis the subjects of disease and medicine as two of the factors among many in the overall process of historical change. In this way, the roles of disease and medicine are fully integrated in historical explanation. A decision to limit the topic for investigation to either disease *or* medicine would result in quite different discussions.

In the mid-1970s, historians of Africa began to take into account the roles played by disease and medicine in the human past.[2] The historical studies have been accompanied by an increasing number of anthropological or ethnomedical studies. This approach was given great impetus in 1977 when the Thirtieth World Health Assembly adopted a resolution to make traditional medicine a focus of research and study and urged governments to give 'adequate importance to the utilisation of their traditional systems of medicine.' The aim was to bridge the gulf between traditional and Western or biomedical systems in developing countries. In the same decade, taking their lead from scholars of European history, notably the 'Annales School' in France, African social historians examined topics such as malaria, smallpox and sleeping sickness. Several conferences were held on the subject with resulting publications.[3] It was no coincidence that such themes came under scrutiny in the decade which also witnessed the devastating droughts, famines and health disasters which continue to the present. It became obvious that no serious assessment of the African past could neglect the fundamental roles of health and disease and the responses to these phenomena by all those concerned.

This study of one disease, human trypanosomiasis, and the responses of both Africans and Europeans has resulted in a richer understanding of the social history of the former Belgian Congo.[4] Between 1890 and 1930 severe disruption of this region and dislocation of its human populations caused by intruding Azande, Afro-Arab traders and Europeans seriously affected ecological relationships. One result was outbreaks of epidemic sleeping sickness.

The human responses to this disease are an essential part of the history of the region. Firstly, this is true because of the observable effect of the disease upon demographic patterns. Secondly, but no less significantly, it is true because of the direct effect of sleeping sickness upon the formulation of early colonial administrative policy. The full brunt of public health policy fell upon northern districts which were perceived to be gravely threatened. For instance, Uele district had been identified early as an economic asset with great potential because of its natural and human resources. Important deposits of gold were discovered between 1903 and 1906 and most early observers commented upon the density of the population which would be an important labour reserve. The north was often referred to in glowing terms such as one of the most rich and interesting regions in the colony, or a vast garden. The British Consul at Stanleyville reported that the region was 'well-populated, [the people] more intelligent than usual and rich in products which attract traders' while another observer noted that 'The Welle basin belongs to the best watered and most fruitful of the countries of the Congo.'[5] The colonial administration believed that a demographic crisis brought about by epidemic sleeping sickness could seriously affect the future exploitation of the district, for which a plentiful supply of labour would be vital. Thus, while most of the north never experienced epidemics of the magnitude of those in parts of Uganda or western Congo, it experienced the full shock of colonial efforts to contain and eliminate sleeping sickness.

As in other regions of Africa experiencing the often brutal colonial conquest during the same period, the disruptions inflicted upon African societies in northern Congo resulted in ecological crises which affected every aspect of life including food production, social relations and individual existence. Often the result was devastating epidemic disease as well as increased incidence of endemic diseases. Sometimes the epidemic diseases were totally new to the environment while in other cases the epidemics resulted from disruptions to the environment which allowed endemic diseases to flare to epidemic proportions.[6]

Thus a study which deals with social upheaval and ecological disruption, the subsequent outbreaks of human sleeping sickness, and the responses to that crisis in northern Congo is an important contribution to an understanding of the history of early colonialism. For many peoples in northern Congo, their first and perhaps most vivid meetings with the new European colonial administration were directly related to the issue of sleeping sickness.· Those early confrontations were often accompanied by an array of regulatory measures with which the administration hoped to avert what it considered to be a potential disaster. The regulations often in turn profoundly disrupted the lives, practices and beliefs of local African societies. This one disease and the responses to it by Europeans, both the colonial administration and the new group of tropical medicine researchers, is a fundamental part of the social history of northern Congo. It is not surprising that by the early twentieth century, many African peoples perceived the increased incidence of disease as a kind of biological warfare which was part of the recent overall upheaval and chaos brought about by European military conquest and the roughshod tactics which accompanied early implementation of colonial authority.[7]

Rarely, if ever did early colonial authorities consider the possibility that Africans not only possessed some ideas about the ecology of sleeping sickness but had gained fairly effective control of their environment.

It is a curious comment to make upon the efforts of colonial scientists to control trypanosomiasis, that they almost entirely overlooked the very considerable achievements of the indigenous peoples in overcoming the obstacle of trypanosomiasis to tame and exploit the natural ecosystem of tropical Africa by cultural and physiological advancement both in themselves and their domestic animals.[8]

The European colonials assumed that they would succeed where Africans had failed and that they would transform the continent by conquering the problem of tsetse and the trypanosome. Most colonials believed that much of the backwardness they saw in African society was attributable to endemic diseases such as sleeping sickness, a fact they thought could help to explain the lack of the use of the wheel and the attendant need for human porterage, or the lack of animal-powered ploughs, mills and the like. Such an understanding had important implications. The present recrudescence of sleeping sickness in epidemic proportions in several foci touched upon in this study is a sad reminder of the continuing problem of the tsetse and the trypanosome. The warning is repeatedly made that surveillance is the key to preventing

the tragic resurgences of disease as have occurred over the past two decades [since independence] in Zaire, Southern Sudan and more recently Uganda. The history of epidemics at the beginning of this century alone indicates the potential threat which the disease poses today.[9]

We can learn much about the contemporary reappearance of this disease by examining its history in a specific region which was highly prized for its potential food production and for its numerous labourers. Five main themes are illustrated in this study. The first examines disease as a cause of historical change. Historians seek to identify wider patterns in human history and in that way they hope to make sense of the otherwise bewildering range of empirical data which they amass in their studies. It is particularly tempting to cite causes and their effects within a series of events and thereby to attempt to find satisfying explanations for the jumble of events which make up life. Disease as a factor in historical change is an attractive explanatory device as it often provides an apparently logical sequence of circumstances and events following one another as cause and effect.[10] By focusing on sleeping sickness in the history of northern Congo, I have been able to reveal wider patterns in the political, economic and social history of the region and show how disease affects the totality of human experience.

The second theme concerns epidemic disease as a 'mirror' of history. Is it a means by which to examine the essential strengths and weaknesses or social structures, such as classes, and their relations? It has been argued that at times of severe stress, as during disease epidemics, both the structures and relations of a society are sharply reflected in the varied responses of people to the crisis situation.[11] This view holds that during an epidemic the true nature of social relations in all their subtlety is clearly revealed. The present crises in many societies occasioned by the AIDS pandemic are a startling example of the ways in which a disease can unmask otherwise imperceptible class relations. Epidemic sleeping sickness in colonial Africa, like cholera in nineteenth-century Europe and plague in the Middle Ages, gave occasion for the reflection of a whole gamut of relationships among Africans and Europeans.

The third theme, medical imperialism as a facet of colonialism, forms the thesis of a number of recent studies.[12] For instance, Martin Shapiro asserts that Portuguese colonialists quite consciously used medicine as a 'tool for domination'. Based upon his Algerian experience, Frantz Fanon propounded this view of Western medicine within the colonial situation. It was his contention that colonised peoples often rejected proffered medical assistance simply because acceptance was too costly in terms of personal and group identity. Nancy Gallagher has shown how there was an inevitable power struggle among medical specialists as those with power and authority in matters of health in Tunisia came into conflict with the Western, biomedical tradition of the French.[13]

Another strand of this theme to be tested in the Congo case is the suggestion that 'the development of tropical medicine was undoubtedly seen as one of the most important initiatives in "constructive imperialism"', an idea closely related to the view of medicine as a 'tool' of suppression. The significant difference is that while it might be sensibly argued that 'constructive imperialism' was not the primary motivation of European presence in Africa, colonisation was accompanied by undeniable benefits for many African peoples. Western biomedicine must be considered an outstanding example of such benefits. In the Congo, where religious missions were obliged by the State to provide education and medical care, the theme of medicine as a form of imperialism offers rich possibility.[14]

The fourth theme concerns the conflict between prevention and cure in public health planning. This takes us into the wider realm of the political economy of health. What political and economic factors affected the development of public health provision and policy in the Belgian Congo? The issue of prevention versus cure remains to the present an often emotional topic of debate in *both* the developed and the developing world. This debate naturally leads to analyses of the 'political economy' of disease and medicine and it, too, plays a major role in the story of sleeping sickness in northern Congo. Thomas McKeown's provocative study best sets out the major thrust of this approach by raising and examining the propositions that 'the improvement of health during the past three centuries was due essentially to provision of food, protection from hazards and limitation of numbers' and 'improvement in health is likely to come in future, as in the past, from modification of conditions which lead to disease, rather than from intervention in the mechanism of disease after it has occurred'.[15] For instance, it has been suggested that the retreat of plague, cholera and leprosy from temperate areas was more often than not due to economic development and changes in standards of living rather than to any specific measures taken against them.[16]

Tensions between proponents of preventive versus curative tactics manifested themselves in the early Belgian Congo in response to sleeping sickness. That tack leads naturally to a consideration of the impact of the nineteenth-century European public health movement on new African territories. Concern by the state for the protection of the health of its citizens had become an important aspect of public administration in Europe. Examination of the factors involved in the health and disease of a society can assist in the attempt to understand the social production of disease as well as medicine. Again, this is seminal to an understanding of the sleeping sickness epidemics and medical responses in the Congo.[17]

The fifth theme concerns the ecology of disease, a most important subject today for development agencies, agricultural and health experts concerned with sub-Saharan Africa. As mentioned earlier, the relationship between man and his environment is germane to any understanding of the epidemiology of trypanosomiasis. Ecology is the science of the habitat while medical ecology is the study of the 'web' of relationships formed by a disease or a disease complex in its physical, biological and social environment. 'Each element in the disease complex, including man himself, is inescapably bound up with the geographical environment.' The ecology of disease is inextricably linked to the political economy of health and the occurrence of 'crises' in history. Andrew Learmonth finds it useful to analyse the total ecology of disease in order to avoid a too anthropocentric view. Man is thus seen in his relation to disease pathogens, other hosts and the physical environment.[18]

While this approach places man within the total context which may also include disease, most importantly it regards man as a participant whose actions affect and sometimes radically alter the balance of relationships. Thomas McKeown underscored this important point with his central thesis that medical science and services have been misdirected because of their fundamental assumption 'that the body can be regarded as a machine whose protection from disease and its effects depends primarily upon internal intervention'. He continued: 'The approach has led to indifference to the external influences and personal behaviour which are the predominant determinants of health.'[19] It is clear that a study of disease patterns must take into account the cultural, social, political and economic context as well as the natural history of the organisms concerned. This concern with the total ecology of disease is not new. Indeed, since antiquity, there has been observation of the relations between geographical location and disease. However,

studies on medical geography were practically neglected when with the discovery of bacterial infection it was erroneously believed that to understand the epidemiology of an infection all that was needed was to know its causal germ, no importance being ascribed to the study of the environment.[20]

This was a view with important consequences for Congo history, as we shall see. First, let us turn to a brief survey of the unique origins of the Belgian Congo and a look at the broad outlines of its political economy.

2

From private empire to public colony

The Belgian conquest of northern Congo was brutal and protracted, taking several decades as African populations strove to retain their independence. The systematic and ruthless exploitation of the land and people which had begun with Afro-Arab traders in the 1860s and 1870s was further developed by the Belgians, first under the flag of the Congo Free State and then under that of the Belgian Congo. This chapter will provide the background necessary to understand how disruptions to African populations and their physical environment resulted in an 'ecological disaster' in northern Congo early this century. Beginning in the late nineteenth century and continuing for some decades into the twentieth, African populations located in what are today the southern Sudan and northern Zaire were subjected to a series of frightful events which, for many of them, resulted in severe malnutrition and lowered resistance to disease. For many, sleeping sickness increased in incidence becoming epidemic in large areas of the north. During the period of their occupation of the Congo, the Belgians believed that most of the northern region of the territory remained free of epidemic sleeping sickness unlike other parts of the colony. This was not true and I will show that for many years a large portion of the north was severely afflicted by epidemic sleeping sickness.

There is no doubt that Belgian conquest and occupation of the Congo was violent and destructive in the early decades of this century and that for many residents of the north the violence continued well into the 1920s. It is no exaggeration to state that the history of the first European administration, that of the Congo Free State between 1885 and 1908, exemplifies nineteenth-century capitalism and unadulterated imperialism in Africa. In the words of Professor Jean Stengers, Belgian historian, the 'Congo State in its genesis, as well as policy of expansion, represented imperialism in its truest form . . . its sole principles were those of greed'.[1] In 1908, a year before Leopold's death, the territory was transferred to the jurisdiction of the Belgian parliament and became a colony more like those under British, French, Portuguese and German administration. One sad result of that greed was that northern Congolese populations, in common with Africans elsewhere on the continent, experienced greatly increased morbidity and mortality. The increases were such that it would have been difficult for most Africans not to have associated these misfortunes with European conquest itself.

The Congo epidemics [of sleeping sickness] had their origin in the social disruption produced on the one hand by Arab slave traders in Eastern Congo and by the brutalities of concessionaires of the Congo Free State and Leopold II and eventually, the conflict between the Europeans and the Arabs.[2]

Previously endemic in small, isolated foci, sleeping sickness increased in incidence early this century becoming epidemic in some regions. First noticed by Europeans in epidemic proportion in Lower, or western, Congo, the disease was later thought to be epidemic in the districts of Kasai, Bangala (presently Equateur and Sud-Ubangi) and Katanga (presently Haut-Shaba) (Map 2). Early epidemiological maps showed the disease present along many of the rivers which crisscross the massive Congo basin.[3] Until the late 1920s, however, north-eastern Congo was generally considered by the authorities to be free of the disease except for isolated cases, most often believed to have been imported into the region. This was not in fact the case. There was a major epidemic in north-central Uele district around the Gwane, Bili and Uere rivers, an area of some 23,000 square kilometres (Map 3). First *noticed* in 1912, this epidemic can be clearly related to a series of earlier disruptions to the region and its residents.[4]

Traders

Between 1867 and 1887, the region later to become the Belgian Congo suffered from the predacious activities of numerous representatives of two trading networks, one based in Sudan and the other on the east coast of Africa.[5] These traders were after slaves, ivory and other commodities carried thousands of miles to ports on the backs of the slaves themselves. By the third quarter of the century, the region was dotted with *zeribas*, or permanent posts, to which local African populations were required to bring their quotas of men and commodities in the form of levies.[6] One estimate for 1870 puts the number at 2,700 merchants and their servants operating between the Ubangi and Bahr-al Ghazal rivers. Between the mid-1870s and the early 1880s the traders had become the backbone of a new administrative network imposed as far south as the districts of Monbuttu and Makaraka by the Turko-Egyptian Empire which had recently imposed its rule.[7] Its hegemony had been extended to the Mbomu-Uele region in Equatoria province administered from 1878 to 1888 by Eduard Schnitzer, more familiarly known as Emin Pasha. The brutal activities of that administration were remembered decades later by local residents.[8] The push from the east coast was no less impressive. According to an estimate in March 1887, one powerful Afro-Arab trader from the east coast, Tippu Tib, was believed to have had 3,000 men raiding and trading out of Stanley Falls.[9] Over time, numbers of the more powerful traders were co-opted into the service of the Turko-Egyptian government. Acting as its representatives and condoned by the administration in distant Egypt, traders now exploited the region for its natural and human resources with intensified vigour.

The *Mahdiya*

In 1881, a Sudanese holy man, Muhammad Ahmad, proclaimed himself the Mahdi and called for *jihad*, holy war, with remarkable effect. Many Danagla, already considerably incensed by the repressive policy of the Turko-Egyptian government as represented by Emin Pasha, rallied eagerly to the call of the Mahdi. Between 1884 and 1898 Mahdist forces conducted sporadic expeditions deep into the southern Sudan and what was later to become the northern Congo Free State forcing the withdrawal of the Turko-Egyptian government. By 1885 the Mahdist government had secured its rule in the Sudan, and was to continue until 1878. Many of the new authorities representing the Mahdi were in fact the same Danagla traders who had served the recent government as agents. Their former trading *zeribas* were now simply transformed into government posts. The full history of the socio-economic impact of that period upon the societies in northern Congo and southern Sudan is yet to be written. It is clear, however, that the region suffered enormously as numerous factions warred and raided.

The relationship between intrusive upheavals and outbreaks of sleeping sickness in the region was noticed, for perhaps the first time, by Europeans in October 1891 upon the conclusion of a major battle between Mahdist and Congo Free State forces near the Bomokandi river, when the Belgian commandant commented on many victims of sleeping sickness among the fallen enemy.[10]

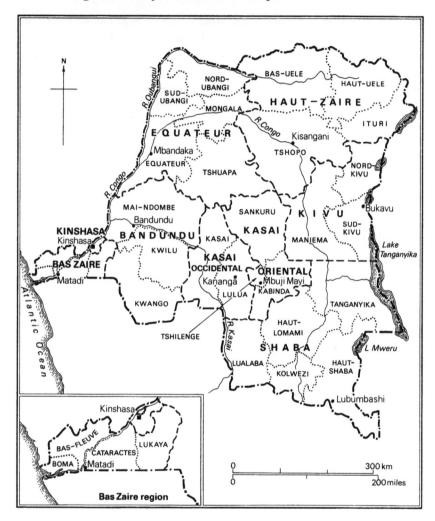

Map 2. Zaire: administrative divisions.

Congo Free State forces and colonial conquest

The last invaders of the area in the nineteenth century were the Belgian expeditionary forces who began in 1886 to make a reality of Leopold's dream of extending his empire to the banks of the Nile. Conquest of the region was harsh, lasting many years during which the repeated military and euphemistically phrased 'police' actions smashed African resistance. Belgian conquest of the Uele district, created as an administrative division of northern Congo Free State in 1888, began dramatically in 1891 with the Van Kerckhoven expedition and continued over nearly three decades if we take into account the concerted resistance of large segments of the population, in particular the Azande, Ababua, Lugbara and Momvu peoples (Map 12). The initial stages of Belgian conquest and the imposition of basic administrative mechanisms were indeed a time of severe trauma for many northern Congolese.[11] In the words of Jan Vansina, pre-eminent historian of Zaire, 'the period of the Congo Independent State is remembered [by Zaireans] in the Equateur Province as "the wars" and the whiteman as the "destroyer of the country" . . . who brought sleeping sickness'.[12]

Leopold's empire

Unique in colonial Africa, the Congo Free State was a private empire which involved no European metropolis in its administration but which was, instead, controlled by one man. The Congo Free State had come into being through the will of a single individual, King Leopold II of Belgium. It must be pointed out that opportunities for investment were great and numbers of ambitious entrepreneurs flocked to the Congo Free State, which became truly international in character with investors ranging from East African trading firms to European and American individuals and companies. Leopold, however, remained firmly in charge of the Congo Free State from 1879 until 1908 and his policies had a profound impact upon African lives for decades to come. A young Canadian scientist who visited the Congo Free State has left us this candid description.

The King of the Belgians is absolute sovereign here and this is not a Belgian colony in the proper sense of the word . . . He is boss of the state both as ruler and in the same way as some of the big mine owners out West are sovereigns of certain towns.[13]

The brutality of administration and the exploitation of its human and natural resources brought condemnation from humanitarian groups in the wider international community. The Leopoldian system was an infamous model which succeeding colonial administrations were anxious to avoid and there was a strange irony for later public health policy. Anxious to avoid any comparisons with the scandalous Leopoldian era, later colonial administrators were forced to be more alert to African social conditions and ahead of many other colonial administrations, the

Belgians declared African social welfare to be an important priority. Much rhetoric emerged concerning African health yet there were real advances in health policy and practice. Public health in the Belgian Congo was born in the impressive campaigns mounted against sleeping sickness.

Prelude to conquest

At the instigation of Leopold, the great powers of Europe sent representatives to a conference in Berlin in 1885. There they divided the African continent into 'zones of influence' which became their new possessions, or colonies. Germany, Portugal and Britain shared most of East Africa while West Africa was apportioned among Britain, France, Germany and Portugal. That left the vast region in the centre of the map, the great Congo basin. Acting on his own initiative, as a private entrepreneur, the king of Belgium sought and received recognition for a private state, albeit named the Congo Free State: 'Free' because recognition was obtained from the other powers on the understanding that the territory would be open to free trade.

After years of plotting, King Leopold had satisfied his combined ambition to increase the status of tiny Belgium and to acquire a vast foreign estate which would enhance his personal wealth and status. 'I would like to make out of our little Belgium with its six million people, the capital of an immense empire.'[14] The fate of a continent was altered profoundly as a result of the Berlin conference. The conference, however, merely formalized a *fait accompli* for in 1876–7 Leopold had begun seriously to acquire the territory, and since 1879 the explorer H. M. Stanley, another man of iron will with obsessive energy, had been exploring central Africa and extending the king's empire.

Leopold's sentimental ambitions to increase the prestige of Belgium did not distract him from the more important goal of organising a commercial venture. A model of the nineteenth-century capitalist, the king set into motion his plans for commercial exploitation which came to be known, notoriously, as the 'Leopoldian' system. During his explorations of the Congo basin Stanley had reported rich human and natural resources which unleashed enormous greed in the king and his business associates. Stanley himself explained that 'the driving force of the Congo Free State was enormous voracity'.[15] In addition to humans, there was ivory, palm oil, copper and cash crops such as tobacco, cotton, cocoa and coffee were added to the list of profitable

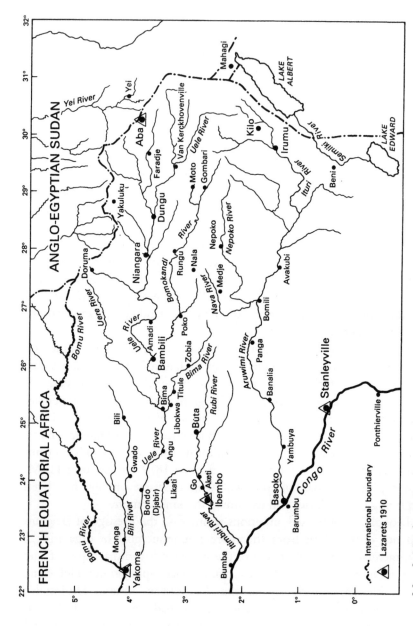

Map 3. Northern Congo (Uele District), *c.* 1910.

resources. The social cost of production was, however, devastating for the Congolese.

Belgian conquest of northern Congo

The late 1880s and early 1890s brought further changes to the lives of northern Congolese. The Congo Free State had been administered under widely varying policies but in 1891–2 Leopold implemented new policies which greatly affected the territory and its African populations. Desperate to cover mounting financial losses, the king issued two 'secret', or unpublished, decrees[16] which systematised the exploitation and established almost total monopoly. Before 1891, several trading firms and numerous African middlemen and traders had been tolerated in the Congo basin in accordance with the Berlin conference agreement. But the new decrees eliminated competition and established a virtual monopoly by specifying huge portions of the State as the king's private domain, which meant that only his agents were allowed to purchase ivory and rubber in those regions.

A second major event affecting northern Congolese was the decision by the king to extend the northern portion of his empire to the banks of the Nile. This task required the deployment of a special military expedition to quash the fierce resistance of Africans and Mahdists. The numbers of people involved in the conquest and occupation of the north were impressive and give a clear idea of the amount of resistance to European conquest encountered in the region. The campaign begun in 1891 numbered on most occasions between 1,000 and 2,000 people. Dungu, one of the military posts established during that campaign, was reported in 1894 to have between 1,000 and 1,500 well-trained, 'elite' troops with six cannons. In 1900, intelligence officers in the British Sudan reported that some Africans said that they 'preferred' the Dervishes (Mahdists) rather than the Belgians as enemies, for the latter with their breech-loading weapons and limitless supplies of ammunition were indeed a superior force.[17]

There is ample evidence for the harshness of the conquest and occupation of northern Congo although it was not always a simple case of European brutality towards African victim. The truth was in fact far more complex. The situation was complicated by a variety of long-standing local disputes. In addition to the disruption and upheaval of the Belgian invasion itself, there were conflicts between already-conquered populations and the foreign soldiers introduced by the Belgians. Two reports, in November 1892 and December 1893, by a Belgian officer with the military expedition described the uncontrollable activities of his own men who spent much time 'plundering' the local populations, who as a result increasingly moved inland from the waterways to avoid the invasion forces. Years later, in 1913, an observer commented on the local people's 'inordinate fear of the Belgian soldier, who', he said, 'loots at will'. And in April 1891, a member of the avant-garde commanded by Ponthier described how the Hausas and other West Africans used in the campaigns exhibited scorn towards the local populations, whom they labelled 'bushmen'.[18]

The initial conquest was followed by long years of reprisals by the colonial army, the Force Publique,[19] against African rulers and northern populations who refused to submit to the new state. A territory in which resistance persisted was placed under *régime militaire spécial* which removed it from the jurisdiction of civil law and placed it under that of military rule while 'mopping up' operations were carried out. In 1891 the basins of both the Uele and Rubi rivers were 'temporarily' detached from the Aruwimi-Uele district and placed under such a *régime militaire*. This region was then subjected to the shocks of a massive military expedition. While not all military expeditions were as large as this one, there was a most significant number of them before World War I, and the relationship between those military expeditions and the consequent hardship, suffering and disease among the African populations cannot be overlooked in an analysis of the history of the health of the entire region.

Leopold and the Van Kerckhoven expedition

Afflicted with 'Afromania', King Leopold's imperialist vision exceeded that of any of his contemporaries. His plan to extend the Congo Free State as far as the banks of the Nile was one of the ways this obsession was expressed. Early in 1884 Emin Pasha, the governor of Equatoria province under Turko-Egyptian rule, had been forced by Mahdist victories to abandon his recently established administrative posts in the Uele valley, and contemporary European observers feared that the retreat of his administration eastwards would create a power vacuum allowing a nasty 'free-for-all' among the numerous Afro-Arab traders in the region. Giving substance to the fears was the case of one trader who, having learned that the station of Lado might surrender to the Mahdists, pillaged the State warehouses and plundered neighbouring Makaraka, reportedly enslaving many women and children. Other traders then apparently followed his example.[20]

Whether or not Leopold could succeed with his dream of expanding his empire, he was extremely anxious to maintain the existing boundaries of the Congo Free State. He believed this goal could only be accomplished through the creation of a cordon of fortified posts along the Uele river as a line of defence against the Mahdists. The military idiom of a defence cordon was to be echoed years later with the attempt to erect a 'sanitary cordon' against another foe, sleeping sickness.

Boula Matendé: *the 'Hurricane'*

So, in 1889, Leopold put into action his plans to enlarge his empire. He found an able agent in Commandant Guillaume Van Kerckhoven (1853–1892). Promoted to state inspector in 1890, Van Kerckhoven was given command of a strong expeditionary force with a brief to 'explore and occupy' the north-east and to push the state frontiers to the Nile. Leopold believed himself to be fully justified in this step by the implicit recognition of the Berlin Congress that the 'débris des provinces égyptiennes occupées par les Mahdistes' was fair game for a European occupation force. Ostensibly, Van Kerckhoven was to gain control of the region by forming alliances with powerful Azande rulers, or 'sultans' as the Belgians called them. He was to do this in much the same way that Stanley, beginning in June 1880, had collected his infamous 'acts of submission', or so-called treaties, from Africans along the path of his explorations.[21] With their X marks in lieu of signatures, African authorities unwittingly accepted the absolute authority of a ruthless European monarch and his agents whose only interest was economic gain.[22]

Setting out from Leopoldville in two groups, on 24 October 1890 and 4 February 1891, the avant-garde commanded by Captain Ponthier consisted of 16 European officers, 500 Hausa soldiers, 6 cannons, and 6,000 porter-loads. In addition to Africans recruited *en route*, foreign troops were brought up as reinforcements from time to time. In late 1892, for example, a British steamer delivered to Boma 600 'Abyssian' [*sic*] soldiers who had been recruited at Massawa and Keren in Ethiopia. Mortality among the Europeans was high; of a total of sixty-three Europeans who eventually took part in the expedition, eighteen died, fifteen of illness. With an additional fourteen who were repatriated because of illness, a total of forty-six per cent fell seriously ill or died.[23] There are no statistics for the morbidity and morality rates of the non-Europeans but given their reduced immune status, we can only surmise that the rates most probably exceeded those for the Europeans.

Consequences

The major accomplishment of the expedition during its first twenty months was the establishment of a line of fortified state posts from Ibembo across Uele to the Nile. Temporary alliances had been formed with prominent Azande rulers and most Afro-Arab trade interests had been eliminated from the region. According to one expedition commander, the Congo Free State had 'operated along the watershed, bribe by bribe' and played off one African ruler against another.[24]

This often proved to be immediately profitable for the Belgians. In September 1891, Van Kerckhoven informed the secretary of state that he could count on an annual production of fifty to sixty tons of ivory from the north-east. The Van Kerckhoven military campaign was, in fact, a 'veritable ivory hunt'. From one trader alone, he confiscated 1,400 tusks valued at half a million francs, while another impressive booty was taken from defeated traders after the battle of October 1891 at the Bomokandi river. In 1892 the Belgian public learned from the popular Belgian journal, *Le Mouvement Géographique*, that the expedition had been in the Uele basin for two years and that 'important cargoes of ivory have not stopped arriving along the Itimbiri to the state post of Bumba'. Tons of ivory worth several million francs had passed through Bumba by then.[25]

Guillaume Van Kerckhoven, or *Boula Matendé*, the 'Hurricane', to the Africans, was long remembered by northern Congolese for the violence of his passage. One eyewitness along the Itimbiri river, deserted by its inhabitants, recalled how in 1893 the people had fled when they learned of his approach as word of the brutality of Van Kerckhoven's conquests preceded him. The British Vice-Consul in the Congo, Roger Casement, has left us this harrowing vignette.

Captain Van Kerckhoven told me during the course of this journey [1887] that he used to pay the native soldiers five brass rods (2½ p) per human head they brought him during the course of any military operations he conducted. He said it was to stimulate their prowess in the face of the enemy.[26]

The American consul, Dorsey Mohun, who voluntarily took part in the expedition corroborated the unanimous 'testimony of Arabs, State agents and traders concerning the disastrous effects of the Van Kerckhoven expedition'. And much later, the Honorary Governor-General, Camille

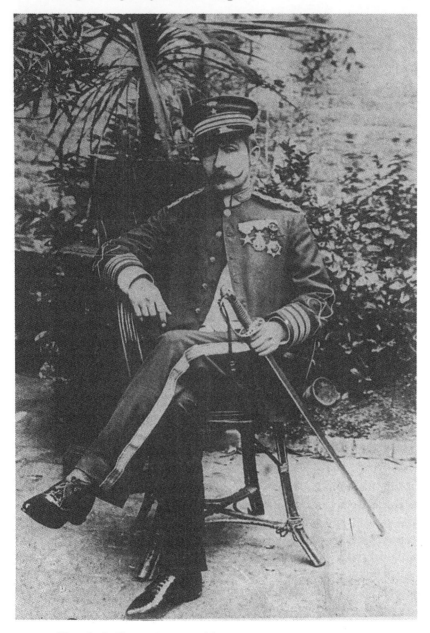

Plate 1. Guillaume Van Kerckhoven.

Janssen, expressed his disgust with the expedition which, he explained, had been an example of 'detestable colonial politics'. It had been 'a hurricane which passed through the country and left ravages behind', and he compared it to another destructive invasion suffered by Africans, that of the Emin Pasha relief expedition.

Quand une masse d'hommes passe . . . dans un pays relativement pauvre, il est évident que la devastation doit en résulter, non parce qu'on veut faire du mal aux populations, mais parce qu'il faut vivre et se procurer par la force la nourriture nécessaire.[27]

Like H. M. Stanley, known to Africans as *Bula Matadi*, 'breaker of rocks', Van Kerckhoven found brute force to be a most useful instrument for state-building.

It is clear that behind Leopold's dream of extending his empire to the banks of the Nile was the more prosaic motive of tearing riches from the Congo Free State. The Belgian prize was a devastating loss to northern Congolese, who suffered famine and disease in addition to the degradation of exploitation by a foreign power. While the Van Kerckhoven expedition marked the beginning of conquest in the north-east, for many decades to come, defiant and resistant African populations continued to suffer military repression. Accompanied by severe stresses occasioned by interrupted food production, frequent displacements and increased demands for labour, Africans with reduced immunity status succumbed more quickly to diseases.

Conquest and commerce

While the conquest forces were often large and well-armed, the same was not always true of the occupation forces. Because of their limited manpower, post administrators attempted to make severe examples of those Africans who hesitated or resisted cooperation with the new colonial state. The Babua, for instance, became a particular target for much Belgian repression during the first decade of Congo Free State administration in the north. In August 1898, the administrator of Aruwimi district reported that with eighty soldiers he had carried out an 'armed demonstration' in Babua territory as a 'deterrent' to further resistance by these people. Apparently they remained undeterred. During the first three years of this century the Belgians often referred to serious 'rebellions' among the Babua and after a massive battle on 5 July 1902 they believed they had finally conquered these people.

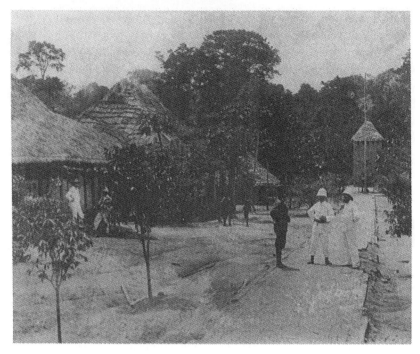

Plate 2. Buta state post, Uele, 1905.

Nevertheless, 'punishment' expeditions continued for years.[28] In the meantime, business began.

'Commerce', a euphemism for enforced collection of commodities, took place at state military posts the first of which had been founded by Stanley in 1880 at Vivi near the mouth of the Congo river. By 1888 there were 132 posts and by 1900 they numbered 183. Ostensibly administrative centres, the posts were virtually trading depots to which Africans were at first encouraged, and later forced, to bring ivory and rubber to exchange for cheap manufactured goods such as cloth, beads and brass rods.[29] Agents of the state were under enormous pressure to collect ivory and rubber from the regions surrounding their posts. In the early days, methods of obtaining desired commodities from African populations included burning villages to set examples, holding wives or other family members to ransom, and attacking uncooperative populations.

We have one vivid description of the manner in which a new state post was typically established. According to Captain Gage, a British eye-witness in 1900, 'the Belgians are quite frank about their methods'. Local chiefs were summoned and informed that the new state required their promise of obedience as well as food supplies for the garrisons. At any sign of resistance, troops were sent early in the morning to surround a village, capture the cattle and women and shoot resisting men. The chief would be captured as well and then instructed to order his people to bring provisions in exchange for the release of the hostages. Sometimes villages were demolished. As a consequence of this policy, Gage continued, the territory for ten days' march round the post would be deserted forcing the garrison troops to travel long distances on their food-raids. Another eyewitness reported in 1902 that the administrator of the post of Dufile in the Lado enclave always kept 50 of his 250 soldiers 'out looking for food and/or porters'. In other words, the Congo Free State simply followed the precedent of the Afro-Arabs and Sudanese of *razzias*, leaving behind them impoverished populations.[30] Another eyewitness in the north, J. C. McLaren, a representative of the East Africa Trading Company, reported in 1905 the widespread Congo State practice of commandeering food supplies from local populations without payment. People not only had to give up vital food supplies, they were forced themselves to carry the provisions on their backs to the state posts and camps. Chief Baduli at Buta complained to McLaren that only a few days previously all of the young men and boys had been swept from his village for a *corvée* – an unpaid labour gang. Post administrators were nagged incessantly by their superiors to increase rubber and ivory collections in their areas and McLaren reported how state agents took hostages in order to force even more rubber and ivory from the people.[31]

Upon their arrival in northern Congo Free State, the Belgians had described the Azande rulers as formidable and well-armed foes and by October 1902, it was clear that the Force Publique had only tenuous control of Zandeland and that a number of rulers, Doruma, Semio and Sasa among them, remained serious threats. They resisted the 'leopoldian system of rubber exploitation' even to the point of open revolt. Inspector of State Leon Hanolet complained that one of the defiant rulers, Sasa, was 'as unconquered today as during the time [of] Van Kerckhoven . . . '. The military campaigns mounted to crush Sasa (c. 1845–1915) are especially important for this study since it can be shown that the disruptions caused by those campaigns were directly connected to the increase and spread of sleeping sickness in north-central Uele district.[32]

In keeping with their habit of characterising African populations as 'cooperative', 'passive', 'defiant', etc., the Belgians were quick to denounce peoples like the Abarambo and Mamvu who from 1905 had fiercely resisted conquest. It was reported that the military reprisals of 1906–7 against the Momvu people around Gombari had still not sufficed to 'suffocate their rebellious spirit'. In June 1907, the British Acting-Consul at Stanley Falls described 'general unrest' throughout northern Congo – in the areas of Aruwimi, Medje and the Uele 'as far as Jabir' (Bondo) – a sweep indeed. He continued, 'It would seem that the feeling of crisis which I noticed everywhere on my journey in the Aruwimi and Ituri Districts last autumn is becoming acute'.[33] As late as 1911 another British agent reported that the Mamvu were 'far from being conquered in spite of the government's presence for many years'.[34] The year before, in 1910, the district commissioner of Bomokandi claimed that most of the zone was 'out of control' with complete anarchy in the east where he said the situation was particularly bad among the Abarambo people. The *chef de poste* of Bomokandi zone, describing the continuing existence of that situation, declared in January 1911, 'We are forced to make military missions but the Africans know we cannot stay and that we are undersupplied so they "patiently wait out the storm"'.[35]

Throughout World War I, the state was faced with serious rebellion of the Lugbara in the eastern portion of Uele district. References to the revolt's 'unexpected proportions' and 'alarming spread' indicated that the Belgians were not prepared for such concerted resistance. It was reported in February 1915 that, around the posts of Aru, Aba and Faradje in the far north-east, African resistance was 'taking on a permanent aspect' but because of the war, the district commissioner could not spare troops to send to the region. During that year there were a number of requests from Uele district for armed forces to be sent to the east to deal with the Lugbara revolt. Three years later, in June 1918, the vice governor-general of the province insisted that the military operations had to continue until the area was 'reorganised into *chefferies*' and tax collections began.[36]

World War I drew many administrators and medical personnel away from the north, a situation which some African peoples turned to their advantage. In December 1918, the administrator of Bambili post in Lower Uele complained of the 'independent character' of the Babua in his region who, seventeen years later, still 'had engraved on their memory the events of the major rebellion of 1900–1'. Mopoie Bangesino, like a number of other Azande rulers, made great use of the boundary between Belgian and French territory in his efforts to remain independent. As late as May 1931 the sleeping sickness service reported that the Azande in the north of Uele district still 'considered themselves to be unconquered' and freely traversed the border with French Congo refusing all attempts by the state to 'regroup' them into villages.[37]

By the time the Congo Free State was surveyed for sleeping sickness early this century, the prevalent view of the epidemiology of most infectious and contagious diseases was based upon the assumption that the movements of populations, sometimes only a few individuals, caused outbreaks and the spread of disease. Thus far, this chapter has presented some of the notable causes of severe disruption to both the environment and human populations of northern Belgian Congo. While the movements of populations undoubtedly contributed to the spread of disease, it is no less true, and perhaps more significant, that the upheavals of ecological relations among men, vectors and parasites were of enormous importance in the outbreak and spread of sleeping sickness. Nevertheless, it was the movements of populations thesis upon which the colonial medical authorities firmly based their policy and practice. Diseases were imported. Humans were agents. Therefore, humans had to be strictly monitored in order to control disease. As recently as 1963, an alluringly convincing argument was offered to explain the epidemiology of sleeping sickness right across the continent moving from west to east early this century. It seemed impossible to deny the 'spread' of the disease in the wake of the clearly disruptive invasions of regions by the exploring and conquest expeditions around the turn of the century. It seemed all too true, as many thought, that 'Stanley became the unwitting harbinger of death and disease . . . '.[38] But the initial exploration and conquest was not the end of the disruptions.

3

Mise en valeur: economic exploitation

Belgian colonials produced much rhetoric on the subject of their 'civilising mission' in Africa and they often rationalised, even justified, their presence in the Congo by referring to their duty to instill and nurture in Africans the European, bourgeois values of education, hard work, moral duty, selflessness, courage and patriotism. These values were not only to be taught in the abstract in schools but were to be acquired by Africans in the process of practical works. Congolese would become civilised by labouring for Europeans. But it was often to prove difficult to obtain African labour, the supply of which remained a major issue during the entire colonial experience. This was an enormous problem as the *mise en valeur*, or economic exploitation, of the Congo in the early decades of its existence depended almost entirely upon obtaining sufficient numbers of African labourers. The earliest instructions to state agents had stressed the significance of labour as the pivot of the Belgian 'civilising mission'.[1]

As we have seen, the conquest of the northern Belgian Congo was protracted and costly for African societies, but military conquest was only the beginning of many decades of real stress for many people. Administrative policies strained societies in ways which for some populations culminated in famine, disease and death. State demands for labour and tax were particularly onerous and began almost immediately upon establishment of each state post. The relationship between labour recruitment and deployment and the overall upheaval experienced by northern Congolese, especially before 1920, is crucial to an understanding of outbreaks of sleeping sickness.

From 1905 medical staff and researchers voiced their concern to protect northern Congo from the much dreaded sleeping sickness. Experts from the Liverpool School of Tropical Medicine had recently surveyed the Congo Free State and concluded that the northern sector was free of sleeping sickness except in small areas.[2] However, they

warned, labour recruitment and demands for tax were particularly grave
dangers as they involved great movement of population throughout the
region. The physical movement of Africans was for most administrators
and medical specialists the primary cause for the spread of sleeping
sickness. Another team of experts sent in 1926 by the League of Nations
to survey the situation *vis-à-vis* sleeping sickness in Uele stressed the
point that of all of the causes behind the frequent movements of Africans,
labour recruitment was an outstanding factor.[3]

Africans were required by every administrative department: the army,
transport (as porters and paddlers), woodposts (to cut and load fuel for
State steamers), construction (of administrative posts, roads and railways),
agriculture and mining, but there never seemed to be enough workers.
Women and children were not exempted. Considerable numbers of
women were required to work on roads and plantations, while until the
end of World War I many children were sent to the Kilo-Moto
goldmines. An idea of the numbers involved in labouring for the State
from the outset of colonisation is provided by the boast of one military
officer that between 1892 and 1895 with sometimes 1,000 troops and
300 'auxiliaries" involved daily in the Van Kerckhoven expedition, he
had been able to 'find' all the labourers required in the Rubi-Uele zone.
He reported that for two years he had successfully provisioned the huge
expedition in its operations throughout Uele. He claimed that he had
been able to replace daily the three hundred men required to paddle his
thirty canoes. At one post alone, he had 'recruited' up to 4,000 porters
in one month alone. That surely must have sorely depleted the food
resources in a subsistence economy.[4] In effect, peoples forced to labour
in this fashion – rounded up in raids when required – were slaves but
usually were referred to in administrative reports as 'labourers'. The
demands for labour accelerated steadily as the State entrenched itself and
concentrated upon economic development, which the Belgians referred
to as the *mise en valeur* of the Congo.

Before 1912 or 1913 the recruitment and deployment of labourers was
especially crude and *ad hoc*. People were simply rounded up – war
captives, for instance. In October 1893 one commander, disappointed by
the small amount of ivory he found after defeating Budu-speaking
people in Lower Uele, was nevertheless very pleased to capture 'many
women to work in his plantations'.[5] In another case, the administrator of
the post at Yakoma in October 1898, explained that in 1894–5 it had
been impossible to find volunteers and that it had been only gradually,
with persuasion, that the situation had altered; although in the present

year it was still difficult to collect the 'crops' of the Congo Free State – ivory and rubber. Indeed, he only managed to achieve this through the use of force![6]

Between 1912 and 1917 a labour policy gradually evolved. This was in part a response to efforts to reap profit more systematically from the colony and in part a reaction to the earlier anti-Congo State campaign in Europe. It quickly became apparent that the understaffed territorial administration required the cooperation of Africans. Various means were used to force people to work. For instance, Africans who defaulted on their tax were pressed into state service, a condition known as *contraint*. Most often, a post administrator obtained the labourers through the offices of an African middleman, a *capita*, who was the village chief or sentry, newly appointed by state administrators. Labourers obtained in this manner were not always satisfactory to European companies. The management of Forminère, Uele, complained to the *chef de zone*, Buta, in April 1911 that 'so-called labourers' they had received from the local administrators ' . . . refused to work . . . fought with the *capitas* . . . and feigned illness'.[7] Forced labour for public works such as road construction and brush clearance for purposes of hygiene was also obtained in the form of *prestations* or *corvées*, and the district commissioner set quotas for this purpose to be met by each *chefferie* in his region. This was a major task for all administrators. Chiefs were frequently exempted from tax obligations and were offered bonuses for their cooperation in providing labourers for the state. Eventually, recruiting agents regularly toured Uele district contacting administrators, chiefs and *capitas* in the ceaseless search for more labour.

Territorial administrators continued to find themselves under great pressure to find labourers to meet quotas set by the central administration. The administrator of Titule post was required during 1910 to 'press into service' a total of 4,300 people. He complained that state 'occupation', a euphemism for conquest, was not yet effective around the post of Titule because the *chefferies* had not been properly organised to provide labourers. The district commissioner then proceeded to designate tasks to specific peoples: some to transport loads of rubber to collection points on the rivers or roads, some to act as porters for European travellers, others to transport post provisions, etc.[8] Table 1 gives *some* idea of the numbers of people who were forced to labour as late as the third quarter of 1918 in parts of the district of Lower Uele. In addition, a further 1,779 people were forced to labour on State plantations. Thus, in a period of three months in parts of the district of Lower

Table 1. *Forced labour in Lower Uele, 3rd quarter 1918*

Territory	Public works	Porterage	Hygiene
Bumba	3,144	—	—
Mandungu	332	158	—
Zobia	1,237	607	814
Bondo	4,641	656	2,718
Monga	2,928	—	276
Lebo	1,832	186	200
Titule	1,960	—	522
Bili	254	400	800
Bambili	700	750	1,850
Dakwa	1,140	660	1,200
	18,168	3,417	8,380

Uele, not counting the administrative headquarters, Buta, and the two major centres of Ibembo and Gwane, a total of 31,744 Africans were forced to labour for the state as *contraints*.[9]

Large numbers of people from the Uele District were made to labour in both state and private enterprises. Time spent working for the state meant a loss of productivity within African societies. Food production was seriously affected as people were siphoned off to perform tasks for the new colonial power, and the reduction in nutrition levels exacerbated existing stresses. An important result was impaired resistance to endemic diseases such as sleeping sickness, which in some instances became epidemic partly because of the weakened condition of so many people.

Kilo–Moto goldmines

Important deposits of gold were discovered in Kilo in 1903 and in Moto in 1905 and mining began in 1905 and 1911 respectively. The mines, which soon proliferated, required large numbers of workers, many of whom in the early decades were forced to walk hundreds of miles across Uele district to the sites. Kilo–Moto gold mining was labour-intensive because all extractions were performed by hand. Conditions were brutal and fully sanctioned by the Force Publique and civil administration which were deeply involved in the functioning of the state-owned mines before the early 1920s. The historian of the mines described the camps in the early decades as 'hell' for the Africans who were forced to stay in them.

Before the early 1920s, when as a result of the investigation of alleged malpractices many changes were implemented, the policy of labour recruitment and employment at the Kilo-Moto mines was scandalous and, needless to say, most deleterious to the health of Africans. District commissioners and territorial agents were, in fact, recruiting agents for the mines, which were totally owned and managed by the state until the 1920s. State administrators thus found themselves in the contradictory positions of supposedly protecting Africans while at the same time being responsible for labour recruitment for dreadful work.[10]

By 1913, Moto and Kilo already required more than 2,000 and 3,000 labourers annually, and most of them were drawn from Uele district. People travelled, often on foot, more than 500–600 miles to the goldmines. In December 1914 the district commissioner of Upper Uele informed his counterpart in Lower Uele that although he had already furnished some 3,000 labourers for Kilo-Moto, he was now required to send even more people. Mine management hoped that as labourers finished their contracts on road construction, they would 'without difficulty' agree to work in the mines. To assist with recruitment, African chiefs were offered bonuses of ten francs for each labourer they furnished, or twelve francs if the wife agreed to go as well. Six months later the district commissioner of Lower Uele, Van Landeghem, informed the vice governor-general that Moto mines wanted still more men in order to meet increased quotas of gold production. All agents in the district were instructed to push recruitment. The demand for workers at the mines continued to grow. By 1919, Kilo mines operated over 160 sites and employed over 5,000 people while Moto employed 6,851. By 1931 Kilo mines alone employed 19,551 labourers.[11]

The statistics shown in Table 2 are derived from the annual reports of the Kilo-Moto mine management for the years 1921–30. While the figures show the numbers of men employed full-time at each of the two mine centres, they do not represent other substantial categories of workers, namely part-time men, all women, and children. Following these 'official' statistics, I have included the figures given for one year, 1919, by Charles Scheyvaerts, the special investigator who between October 1918 and January 1919 inspected the reportedly atrocious conditions at the mines. Using his statistics as a guide, we can infer that quite significant numbers of labourers were not represented in the mine management's official figures. The mine's figures should be regarded as

Table 2. *Kilo-Moto goldmine labour, 1921–1930:*
management's statistics

	Kilo	Moto	Total
1921	3,159	5,189	8,348
1922	4,856	7,270	12,126
1923	6,733	7,753	14,486
1924	7,471	11,238	18,709
1925	7,211	10,913	18,124
1926	9,359	13,524	22,883
1928	8,416	11,906	20,322
1930	10,382	9,680	20,062

Scheyvaerts' figures for Moto mines alone in 1919 were:[12]

Full-time men	3,409
Part-time men	1,260
Women	1,675
Children	487
Total	6,831

only a basic guide to the total numbers of labourers involved. We must add estimates of the numbers of women, children and part-time men. It is most likely, however, that following the investigation and reorganisation of the mines in 1919–20 the number of children actually employed in labour would have decreased.

The labourers

The poor physical condition, morbidity and mortality of the African labourer was a common theme in many company reports. Africans put to work at agricultural posts were said to be 'demoralised' and succumbed quickly. At Kilo mines, Dr Abetti in 1909 considered Uelians to be 'sickly' and the managers complained that they were often 'done for' in only seven months. Uelians, they said, could not cope with the climate, the food and the long forced marches. Abetti reported that 60 per cent of the hospital patients were Uelians from the Nepoko region, and the majority of those were children between 8 and 10 years of age with tuberculosis. He continued that 'true men' were from the Kilo region and advised against further recruitment from eastern and central Uele. Intense recruitment continued, however, for nearly two decades. Until the late 1920s, conditions in the Kilo and Moto gold-mines remained dreadful. In 1923, for example, 33 per cent of the labour force at Kilo and 10 per cent at Moto were discharged because of ill-health.[13]

Northern Congolese, then, were confronted with sustained conditions of stress. Psychological stress frequently added to physical stress of labouring for the Europeans. One great fear of many people concerned their eventual destinations as porters. In May 1915, for instance, a rumour spread among *contraints* that they were being sent to fight the Germans in the east. In the autumn of 1915, orders arrived from the central administration in the Belgian Congo that 'unlimited numbers' of porters were required for Kivu, and by December some administrators became concerned about the heavy burden of *corvées* which were being imposed upon Africans in Uele.[14]

Cotton

The government also made demands on Africans by requiring them to produce particular kinds of export crops. The ordinance of 20 February 1917 formally instituted the system of obligatory cultivation. The government had decided already in 1914 to promote cotton in the north, but it was not until 1920 that seed cotton was first introduced in the region. In 1919 preliminary trials had begun in Lower Uele, which by 1921–2 were producing 1,500 metric tons of cotton.[15] In response to a request from the colonial minister, the Société Générale in 1920 assisted with the creation of the Compagnie Cotonière Congolaise, or Cotonco as it was known, and by 1925, that company traded 80 per cent of the total cotton crop of the colony. In that year Uele produced 3,508 tons; by 1930 its production had increased to 13,455 tons. Cotonco had thirty-four 'plants', or purchasing and packing stations, to which Africans brought their cotton to sell at prices set by the state. All told, there were six cotton companies with some fifty plants operating in the north in 1927. By 1930 cotton constituted the *only* resource for African taxes in some regions such as the Uele-Nepoko district.[16]

To further its economic aims, the State requested religious missions to educate Africans in agricultural techniques relevant to the production of cash crops. In Buta the Marist Brothers' school undertook such training. Trained African agriculturalists became 'monitors', state employees who supervised the mass of African cultivators. Under the direction of European agronomists, 10 or 12 such monitors would oversee some 300 cultivators each. One retired official of Cotonco noted that when he began working for Cotonco in the region of Dili in 1927, the Africans in that area were involved in cotton cultivation, and he was responsible for about 3,000 people who tilled their own fields. The initial requirement from each African cultivator was 200 kilograms of cotton.[17]

The central government had been reluctant to formally oblige Africans to cultivate certain crops. Such sensitivity grew out of a concern to avoid policies likely to remind the world of the notorious Leopoldian misrule. In the event, the circumstances of World War I led to the issuing in 1917 of an ordinance which one historian feels allowed 'abuses without name or number'. It is interesting that the colonial authorities repeatedly referred to obligatory cultivation as an 'educative' activity, forming a part of their 'civilising mission'. Bertrand reported in 1931 that obligatory cultivation was usually 'slight' in those areas where there was no nearby European business or enterprise, but it was heavy in the cotton areas and around Kilo-Moto goldmines where the people were forced to provide food for the mine workers. In Dungu territory, for example, the Africans were exempted from cotton production at the request of the mine management who needed food crops with which to feed the workers.[18]

Tax

Another area of administration which severely affected the populations of the region and which was directly connected to the increase of sleeping sickness was the demand for tax. As already explained, a principal function of the state posts was the collection of 'tax' which, in the northern district of Uele until July 1912, consisted almost entirely of wild rubber. After July 1912, although tax was ostensibly collected in the form of currency, the main source of cash for most Africans remained for many years rubber. As with labour, an examination of the 'rubber tax' would take far too long to seriously discuss in this book, but as this facet of colonialism was so directly related to the whole issue of sleeping sickness and public health legislation, some details must be presented here. As soon as a region was conquered and submission obtained from some of the inhabitants, state agents were expected to begin the collection of tax. Conquest was inseparable from tax because conquest was *for* tax.

Just prior to the despatch of the Van Kerckhoven expedition, the Congo Free State administration had been notified of Leopold's decision to create private zones from which all rubber and other products would belong directly to the state, that is, Leopold. 'Capable' agents were to survey the private domains for rubber, gum copal and all other potentially valuable products. With regard to the north, the state administration was informed that 'the King thinks that a series of little "fiscal" military posts ought to be established at judicious points and besides their political action they should initiate natives into the collection of rubber, and eventually other products, and they should oblige the natives to bring their collections to the posts'.[19] Travellers in northern regions often reported in much the same vein as Alexander Boyd in 1906, that 'the natives as a whole do not like "Bula Matari" who grinds him for rubber, the collection of which is the one great underlying principle of the Belgian Government . . . "collect rubber, collect rubber" is the cry of the Belgian commander and *chef de poste*'.[20]

One effect of the state's demands for 'tax' was the enormous pressure upon African authorities. A vivid account of the effects of the state in the north is contained in the *Report on the Condition of Natives in the Uele District* compiled by Jack P. Armstrong, acting British consul, who toured the region for six months in 1910. During his long tour Armstrong observed that Azande chiefs were in the difficult situation of having to maintain their authority while fulfilling state demands for tax in the form of wild rubber.

The sultans are completely in the hands of the people. They are quite aware that any attempt to compromise the present situation (which is one of passive resistance to all government demands) by submitting to any Government proposals to supply food or porters in lieu of rubber would mean their immediate assassination.

He then described the system of tax collection and its effects which reminded him of the situation in 1906 in the infamous Anglo-Belgian India Rubber Company (ABIR), perhaps the most brutal of the private concessions in the Congo Free State. Generally, each collector was obliged to deliver one kilogram of rubber per month. An official informed Armstrong that it normally took forty-seven hours to collect that amount, although the people usually had to spend twenty-one to twenty-five days per month in the forests, far from their homes, seeking wild vine rubber. Other people were driven from their villages and not allowed to return without a specified quota of rubber. If they broke those rules, they were severely punished with fines and imprisonment. He explained that the people 'suffered hardships of exposure and insufficient food' while in the forests. Chiefs were paid by state agents according to the amount of rubber they had collected. Thus many chiefs abused this new aspect of power over their people, although later they sometimes found themselves charged by the state for those very abuses. When a chief appeared to have lost his authority, that is his ability to meet state demands, he was deposed and his territory often divided amongst ex-soldiers, who with their own men and guns could meet the state's demands for rubber 'tax'.[21]

In the north-east, throughout the period of this study, the issue of rubber collection was intimately related to public health policy and sleeping sickness. Increasingly the people found it necessary to search farther and farther afield for rubber. As the public health policy evolved into a clearer set of practices, with strict sanitary cordons thrown around regions which happened to contain gallery forests rich in wild rubber, there was increasing incidence of conflict between the policies of public health and territorial administrations, while the victims, as usual, were the African populations.

Increasing demands for both labour and taxes induced many Africans to flee across colonial frontiers as well as to travel long distances within the colony in order to satisfy the demands of the new rulers. In the far northern regions of the Gwane, Uere and Bili rivers in particular, there was much movement of people. As wild rubber became more difficult to find south of the Uele river, many people were forced to make the long journey north. This particular type of uncontrolled population movement was to become a major issue of the sleeping sickness campaign during World War I.

Rubber tax and sleeping sickness

Because of war demands, the government applied pressure upon territorial staff to increase the collection of rubber in their districts. The war ended the slump in the world market of 1913–14 and by 1915 world demand was again high and the British particularly needed rubber from the Belgian Congo. For instance, on 13 July 1915 the vice governor of Province Orientale, Malfeyt, instructed all his administrators that

Le moment est . . . favorable pour ramener les indigènes à la récolte de la gomme . . . je vous prie d'user de votre influence surtout à l'occasion de la collecte de l'impôt et de l'application de la contrainte pour stimuler les natifs et les décider à reprendre le travail.[22]

But increased pressure on administrators to substantially increase their quotas of rubber for the European war effort resulted in the increase and spread of sleeping sickness in Uele district. By April 1917, Bertrand was commenting that the collection of rubber had become, perhaps, the principal factor in the spread of the disease.[23] As with gold production, people were forced to move long distances, travelling to tsetse areas to seek rubber for the obligatory tax. Here again, the administration directly contradicted its own public health policy of a *cordon sanitaire*. The administrator at Zobia reported in 1915 that Africans in his territory were forced to walk four days each way to the Rubi river in order to find rubber to collect. He very carefully illustrated that it took a *minimum* of seventy-seven days' labour for one man to collect enough rubber in order to obtain the required 12 francs for tax.[24]

Administrators were ordered to use their powers of detention to 'enliven' local production. Africans placed in detention were *contraints* and while put into that category through failure to fulfil tax demands (most often obtained through sale of rubber), they were, nevertheless, still exploited by the state. For instance, in June 1915 a new state transport service – human porters – began functioning between Buta and Niangara and Buta and Poko. The porters were all Africans who had been unable to meet their tax demands. To provide an idea of the numbers of people who were made *contraint*, during the first half of 1918 alone, it can be noted that in Lower Uele 27,722 man-days' labour was used by the state as follows:[25]

porterage	4,875
hygiene works	7,401
'other'	15,446

The new porterage service was available for a fee to the private sector: 50 centimes per 30 kilogrammes per day plus 50 centimes per day for the 'accompanying territorial police'. Thus, failure on the part of a resident of Uele to collect enough wild rubber to pay his tax *still* benefited the state.[26] Sometimes the state benefited in another way from its policy of *contrainte* when kin paid for the release of the unfortunate detainee. In May 1915 the Buta administrator reported that almost immediately following the arrest of thirty men for failing to pay their taxes, their 'friends and relations' came forward to make payment for them.[27]

In summary, the military campaigns conducted in parts of the north, until after World War I in some cases, and the Belgian reprisals for African resistance, were harsh. The issues of labour recruitment and taxation lay at the heart of what the colonials euphemistically referred to as their 'civilising mission' and, in their typically paternalistic style, the colonisers felt justified in their heavy-handed attempts to transform African socio-economic conditions, dragging African societies 'into the twentieth century' and the world economy. Unfortunately, the upheavals to African societies which accompanied 'the civilising mission' brought sleeping sickness to some areas in their wake. John Ford explained that 'the determining factor of the epidemics resided essentially in violent change in the human ecology' of regions, resulting in stresses such as famine and exhaustion. However, he added, 'In most medical thinking, these initiating factors were overlooked and epidemics tended to be ascribed to the arrival in an area of people, or even one person, with trypanosomes in his blood.' A few administrators were aware of the disastrous effects of Belgian colonisation. For instance, a senior administrator with years of experience in the north explained:

The life of the blacks in the centre of Africa has become a tragic thing. It is only a generation since we have established ourselves among them, stepping on feet or repressing with a scornful ignorance, when it was not with pitiless harshness, their customs, beliefs and all which made their existence valuable . . . We did not even protect them from the scourges that we have propagated in the necessity of occupying the country and the imperfection of science during that epoch . . . [28]

4

Epidemiology and ecology of human sleeping sickness

Late-nineteenth-century European concepts and practices concerning epidemic disease deeply affected the lives of millions of colonised Africans early this century. This was especially true in the Belgian Congo. The term 'epidemic' can be highly emotive, even political, evoking images of catastrophic mortality involving millions of deaths such as those caused by plague in early modern Europe and by the great influenza pandemic this century. Between 1901 and 1905 a sleeping sickness epidemic caused the deaths of over a quarter of a million people in Uganda. Depopulating entire regions of the country, that devastating epidemic altered for many decades the demographic pattern of the northern shores of Lake Victoria.

The decision to declare an epidemic is influenced by political factors as much as purely scientific ones as it is most often the state which declares a disease to have reached epidemic proportions. This fact was borne out in the early colonial history of parts of sub-Saharan Africa. For instance, the declaration of an epidemic could provide a new and under-staffed colonial administration with important control mechanisms as there would be a rationale for the introduction of a range of highly authoritarian measures. In the Belgian Congo, sleeping sickness legislation became, in fact, a clear example of an attempt at 'social engineering' in Africa.[1]

The impressive discoveries of the mid- to late-nineteenth century in the fields of bacteriology and antisepsis had a profound impact on the prevailing theories of the epidemiology of disease which had evolved over the long centuries of plague and more recent cholera epidemics. However, the lengthy debate between supporters of the two major theories of epidemiology, the 'miasmists' and the 'contagionists' was still unresolved when human sleeping sickness was declared to be epidemic in the Congo. In the mid-nineteenth century 'epidemic' disease was not believed to be transmitted from sick to healthy people but was, instead, believed to simultaneously affect large numbers ' . . . under the influence of certain atmospheric, climatic and soil conditions to which "filth" was often added and the whole known as "epidemic constitution" '.[2]

The 'pythogenic' theory, widely held among both the public and medical circles into the 1880s, was that disease arose spontaneously from the miasma, effluvia or noxious gases emanating from decaying organic matter. It was a very old idea first expressed by Hippocrates and developed by Galen. The Italian term for fever, *mal'aria* (bad air) obviously derives from this. It was believed that miasma harmed all living creatures. An alternative theory of the spread of disease was that held by contagionists, who propounded that disease was spread through direct contact with infected individuals.[3]

Public health measures

By the late-nineteenth century the main methods employed to protect the health of the public were quarantine and isolation. Medical and public health authorities generally concurred that the only defence against epidemic disease was the quarantine of suspects and the strict isolation of infected victims, public health measures which required extensive intervention by state authorities. These methods had evolved in response to the dreaded plague and cholera epidemics. From 1840 until the 1860s and Pasteurian bacteriology, public hygiene had consisted mainly of segregation and sanitation. Sanitation (or disinfection) was generally achieved by means of acrid smoke or strong fumes such as sulphur and vinegar and it involved the energies of engineers and architects as much as those of medical authorities. For instance, water supply and sewage disposal increasingly became matters of concern in the growing population centres of Europe. In the late 1880s the first widespread labour protection and hygiene legislation was passed in Belgium, and by 1893 a survey of hygiene in Western Europe reported that Brussels possessed the 'most complete sanitation administration of any continental town with a staff of twenty-one'.[4]

In Europe, the practice of segregation took two forms. People arriving from regions where disease was epidemic were submitted to quarantine which most often lasted forty days. Those people *believed* to be infected (often symptomless!) were isolated in lazarets in the hope of preventing contagion. Gradually, in the African colonial setting the practice evolved of permanent segregation of races and social groupings. Ordinances in the Congo of 14 September and 12 February 1913, for instance, created *quartiers agglomères* for Africans resident in the urban areas. Contagionists were very unpopular in the business community as their theory of the spread of disease required the state to impose quarantine and isolation, which could be most unpropitious for business interests! So by the turn of the century it was widely believed by many that diseases were caused by bad air while others were convinced that diseases were spread through contact with victims. Long after scientists discovered the aetiology and pathology of human trypanosomiasis early this century, popular ideas persisted on the spread of disease.[5]

The new scientific understanding of the spread of disease based on the 'germ' theory had an unfortunate corollary. As the theory of miasma had been intimately related to the subject of the geographical location of disease, and as bacteriology appeared to 'sweep away' the miasmatist thesis, other important aspects of geographical medicine were ignored for several decades. (This oversight had serious implications for the conclusions and advice of researchers working on sleeping sickness in the Congo.)

Circumstantial epidemiology

There is another way to discuss nineteenth-century ideas of how diseases spread. It was commonly believed that disease epidemics appeared within a setting of specific physical circumstances. This belief is known as 'circumstantial epidemiology'. Once the circumstances were identified, the further spread of a disease could be halted, or at least hindered. It was widely believed, even assumed, that diseases in Africa could and would be controlled, even eliminated, with techniques and technology developed in Europe. The powerful notion of the transfer of Western technology to solve problems in Africa survived in the area of health policy until quite recently.[6]

It was not until the 1970s that the influential World Health Organisation acknowledged the need to include analyses of local socioeconomic factors involved in the production of *both* disease and health instead of relying exclusively on the delivery of health-care systems as a solution. During the colonial period, however, the attention of the authorities was directed almost exclusively on the visible circumstances of epidemic sleeping sickness. And many of those circumstances were, indeed, closely connected to the ecology of the disease. It was sadly ironic that the discovery of a portion of the larger web of relationships which together resulted in epidemic sleeping sickness in fact prevented the more important discovery of the entire set of relationships. For example, some authorities observed the correlation between the incidence of sleeping sickness and the importation of labourers from outside the region. It seemed logical that the imported labourers had carried sleeping sickness with them since it was they who most often succumbed. It was not immediately obvious to the colonialists that the newcomers fell victim to dangerous new pathogens *already* present in the environment.[7]

Liverpool epidemiological map

With the foregoing in mind, it is not difficult to understand the epidemiological map of sleeping sickness in the Congo Free State which was drawn by J. E. Dutton and J. L. Todd, the scientists who were invited from the Liverpool School of Tropical Medicine to survey the State between 1904 and 1905. Regions inhabited by numbers of sleeping sickness victims were labelled *non-indemne*, infected, while those with very few victims were considered to be *indemne*, or uninfected. In 1905, most of north-eastern Congo State was declared to be free of sleeping sickness, a *région indemne* on the epidemiology maps, and for decades very considerable effort was exerted by the authorities to protect this highly valued and uninfected triangle of territory from an 'invasion' of the disease. The judgement and advice of the Liverpool scientists had far-reaching effects in the history of the Congo. In addition to the older theories, the conclusions of the Liverpool scientists were also based upon the most recent research in parasitology, a new and rapidly developing field of medical science which was to greatly affect all of the new colonial administrations in Africa.

Population movements

It was believed for a long time that the primary cause of the spread of sleeping sickness was the movements of African peoples.[8] Northern Congo and the region of the Congo–Nile divide have experienced a long history of population movements and socio-economic changes some of which involved considerable upheaval. Over a century of Azande expansion and assimilation of peoples had preceded the late-nineteenth-century incursions of the Danaqla and Waungwana traders. Then the end of the century witnessed the disruptive arrival of the

Belgians. Each of these incursions led to very considerable demographic alterations which were directly linked to changes in African socio-economic structures and relations. In turn, the demographic shifts often unbalanced the delicate relations between the peoples and their 'disease environments'.[9]

A British colonial administrator, Sir Harry H. Johnston, was one of the first influential proponents of the idea that sleeping sickness had been either introduced or reintroduced into the Congo Basin and hinterland through the movements of peoples. He cited in particular the upheavals attendant upon the explorations of Henry Morton Stanley and the European campaigns against the Afro-Arab traders who dominated the region at the turn of the century. Johnston believed that the Sudanese auxiliaries and their families left behind during Emin Pasha's withdrawal from Equatoria in the southern Sudan were directly responsible for the introduction of the disease to the peoples in Busoga (Uganda) around the northern shores of Lake Victoria in the late-1880s. Johnston's views were then picked up by other observers and passed through the literature practically unquestioned.[10]

The Congo colonial administration was generally concerned to limit and control movements of Africans for political and economic reasons. The perceived need to control movement as a public health measure to protect the potential labour reserves fitted neatly into the paradigm of a paternalistic authority. Touring several colonies in 1929, the Chief Medical Officer of Nigeria, W. B. Johnson while in the Belgian Congo commented on 'the absence of native travel [which] is a noticeable feature . . . especially after one's experience in Nigeria . . . '.[11]

There were occasional suggestions by the Belgians verging on a more ecological approach to understanding the epidemiology of sleeping sickness. For instance, in 1912 Dr Emile Van Campenhout, a prominent colonial scientist, later director of the Belgian School of Tropical Medicine, advocated the destruction of wild game around African settlements in line with British recommendations in Rhodesia. In 1913, he carefully considered the proposal that a particular spider, the *nephila*, which was a natural predator of the tsetse fly, be used in a campaign to eliminate flies. In 1914, a colonial administrator suggested the destruction of tsetse-sheltering palm groves near African settlements although he added that he himself dare not impose such a measure which would so radically affect the local African economy.[12]

In the 1920s, a prominent Belgian researcher, Dr Van Hoof argued for the critical socio-economic factors of famine and profession of victim, along with population movement and labour recruitment. He also showed that the number of flies in an area was less important than the occupation of the victim. These important observations did not, however, induce the Belgians in the early days to study the ecology of sleeping sickness. First, as has been mentioned, such an approach was not generally in fashion at that time. Secondly, and ironically, the ecology of sleeping sickness in most of the Congo State prevented the Belgians from researching in this direction. When the ecological approach did develop in British colonial territories, it was almost synonymous with an attack on the insect vector, the tsetse. Since much of the area affected by sleeping sickness in the Belgian Congo was geographically unsuitable for an attack on the insect vector, the ecological approach was ignored.[13]

The disease: aetiology, epidemiology, immunology

Les trypanosomiases africaines ne représentent pas un fléau commes les autres maladies, elles constituent la calamité de l'Afrique.[14]

Human trypanosomiasis, or sleeping sickness, left untreated, is a fatal disease caused by a protozoan, haemoflagellate parasite, the trypanosome. It is transmitted through the bite of a tsetse fly, the vector, which for the region under discussion in this study is the riverine *Glossina palpalis*. The gallery forests found throughout most of the region in this study are an excellent biotope for *Gl. palpalis*. While tsetse flies occupy about one-third of the sub-Saharan African continent, not all regions are in fact infected with the parasites which cause the disease and no sleeping sickness is found above 1,000 metres altitude. The flies are active only during daylight hours and the *Gl. palpalis* variety prefers to feed on man and large reptiles such as monitor lizards and crocodiles. This fly transmits the *gambiense* variety of the disease caused by *Trypanosome brucei gambiense*, a form of the parasite adapted almost solely to humans and the variety relevant to this study.[15] *Gambiense* sleeping sickness is a slower-acting, chronic disease distributed across western and central Africa.

Manifestation of symptoms is complicated by a number of factors although onset is generally quicker in Europeans than in Africans; symptoms in the first few weeks, sometimes months, include headache, nausea and intermittent fever, among others. Following the bite of an infected fly, local inflammation, or the characteristic trypanosomal

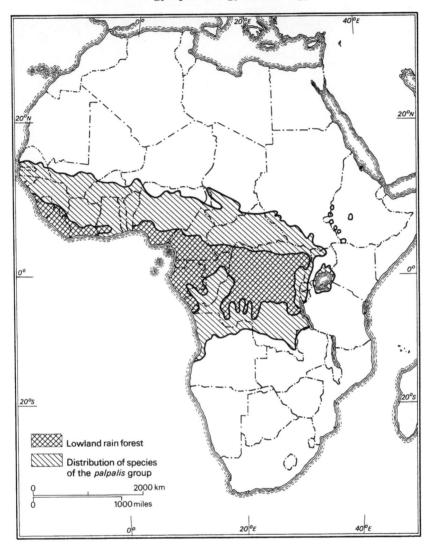

Map 4. Distribution of the *Glossina palpalis* group of species in relation to lowland rain forest.

chancre, occurs in most victims and parasites migrate from this site to multiply in the blood, lymph, tissue fluids and, eventually, the cerebrospinal fluid. In the first stage of infection, trypanosomes remain in the circulatory system, making new victims carriers from which uninfected flies can acquire the parasite and pass it on to other humans. The disease manifests a bewildering, sometimes startling, array of clinical symptoms

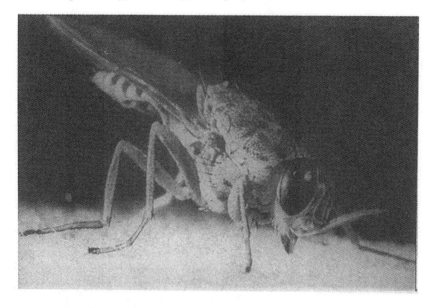

Plate 3. *Glossina palpalis.*

which can vary from place to place and among individuals. In addition to those mentioned above, symptoms can include neurological degeneration with psychiatric disorders such as nervousness, irascibility, emotionalism, melancholia and insomnia. There may be loss of appetite, gross emaciation, sleep abnormalities, stupor and coma. Since some of the initial symptoms of sleeping sickness are also characteristic of early malaria, it can be difficult in field conditions to differentiate between the two diseases. A common, easily recognisable symptom is swelling of the lymph nodes, especially those of the cervical, sub-clavicular and inguinal regions. Another common symptom is the so-called 'moon face', an oedema caused by leaking of small blood vessels. A most common complication during trypanosomiasis is pneumonia which is a frequent cause of death. A disturbing aspect of the chronic *gambiense* form can be its long period of development, sometimes as long as fifteen years after the victim has left an endemic area. Gradually over a period of several months or years the parasites invade the lymphatic and finally the central nervous systems, at which point the disease is diagnosed as second stage. It is in the latter stage when all organs are invaded that the more dramatic symptoms of comatose sleep and death occur.

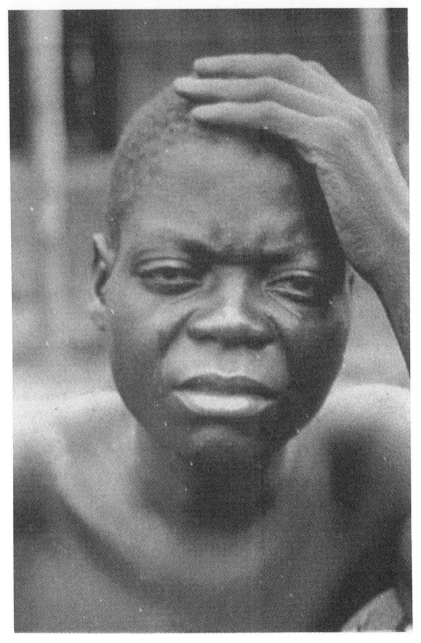

Plate 4. Advanced stages of sleeping sickness, Buvuma Island, Uganda, 1902.

Immunology

The prospect for a vaccine for human trypanosomiasis is bleak because of the trypanosome's ability rapidly to alter surface antigens, apparently the path to evasion of the host's humoral immunity.[16] During *gambiense* infection, trypanosomes multiply and, with increased parasitaemia, the victim suffers fever; afterwards the parasitaemia recedes in apparent response to the production of antibodies. Soon the parasites again multiply but this new generation produces antigenic material against which the previous antibodies are ineffective. In this manner, trypanosomes evade antibodies raised by the host to their previous surface coats.[17] This process repeats itself until, almost always, the patient dies. It is this phenomenon of 'antigenic variation' which greatly reduces the prospect of producing an effective vaccine and by the late 1980s, very little research had been directed to vaccine development.[18]

Nevertheless, it is believed that immune mechanisms may be involved in several aspects of the disease. This is probably the case with endemic *gambiense* disease in west and central Africa; the fact that immune mechanisms may be involved can be taken as an indication of man's long contact with the disease in this region. The palaeogenesis of human trypanosomiasis has been much studied and it is well established that the trypanosomiases are ancient in Africa. It is conjectured that the presence of sleeping sickness explains why the ungulate herds of the African savannah have survived so long. It is clear that the wild-animal reservoir of trypanosomes firmly restricted the boundaries of early human settlement.[19] It has even been suggested that the presence of trypanosomes in Africa may have precluded the development of certain ground-dwelling fauna, which allowed certain more resistant primates, including the early ancestors of man, to fill the empty ecological niches.[20] Thus, it appears that man was exposed to the possibility of trypanosomal infections at the time of his very remote origin. Yet, on the whole, the parasites remain poorly adapted to humans which accounts for the variety of clinical symptoms and ever-changing epidemiological patterns.

The fact that the parasitism of man is still evolving helps us to understand the unpredictable nature of the disease in humans. After all, a perfectly adapted parasite does not kill its host! This fact also helps us to understand why *gambiense* sleeping sickness is most often a chronic and endemic mild disease. In scientific parlance, premunity or premunition is a condition in which the infected victim continues to survive as long as his immune system is capable of producing effective antibodies to each new variation of antigen. It is important to note that premunity may end 'under the stress of other infections or when the challenge of new strains of the parasite becomes too severe'.[21] Early scientists occasionally remarked on what appeared to be the phenomenon of symptomless carriers, and several researchers, like John Ford, have postulated that a few victims may survive very long times as a result of having achieved a 'state of adjustment with the parasite'. He referred to the interesting report of the German parasitologist, Robert Koch who led a research expedition to the Sesse Islands in Lake Victoria at the time of the great Uganda epidemic. Apparently robust and healthy boatmen who paddled heavy, dugout canoes for several hours covering some thirty miles were found to be infected with the parasite! Five years later several of these patients were still alive.[22] What is seminal to this study is the fact that contraction of sleeping sickness is clearly related to far more than simply being bitten by an infected fly. A person's physical condition, immune status and the degree of stress to which he is subjected are crucial in determining his ability to *resist* infection and illness.[23]

The epidemiology of African sleeping sickness is far from being understood.[24] A complex epidemiology makes it most difficult to analyse and predict, thereby necessitating analysis of the total context of the disease pattern. In addition, the epidemiological pattern varies considerably from place to place. Nevertheless, two features of the epidemiology are well recognised. Firstly, it is exceptionally focal, occurring at or around specific geographical locations, and secondly, the number of tsetse flies is apparently not as important for disease incidence as is the nature of man–fly contact. The focal nature of sleeping sickness means that the ecological settings in which it occurs are of vital import-ance in the attempt to understand its epidemiology. Many of the foci in Congo are relatively small and old, with the human populations around them often living in a 'tolerant' relationship with the parasites. Accord-ing to a former director of the Prince Léopold Institute of Tropical Medicine at Antwerp, Professor P. G. Janssens, in the past 'Africans were very well aware of their relationship to particular places and the danger [to them] of displacement'. African peoples were often not only aware of the connection between stress and disease, but were aware as well of the connections between ecology and disease.[25] Seemingly impossible to destroy, many historical foci have continued to flare up in spite of concentrated efforts since the 1930s on the part of surveillance and prevention personnel.[26] This means that very often the same villages and regions affected decades ago remain problem areas today. The disease

involves humans, parasites, tsetse flies, wild and domesticated animals
and the ecological settings which they share. While foci remain at varying levels of endemicity, increasing population movements complicate
the epidemiology.[27]

With regard to the second epidemiological feature, i.e. disease
incidence is not necessarily related to fly density, research has shown that
a small number of flies with good man–fly contact can sustain an
endemic, even an epidemic, incidence.

Sleeping sickness is a disease intimately related to delicate ecological
relationships. The *gambiense* variety of the disease is classically a disease of
the savannah and transitional savannah around river systems; it also
occurs commonly in the zones where man-created habitat melds into
sylvan biotope. It is at this point that tsetse flies and humans come into
close contact, each seeking water.[28] Sleeping sickness can be spread on a
small scale, as most research has demonstrated, by an infected man
introducing trypanosomes into a suitable environment where people in
close contact live next to tsetse-infected aquatic areas. A traveller may
introduce a new strain of parasite into a community which can account
for sporadic outbreaks of the disease. But the movement of carriers is an
insufficient explanation for the great epidemics; to use the words of John
Ford, it is 'so improbable as to be impossible'.[29]

The disease environment

The relationship between humans and the disease-causing organisms, or
pathogens, in their environment is a vital factor in the analysis of
disease in history. All physical environments contain pathogens, both
flora and fauna (bacteria and protozoans) as well as their carriers (vectors)
which can cause disease in humans. All humans reside within a specific
'disease environment' and like all environments in nature, the disease
environment is subject to alteration. Such alterations can either happen
naturally or result from human activities. Often, humans move through
a variety of disease environments during their lives, with differing effects
on their health. The relationship of individuals to the disease environment ranges from complete immunity, through semi-immunity, to total
susceptibility. Certain physical environments are related to particular
disease environments. For example, I shall discuss the relationship
between lateritic soils and tsetse flies. Another example is provided by
the generally humid and hot daytime conditions of the tropical rain
forest which are directly related to a syndrome of respiratory diseases.

Extreme fluctuations of temperature daily – as much as ten degrees centigrade – increase the incidence of diseases. In the same physical environment insect life proliferates; thus it is not surprising to find a higher incidence of insect-borne diseases.

The disease environment of northern Congo during the period of this study included malaria, leprosy, onchoceriasis (river blindness), schistosomiasis (or bilharzia), filariasis and elephantiasis ('filaria volvulus' – hyperendemic in Uele), thyroid deficiency (goitres were common) and pulmonary tuberculosis. These diseases were observed in 1914 in the Uele district of northern Congo by Dr Rodhain who was surveying the region for sleeping sickness. He was an excellent scientist and we can take his observations as a reasonable depiction of the disease environment. His views on tuberculosis, however, are open to question and there is still considerable debate concerning the history of tuberculosis in Africa. Rodhain firmly believed it to have been introduced to Africa from Europe.[30] By 1914, he found it 'definitely established in the large centres of Congo: Boma, Stanleyville [Kisangani] and it had followed Europeans to Ouellé and contaminated natives in certain areas'.[31] Other diseases reported in northern Congo included: yaws (pian); cerebral spinal meningitis;[32] smallpox; bacillary and amoebic dysentaries; influenza (1918–25); respiratory infections (pneumonias, bronchial infections); venereal diseases, especially gonorrhoea and syphilis; tropical ulcer; and in the eastern border regions, bubonic plague and cholera. A researcher who studied Azande agriculture in the southern Sudan in the 1950s noted that

microfauna and microflora are represented in full variety, and the ailments they cause present an almost complete medical catalogue. It is far easier to list the diseases that do not afflict the Azande than to enumerate those that do. Of the common African ailments, the only ones from which the Azande appear to be free are guinea worm, found immediately to the north of their country, and yaws.[33]

Man adapts in a variety of ways to his disease environment, and alterations to that relationship are central to historical understanding. One form of adaptation is biological as referred to above. Over long periods of time, biological adaptation occurs through the development of antibodies which enable humans to resist, combat and perhaps tolerate pathogens. Immunity is full or partial depending upon the degree of protection generated within a human body. Just as a person lives within his natural and disease environments, pathogens must struggle to survive in their environment which might be a human body.

Another form of human adaptation to pathogens is social. Societies develop mechanisms to deal with disease-causing pathogens. For example, African peoples informed David Livingstone that he must travel with his oxen through certain regions only at night if he wished the animals to survive. The tsetses which cause *nagana* (livestock trypanosomiasis) bite during daylight hours. Some African societies were fully aware that when enervated by stress they were far more likely to succumb to disease. One form of African social adjustment to pathogens was the practice of isolation of infected individuals in order to protect the group. This practice was widespread in the Congo State for diseases such as smallpox and sleeping sickness. The Liverpool scientists were informed in July 1904 of such a practice among local African residents.[34] Thus, biological and social forms of adaptation to the disease environment combined to protect humans and enable them to survive.

As noted, the relation of humans to their disease environments is susceptible to change. Changes might be natural, such as variations in rainfall, cloud cover or soil composition which in turn would affect micro-organisms, flora and fauna and all the inhabitants of the environment. Alternatively, and most significantly for this study, the alteration in the relationship to the disease environment can be caused by human activities. We are now familiar with discussion concerning the ways in which man has successfully altered the physical world to suit his own needs. More recently there have been exposés of man's destruction of the natural environment as a result of ignorance of the long-term effects of some of his activities. One of the most disastrous consequences of these activities is their effect on the delicate relations between humans and pathogens in the environment.

This observation applies equally to every period of human history. Activities as apparently beneficial as new agricultural techniques – for instance, a method of irrigation or a new crop – might have disastrous results with respect to disease. In an environment containing the potential for sleeping sickness, any substantial change could result in increased contact among tsetse flies, parasites and humans, thus leading to outbreaks of the disease. For instance, the introduction of banana groves near settlements can provide a suitable environment for the tsetse fly, *Gl. palpalis*, thus bringing the potentially dangerous flies close to people and providing the intimate man–fly contact necessary for a real epidemic. In the 1940s in northern Uganda a colonial administrator introduced a new type of hedge, the lantana, from India. It flourished but unfortunately provided an excellent biotype for the tsetse species, *Gl. fuscipes*, which then introduced *T. rhodesiense* and human sleeping sickness into the southern Sudan.[35]

Serious outbreaks of epidemic sleeping sickness generally do not follow immediately upon upheavals in demographic or ecological relations; rather, they occur some time later. Keeping in mind the complicated ecology of trypanosomiasis, perhaps we can more easily understand the common attribution of an epidemic to more readily visible factors such as newcomers to a region or a disparaged social class. While it is true that peaceful alterations in an environment may result in conditions in which disease can erupt, it is far more likely that such conditions will come about following more violent changes to the environment and its inhabitants such as those occasioned by the events of conquest and colonisation.[36]

Reservoirs of trypanosomiasis

The principal reservoir of *T. gambiense* is man who maintains the typical endemic cycle of the disease. It is now known however that some animals can also act as reservoirs and these include domestic pigs, cattle, sheep and even chickens. The important relationship of human trypanosomiasis to its zoonotic, or animal, origin was often disregarded although the British researcher, David Bruce, had advised quite early on that animals were possible reservoirs of infection and should be either controlled or eliminated.[37] Much research and debate covered this subject, with disagreement concerning possible reservoirs, and highly emotional discussions ensued regarding the issue of the preservation of game animals. Thus, the German scientist, Robert Koch, mistakenly concluded during his visit to Tanganyika in 1908 that crocodiles should be eradicated! Domestic pigs are also 'host reservoirs' of the parasites. In one area, Dutton and Todd learned that Africans knew that tsetse flies followed domestic pigs about – in fact, they were known as 'pig-flies'.[38] Trypanosomes are normal parasites of several species of antelope with no noticeable signs of illness in either fly or host, an indication of an 'ancient, well-adjusted parasitism'. The reader is reminded of the interesting hypothesis mentioned earlier that, since the parasite produced such debility in man and was so devastating, the vast ungulate herds of the African savannahs have survived to the present day.[39] Nevertheless, the early attention paid to animal reservoirs tended to dwell on their role as carriers of infection to be avoided and not on their *relationships* to man and his domestic stock. In any case, the Belgians, like the French, tended to concentrate their efforts on one factor in the epidemiological web, man.

As we have seen, most commonly the *gambiense* variety of the disease is less virulent, although fatal when untreated. It is generally a chronic and endemic disease which evokes some antibody response in infected individuals. The key to understanding the *gambiense* form is its chronicity and the fact that there are usually a very low number of parasites present. In some cases the situation can even reach the state of premunity with rare transmission. More is required than the contiguity of humans and flies to produce an epidemic; a minimum population density and the nutritional and immunological status of people are vital factors. *Gambiense* disease can be maintained by a mere handful of peridomestic flies, that is, those which have invaded bush or cultivations near human settlements. This is known as close man–fly contact. Cultivation practices such as the introduction of banana groves, shade trees, new crops like tobacco and lantana hedges or the creation of new farms can provide fresh ecological niches into which tsetse flies can spread, introducing sleeping sickness through peridomestic transmission. The system of mass prophylaxis which was eventually developed by the Belgians in the Congo was admirably organised and quite effective in protecting people at risk. However, it did not affect the fundamental ecology of the parasites, and at the same time the mass chemotherapy had the effect of removing the store of antibodies from humans which had built up through long contact with the parasites.

Riverine *palpalis* tsetse flies are most commonly found near the low-level brush bordering smaller waterways and pools, and during dry seasons, when humans and flies are brought together through their shared need for water, the flies become particularly infective. Activities such as fishing, bathing, water collection and travel bring humans into daily contact with the insects and in this way an endemic level of the disease can be maintained over long periods. Obviously, the patterns of cultural and social practices become important in understanding the epidemiology of such a disease. For instance, which individuals fish or fetch water and at what times of the day or year are practices carried out? Again, other common foci for the disease are sacred groves for ritual practices which are often small clearings in the forest where the high humidity allows the flies to venture farther from water sources. Much important research was neglected and the zoonotic origin of the disease as well as its origin in the interaction of ecosystems went unnoticed for the most part early this century while circumstantial epidemiology persisted. While this might appear at first to be quibbling over terminology, there is a significant difference between a circumstantial approach to epidemiology as outlined earlier and an ecological one.[40]

The ecological approach

It is clear that the disciplines of 'geographical medicine' and the 'ecology of disease' evolved in part from the scientific research on human trypanosomiasis. The intensely focal nature of this disease and the complexity of its components of parasites, vectors, reservoirs and victims, eventually prompted the search for ecological explanations. Gradually, researchers recognised that both physical and human geography, that is, the total biota or ecosystem, played a major role in the occurrence of sleeping sickness.[41]

The ecological approach to the control of disease takes into account all of the factors in the environment and their relationships to each other in the attempt to explore the pattern of that disease. In the circumstantial approach certain observable phenomena are selected from the complete spectrum as the explanation of an epidemic. Attention is then concentrated upon these factors while research directed toward examining more complex sets of possible causes and their relationships is neglected. Most often the latter approach – the ecological – could not be competently accomplished by a single researcher whose expertise was limited, and it was only very late in the colonial period that the necessary cooperation of entomologists, epidemiologists and parasitologists began to reveal the very complicated ecology of human trypanosomiasis.

An example presents itself in the case of the Congo–Nile divide region of the southern Sudan where a correlation exists between physical geography, the presence of tsetse flies and the occurrence of sleeping sickness. The combined efforts of geographer, entomologist and parasitologist were required to observe and study this situation. Plateaux containing major lateritic deposits are found in the Yei basin, western Equatoria (west of the Maridi–Yei watershed) around Yambio, and south-east of Yei near Kadjo-Kadji. It was precisely in those three locations that sleeping sickness became epidemic early this century and both the Yei and Kadjo-Kadji foci are currently experiencing new and serious outbreaks of the disease.[42]

Epidemic as 'social event'

The study of 'crises' in history is one way to overcome the difficulty of locating adequate source material for the African past. Critics of this approach make the legitimate observation that crises in human history are more likely to be aberrations from the normal current of events, giving a distorted impression. Thus, concentration upon a war, a spectacular social event, or a natural disaster such as a disease epidemic may mislead the historian into misunderstanding the past. On the other hand, crises can make much sharper the contrasts and conflicts existing in societies in more 'normal' times and so assist the work of uncovering the past. And as the French social historian, Emmanuel Le Roy Ladurie, points out, crises can extend over quite long periods of time with 'snow-balling effects' generating various stages. For example, the Hundred Years War and the Black Death of the Early Modern period each produced chains of events which can be viewed as integral parts of an overall crisis.[43]

Epidemics have been described as 'social events': 'illness is now "endopolic", the product not of nature but of historically specific political and economic decisions and processes'.[44] Although the original reference was to the relationship between disease patterns and the changing nature of Western European capitalism in the nineteenth century, it helps us to understand the African disease patterns in the early colonial context as well.

The ecological crisis

There has been some speculation on the nature of pre-colonial African disease environments and the dramatic effects on them of events between 1890 and 1930. Some scholars propound an African 'Eden' before the late-nineteenth century in which most populations experienced better health. According to proponents of this view, around the turn of the century much of Africa suffered an 'ecological disaster" or 'crisis' bringing widespread famine and disease to African populations in large parts of the continent.[45]

John Ford was one of the first to conclude that during the last decades of the nineteenth and first decades of the twentieth centuries large portions of east and central Africa suffered long-term and severe shock culminating in a veritable ecological disaster. He contended that the competition between two ecosystems – the man-made and controlled domestic system and the natural or wild system – had resulted, among other things, in the spread of sleeping sickness which in some regions became epidemic. As the result of a series of developments the intricate balances among people, flora, fauna, tsetse flies and trypanosomes were profoundly disturbed. Ford's important point is that the crisis was very much the result of the activities of one segment of the model – humans.[46]

In a controversial study of ecology and economic history in eastern Africa, Helge Kjekshus states that by the nineteenth century African populations had managed successfully to gain control of their environment.[47] 'Man and beast [domestic livestock] combined to maintain an ecological control situation through the nineteenth century.' It is clear that by the 1890s much of east and central Africa, including northern Congo, had experienced a series of shocks with dreadful consequences for many African populations. The individual events were not necessarily novel or unprecedented, but by the 1890s their combined effects raised the scale of impact to a level which was new.

A recent study shows the many faceted transition of the environment in Equatoria province, southern Sudan, where between 1850 and 1950 the tsetse-fly belt significantly increased. As a consequence of the economic upheaval experienced by many Africans, there were significant changes in the demography of the region, aided in part, by trypanosomiasis.[48] East Africa in the late-nineteenth century witnessed similar kinds of events including the great rinderpest epidemic of the 1890s, the plague of jiggers (*Tunga penetrans*), and famine induced in part by the natural disasters and in part by the depredations of newly arrived European intruders. Kjekshus argues:

At a crucial stage in this decline, a new ecological balance was established in which man was no longer in control and where he suffered the consequences of this through *nagana* and sleeping sickness which erupted in epidemic form in East Africa at the beginning of this century.[49]

If anything, the disruptions at the end of the century in north-east Congo were even more far-reaching and complex. It is not difficult to see a connection between this far-reaching crisis and the onset of epidemics of human disease.

Unaware of the ecology of sleeping sickness, or finding ecological measures impractical or unpalatable, the new colonial authorities of Congo early this century sometimes took public health measures which made the situation worse rather than ameliorating it. Most medical theory neglected ecological factors, and the early sleeping sickness epidemics were generally ascribed to the 'importation' or 'invasion' of the disease. This ascription resulted in the notion that there were non-infected (*indemne*) as opposed to infected (*non-indemne*) zones. Disease was perceived as an enemy which moved about the landscape threatening uninfected regions and against which defences had to be erected. The Liverpool scientists' advice for the Congo State and the resultant sleeping sickness policy of the colonial administration can only be understood in the light of this perception.

Geography and climate

In the first part of this chapter I have discussed the ways in which sleeping sickness can be described as an 'ecological disease'. Therefore, it is now necessary to introduce details of the physical environment of north-eastern Congo as well as aspects of the behaviour of tsetse flies and their parasitical trypanosomes in order that the reader can more readily understand how epidemic sleeping sickness occurred. It has been observed that so many conditions are necessary for an epidemic to take place, that the surprising thing might not be the absence of an epidemic, but its presence.[50]

The northern portion of Province Orientale in the former Belgian Congo and the far southern section of the former Equatoria province of the southern Anglo-Egyptian Sudan can be thought of as a great triangle covering a surface area of well over 300,000 square kilometres. Included are the Uele district of northern Belgian Congo and the neighbouring frontiers with the former French Congo and Sudan.

A major geographical feature of the region is the Congo–Nile water-shed, or divide, which in fact became the political boundary separating the three territories of French Congo, Anglo-Egyptian Sudan and Belgian Congo. This well-watered region is the source of many streams and rivers which flow northwards towards the Nile or southwards to join the Congo. The terrain in the vicinity of the divide is an undulating plateau of gently hilly country between 700 and 1100 metres in altitude, with small brush-covered mountains rising 90 to 210 metres above the plateau. On the divide, small hills define the crest as far west as the point where the Faradje–Juba road crosses the boundary; but from there to the source of the Bomu River, the watershed is a narrow strip of nearly flat bush-covered upland sometimes as much as three kilometres in width, but generally much less.

The well-watered aspect of northern Congo accounts for the relative ease with which the initial European invasions were made as the profusion of waterways in the Congo formed one of its early attractions to all newcomers who used them for communication and transport. The Congo river and its affluents contain about 12,000 kilometres of navigable water. It was not only human travellers who made use of this network of waterways; the riverine species of tsetse fly, *Gl. palpalis*, the most common vector of human trypanosomiasis in the region, also followed the waterways. One river, the Itimbiri, described as 'the highway to the cotton growing and gold producing Uele District and Uganda', is navigable 240 kilometres from the Congo river to the Lubi rapids at Akedi (Port Chaltin). The Aruwimi river can be followed 130 kilometres before the first rapids are encountered. But it was the Uele river (Kibali river in the upper reaches) which became the major route through the region especially during the early period in King Leopold's ambitious drive to extend his empire to the Nile.[51]

The upper Uele river can be considered a frontier between the two major ecological zones of the region each with its own distinctive flora and fauna. This fact was striking to the early European explorers of the region. Emin Pasha visited the 'Mombuttu country' in 1883 and agreed with the botanist-explorer, George Schweinfurth's earlier observation[52] that it formed the transition from north-eastern Africa to tropical west Africa.[53] In the transitional area between the upper Uele and Nepoko rivers, 'ever-wet' forests gradually give way to forested savannah. This transition does not occur abruptly. Rather, there are patches of forest interspersed with natural and man-made clearings or with areas of savannah. Farther north, truer savannah dominates. The region around Isiro, Wamba and Niangara provides an example of this transition south of the Uele river.[54]

As mentioned earlier, sleeping sickness is a classical disease of the savannah and transitional savannah around river systems where tsetse flies and people are forced into close contact by their shared need for water, especially during dry seasons. It has also been labelled a disease of frontier zones as it more generally occurs on the edges of human settlements where the transition from the sylvan, or wild, ecosystem to the domesticated ecosystem of man is in process.[55]

North-east of the Uele river a great undulating plateau descends from 1220 metres in the north to 488 metres farther south. Throughout most of the Uele region the terrain is formed by broad undulations which are barely visible from the surface. South and west of Niangara, in central Uele district, the country retains the same general character but is somewhat less elevated than farther north. South of the Uele river the terrain has a less 'valleyed' aspect but there are numerous streams, most of which are generally broad and shallow (rather than narrow and deep) and descend only gradually, although numerous low falls and rapids prevent continuous navigation. A 'fringe' of forest clothes the banks of most of the rivers. The Uele, then, is the northern limit of the tropical forest, which is most luxuriant farther south in the valley of the Ituri river. Throughout the Uele region, alluvial soils occur in the vicinity of the rivers, and it is in these districts that the most extensive areas of arable land are found.

Stretching north from the former administrative centre, Ibembo, on the Itimbiri river to the Uele river is the tropical or Guinean, evergreen Equatorial rainforest. The average annual rainfall is 1,800 to 2,000 mm (71 to 79 inches) and temperatures average 23 to 26 degrees Centigrade with a more or less even humidity. The forest has been described many times as an awe-inspiring sight with 'cathedral-like vegetation' deep within shadow, shade and silence. Stanley reported in 1889 that 'the Amazon valley cannot boast a more impervious or umbrageous forest . . . than this vast Upper Congo forest . . . '.[56] The trees typically attain thirty or forty metres in height. Importantly, a tropical rainforest produces not one, but a whole series of environments each with its different climate or microclimate. Beneath the towering trees, masses of lianas, tree-like herbaceous plants, palm trees, ferns and lichens proliferate in the humid soil and decomposing vegetation and mosses. The atmosphere is humid and heavy.

Gallery or fringing forests are a distinctive feature of northern Congo and neighbouring Sudan and they are most significant in the ecology of sleeping sickness because they provide an excellent biotope for *Gl. palpalis*.[57] Much impressed by the verdure of these isolated strips of forest after the open savannah country to the north, George Schweinfurth was the first European to describe them when he visited the Uele region in March 1870. There were places where numerous springs restrained within deep-cut channels created a terrain comparable to an 'overfull sponge'.[58] There it was possible for many plants to flourish all year. The trees within such a gallery were twenty to thirty metres tall and were much more imposing from within the gallery than from the surrounding plateaux which themselves supported 'park-like woods' containing lofty rainforest trees. These narrow, but luxuriant, 'tunnel-like woodlands' are a vital feature of the transitional zone between forest and savannah. They make possible projection of the forest biotope far into the savannah which is otherwise a quite different environment. They provide a splendid example of how an apparently hostile environment, here open savannah, can be successfully penetrated by a disease vector, in this case, *Gl. palpalis*. These 'fringes along margins of larger streams . . . are enabled to exist under a lesser rainfall by the more abundant ground water'.[59] According to Schweinfurth, the galleries were a microclimate within the larger macroclimate, a concept much more familiar to us today. 'The air was no longer that of the sunny steppe, nor that of a palm-house. Temperatures could vary between 70 degrees and 80 degrees Fahrenheit [21–27 degrees Centigrade] *but* it was excessively humid and very difficult to endure.' The galleries fairly seethed with life.[60]

Gallery forests are more suitable for human habitation than the virgin forests of the type described earlier. This is in part because the two ecosystems are so interspersed that advantages can be had of both. Large mammals are more numerous in galleries where light alternates with shade whereas in the tropical forest relentless gloom can prevail. Travel is much easier on the edges of the galleries. As one would expect, they contain places with very fertile soil composed in part of humus. As noted, gallery forests provide an excellent setting for *Gl. palpalis*; and since man seeks the same shaded verdure and water, it is within these spots that many foci of trypanosomiasis are to be found. The numerous Azande of Sudan and Congo were particularly fond of settling along galleries, a factor of significance in relation to European sleeping sickness policies.

Climate plays another vital role in the ecology of human trypanosomiasis as it does with all diseases transmitted by insect vectors. The fact that trypanosomiasis requires three participants – parasite, fly and host – involves it closely with the total ecology. Climatic factors affect the reproductive cycle of the fly as well as the degree to which it is receptive, itself, to infection by the parasitic trypanosomes. Climatic factors obviously affect the behaviour of both animal and human hosts of the parasites. Lack of water will force hosts and vector into close proximity creating excellent conditions for outbreaks of disease. It only requires a very small population of flies – quite literally a dozen or so – to feed repeatedly on numerous humans in order to spread the parasite amongst them. (This type of man–fly relation is referred to as 'personal man–fly' or 'intimate' contact.) Surprisingly, an epidemic can occur in a situation containing very few flies indeed. The climate is crucial. During the wet season, the range of flies is not so restricted, so they can enter the villages some distance from their normal habitat. This type of contact is 'impersonal' and *not* to be confused with the type in villages in which there is a permanently resident population of tsetses. In humid areas, *Gl. palpalis* forsakes its riverine habitat and man–fly contact is then impersonal because of the mobile fly population. It is because of the resulting less frequent human contacts by the fly that sleeping sickness can be absent in some areas which nevertheless contain the flies.

The type of cloud cover present over the landscape has also been shown to affect the behaviour of tsetses, a further demonstration that 'the key to a proper understanding of the ecology of a fly community is to be found in climatic conditions'. *Gl. palpalis* requires shade; thus in the presence of the thick clouds known as cumulus, the flies are most active, flying great distances and even crossing clearings of 300 metres or venturing across open water when attracted by a moving object. With cirrus clouds, the flies bite eagerly in the morning and late evening but not during the middle of the day.[61]

Rainfall varies considerably throughout this very large region encompassing as it does several ecosystems. Thus annual precipitation averages 900 mm in the far north at Juba in the Sudan, while it is 1,800 mm in the Equatorial forest farther south in the Congo. Again, while the average at Juba is just over 900 mm, at Loka it is 1,326 mm, and at Yei, 1,438 mm. At the divide itself, the annual average is nearly 1,500 mm with marked increases near the borders with Uganda and Sudan.[62] South-west Equatoria has an even rainfall between March and November with occasional showers in the dry season of December to February. Between the upper Uele and Nepoko rivers, lies a transitional zone stretching 200 kilometres from north to south with very different precipitation rates. In much of this zone, the dry season begins in early November. Between Stanleyville on the Congo river and the Uele river in the region of the forest, annual rainfall ranges between 1,800 and 2,000 mm (71 to 79 inches).

This Equatorial climate reaches right into the Uele region. It is more or less evenly humid and hot throughout the year with average temperatures of 25 to 26 degrees Centigrade. But considerable fluctuation of the daily temperature is also possible. These conditions are directly related to a pattern of respiratory diseases among residents. The daily fluctuations of temperature can be as much as nearly ten degrees Centigrade in some savannah areas near the Congo–Nile divide.[63]

The insect and the disease: tsetse and trypanosome

The life-cycle of the tsetse fly is rather unusual when compared to that of other flies or insects. The adult female fly only needs to mate once in her life to remain permanently fertile and she lives on average 150 to 200 days.[64] During that time, she can give birth to approximately fifteen to twenty larvae. It is actually 'birthing' for unlike other flies which generally deposit very numerous eggs, the tsetse is larviparous which means she delivers at intervals, not eggs, but single larvae. The intervals are governed by temperature but are usually about eleven days, and the larviposition, or birth, must occur in certain conditions. Most often, *Gl. palpalis* will alight on the bottom side of a projecting rock, fallen log or bush and in that shady position, which will be near moderately slow-moving water, she will drop the larva onto shady, loose soil.

When deposited, the larva, which appears like a whitish maggot 6 to 8 mm in length, will burrow out of sight within 20 minutes. It burrows 1–2.5 cm beneath the soil surface where it remains as a puparium for about thirty days. The length of time spent as a puparium is controlled by the temperature and outside the range of 16 to 24 degrees Centigrade development is seriously affected. Thus, the number of flies in a region is again closely connected to climate. Upon emergence from its chrysalis, the young fly leaves the soil and dries its wings for a short period before moving off to find its first meal. This is a crucial event in the life of the tsetse.[65]

Infection of tsetse by trypanosomes

Research has shown that for *Gl. palpalis* to become infected with *T. brucei gambiense*, five conditions are necessary. (1) The fly must be ready to feed within twenty-four hours of its emergence from the puparium. (2) The first host preferably should be a human although occasionally an animal will suffice.[66] (3) That first meal must be infected with parasites and (4) the disease has to be at an early stage with sufficient numbers of trypanosomes circulating in the peripheral blood, i.e. in the extremities. (5) The fly must then live at least eighteen days so that the trypanosomes can undergo the necessary cycle of development in the gut of the fly. After all these five conditions have been fulfilled, the fly can then act as a vector, or transmitter, of sleeping sickness! It should be noted that the chances of a fly becoming infected with its first meal of blood may depend upon the ecological conditions, especially the temperature, in which the puparium developed. A higher temperature in the environment of the puparium ensures that the new fly can more quickly and easily become infected. Furthermore, certain animals (including man) transmit infection to the fly more readily. For instance, pigs make excellent 'transmitters'.[67]

The usual habitat of *Gl. palpalis*, the riverine tsetse fly central to my study, is low-lying bush and fringe or gallery forests along river systems. As noted earlier, these flies, in fact, prefer humans for their blood meals, but they can readily turn to reptiles and other animals which also frequent rivers. Since they live in riverine conditions and only rarely stray far from the water, *Gl. palpalis* by following the galleries are able to penetrate farther into otherwise hostile environments, provided there is water available. Thus, they can survive in relatively well-populated regions unlike, for instance, savannah flies of the *Gl. morsitans* group. This is made possible because people generally do not destroy the vegetation along rivers. In some areas, *Gl. palpalis* has become peri-domestic which means that it lives and breeds in close proximity to man and his domestic animals, particularly pigs. We now know that tsetses can live in vegetation planted by man such as banana, oil-palm, mango, cocoa and sugar plantations.[68]

In the Congo, the palpalis group of flies live along the Congo river and its tributaries, and the flies overflow into the basin of the Nile. They live in the northern half of the Congo basin, both along the river itself, and along the Ubangi, Uele, Aruwimi, Lomani and lower Lualaba rivers. The flies were first mentioned by Gaetano Casati, an Italian cartographer and explorer, while he was in the region which was later to become the Uele district in northern Congo Free State. He reported that 'Cattle cannot be successfully reared by the Mambettu [Mangbetu] on account of a fly called tsetse, the stings of which cause death'.[69] Dr Emile Brumpt, accompanying the traveller, Bourg de Bozas, who followed the length of the Uele river in late 1902 and early 1903, had commented upon the ubiquitous *Gl. palpalis* along that river from the Congo State post of Dungu westwards.[70]

Tsetse and terrain

There has been some debate about the strength of the relationship between the presence of tsetses and specific soils and vegetation cover. In the past, it was commonly believed by some colonial researchers that there was a definite correlation, and this belief must be kept in mind when considering policy decisions in history. More recently, it has been argued that the more important correlation is that between flies and host animals, including man. The effectiveness of bush clearance policies in the past lay in the concomitant removal of animal reservoirs rather than the removal of the fly habitat *per se*. There does remain, however, a view that there are important correlations between the presence of flies and certain geographical features. For instance, a recent study demonstrates a relationship between the distribution of tsetse and laterite ironstone crust soil conditions. Occurring widely throughout the southern Sudan and northern Zaire, these formations are significant in relation to tsetse flies.

Laterites are formed in hot wet climates with hot dry intervals in which evaporation is intense. Under these conditions weak solutions produced by leaching from underlying rocks are concentrated and redissolved. This process extracts the more soluble salts but leaves the less soluble, especially hydroxides of iron and aluminium, near the surface. Here they accumulate as a reddish deposit of laterite which, in contact with the air, becomes very hard and may eventually form a shield several feet thick.[71]

Laterites are important in determining the pattern of tsetse habitats in many areas because the soil over them has been washed away completely or is very shallow. This creates a broken terrain with areas of savannah grassland alternating with patches of shrub and tree-covered land; the Azande referred to such ironstone hills as *gangara*. The behaviour of humans and other host animals of the parasitic trypanosomes as well as that of the tsetse flies is greatly affected by the nature of the terrain. As we have seen, because of their biological needs for water, shade and nutrition, the focal points for all three participants become the shaded patches where food and water will be more likely. Thus, the flies are constrained to remain near the shaded water's edge where they come into contact with man and beast who are drawn as well to these patches by their biological needs. It is significant to point out that the human form of sleeping sickness caused by *T. br. gambiense* and which is transmitted by *Gl. palpalis* from person to person, is quite different from human sleeping sickness caused by *T. br. rhodesiense*. With the latter form, humans are only an *incidental* host of what is in fact a parasite of game animals.

The case of trypanosomiasis demonstrates the importance of understanding the ecological nature of diseases and aptly illustrates Garnham's dictum that 'infections have characteristic natural foci, outside which they cannot spread except under particular environmental circumstances'.[72]

5

'The Lure of the Exotic': sleeping sickness, tropical medicine and imperialism

The elucidation of sleeping sickness has a large bearing upon the development and prosperity of Africa.   Dr Louis Sambon, 1905.

In 1904, sleeping sickness was declared to be epidemic in some parts of the Congo Free State. This was the conclusion of a team of British scientists invited from the Liverpool School of Tropical Medicine to conduct a survey of health conditions in central Africa. They advised the state authorities to take immediate action to control the further spread of sleeping sickness. It was certainly not the first time the disease had been reported. The 'sleepy sickness' had been noted in the region in the early 1880s, and fresh outbreaks were confirmed by missionaries and travellers.[1] But, by 1901, a terrible epidemic had spread around the northern shores of Lake Victoria and neighbouring islands in the Lake in the region of Busoga, in the adjoining Uganda Protectorate.[2]

The declaration of an epidemic was a watershed in the history of public health for Africans in the Congo; for, more than any other one factor, sleeping sickness prompted the development of the Belgian colonial medical service.[3] This medical service was consciously used by the Belgians as a form of 'constructive imperialism', with which they hoped to establish European influence. The provision of health services was considered by the Belgians to be a central feature of what they called their 'civilising mission' in Africa.

In discussing sleeping sickness in Africa in the early twentieth century, there are three important points. First, there was a direct link between sleeping sickness and the rapidly expanding new field of tropical medicine. Second, the epidemic in Uganda, which began in 1901, alarmed all the new colonial powers who feared the loss of potential labour forces. Finally, the European colonisers in Africa were aware of the propaganda potential of public health.

From the earliest days of colonial settlement, it had not been uncommon to find sleeping sickness cited as the cause of abandoned villages and depopulated regions which Europeans encountered during their push into the interior. Older Africans in Lower (western) Congo told a missionary doctor that the disease had arrived in their region in the 1850s.[4] By the end of the nineteenth century, both African and European observers believed that the disease had long been present in endemic form in some parts of Lower Congo; but in the 1880s and 1890s, the decades of colonial conquest, the disease had become progressively epidemic. It was clear from European reports that sleeping sickness was epidemic in Lower Congo in the 1890s. In 1895, state officials Herbert Ward and Alexandre Delcommune reported the disease among riverine populations such as the Bobangi.[5] Another state administrator claimed that there had been sporadic cases of sleeping sickness in the distant Uele district in 1902 and 1903.[6] While sleeping sickness was certainly a factor in demographic change, so was the withdrawal of peoples from troubled areas, including the major paths of communication along the rivers. It was along these routes that most European exploration and conquest took place. Often, it was not sleeping sickness itself, but other causes which were responsible for the distress of African populations. In European medical thinking, epidemics were ascribed to the arrival in an area of people with the disease-causing pathogens, the trypanosomes, in their blood. But colonial Europeans disrupted African societies to the extent that the delicate balance of natural relationships between indigenous peoples and their disease-causing pathogens was thrown into chaos. Violent changes in the human ecology, including famine, exhaustion and disease, resulted in increased stress and lowered resistance. When sleeping sickness came, the result for many Congolese was devastating.[7] By late 1902, the situation had become so critical that the Belgian vice governor-general of the Congo Free State, Felix Fuchs, warned of the need for urgent public health measures to combat the disease.[8]

Early accounts

The aetiology, pathology and epidemiology of human trypanosomiasis were unknown before 1901–3 but the 'African lethargy' or 'sleepy distemper' was well known to Europeans in West Africa from as early as the fourteenth century when good descriptions were given by Arab and Portuguese writers. Sir Harry H. Johnston[9] reported that there were certainly sporadic cases in the Gambia, in Sierra Leone and in western

Liberia between about 1785 and 1840, while it was frequently occurring on the Liberian coast between 1820 and 1870. British doctors described the disease from the mid-eighteenth century on, and in the early nineteenth century Thomas Winterbottom provided a description of the common symptom of enlarged cervical glands at the back of the neck – now known as 'Winterbottom's sign'. But long before that scientific observation, slave traders along the West Coast had rejected slaves with such swollen glands for it was common knowledge that most of those with this symptom sooner or later died in the New World. A British naval surgeon in the eighteenth century, John Atkins, provided a vivid description of the comatose stage of the disease and pointed out that the young more often contracted the 'sleepy distemper' than the elderly, and those from the interior succumbed more than those from the coast.[10]

Tropical medicine in the making

While the field of public health was relatively new in Western Europe, that of tropical medicine in 1902 was even more novel. The London and Liverpool Schools of Tropical Medicine had existed only since 1899, and Germany's Institut für Schiffs-und-Tropenkrankheiten was established in Hamburg in 1901; but Belgium did not establish its own school in Brussels until 1906. A new field of scientific endeavour, tropical medicine offered opportunities for bright young men to win international reputations. Thus the young English scientist, John Lancelot Todd, pleased by the opportunity to study sleeping sickness in the Congo Free State, informed his family in Canada: 'Tryps are a big thing and if we have luck, I may make a name yet!'[11] Research in this rapidly growing field took medical scientists far from their urban laboratories to 'exotic' regions of the globe and immersed them in the adventure of safari in the 'bush'. Partly for this reason, tropical medicine was glamorous and idealistic. One specialist found 'Negro lethargy, or the sleeping sickness of the Congo, . . . a romantic disease, which provided a subject for graphical clinical descriptions'.[12] As *Punch* rhapsodised:

> Men of Science, you that dare
> Beard the microbe in his lair,
> Tracking through the jungly thickness
> Afric's germ of Sleeping Sickness,
> Hear, oh hear my parting plea,
> *Send a microbe home to me!*[13]

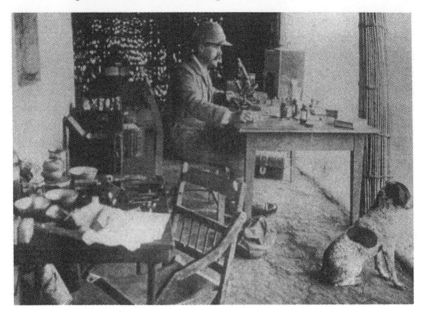

Plate 5. Cuthbert Christy in Uganda, 1902.

Tropical medicine was also intellectually exciting. Successful researchers had to be open to experimentation, ingenious at problem-solving, and innovative in difficult climates – the 'stuff' of missionary medicine. As tropical medicine gradually became more specialised, it incorporated techniques and theories from a number of scientific disciplines. Investigators required knowledge of medical zoology, proto-zoology and parasitology, helminthology, entomology, bacteriology, chemistry and haematology, in addition to traditional medicine and microscopy. In April 1898, Dr Patrick Manson published his manual *Tropical Diseases* which contained the first cogent discussion of what came to be known as 'tropical medicine' in the English-speaking world. Yet, as recently as 1939, H. Harold Scott admitted that there was still confusion over the definition of the term. Tropical medicine did not develop as a full medical specialty, and, as time passed, its development took it further from mainstream Western medicine.[14]

Most researchers concurred with the 'father of tropical medicine', Patrick Manson, that tropical diseases were those prevalent in warm climates. As they were often insect-borne parasitical diseases, climate and entomic forms became important pathogenic factors. The exemplar of tropical disease, according to Manson, was trypanosomiasis. But a few argued that many so-called 'tropical' diseases had occurred in previous ages in temperate climates – diseases such as malaria, cholera, plague, relapsing fever, leprosy, ankylostomiasis and other helminthic infestations, smallpox and typhoid fever. This was, however, a more radical view held by only a few researchers within the British and European tropical medicine research network, and while it was finding more support by the 1920s, it has only recently again been seriously discussed. Supporters of this view maintain today that many diseases labelled 'tropical' are in reality diseases of poverty and when socio-economic conditions are ameliorated, many of these 'exotic' diseases decrease or even disappear.[15]

Sleeping sickness

If colonial administrators fretted about the effects of sleeping sickness upon potential labour supplies, the international scientific community wished to solve the tantalising problem of a mysterious disease. The British scientist, Lieutenant-Colonel David Bruce, who in Natal in 1896 had first seen a trypanosome in the blood of a horse, thus discovering the cause of *nagana*, the animal form of trypanosomiasis, explained in 1908 that

a few years before the opening up of the Congo territories and Uganda, [sleeping sickness] was looked on more as a pathological curiosity than a disease . . . the curiosity is that it *never* spread from sick slaves to their neighbours in America or anywhere else out of its home in West Africa.[16]

Sleeping sickness was a real 'social event', capturing as it did the imagination of colonial authorities in Africa in much the same way that AIDS has today alarmed governments throughout the world. According to one molecular biologist working on trypanosomes, 'sleeping sickness was the AIDS of the turn of the century' which, he adds, 'made AIDS look like nothing'.[17]

The London and Liverpool Schools of Tropical Medicine responded by sending research expeditions to conduct studies of the diseases threatening colonial territories. Malaria was the first disease to evoke such a response, but with the news from Uganda, sleeping sickness soon dominated research calendars. The Liverpool School's Sixth Expedition, of 21 September 1901, consisted of Drs Joseph Everett Dutton and J. L. Todd who were sent to Gambia in West Africa to study trypanosomiasis. (At this time, they still doubted any connection between this condition and sleeping sickness.)[18] That expedition actually 'melded' into the School's Tenth Expedition to Senegambia, which began on 21 September 1902, and the Twelfth Expedition to the Congo Free State, beginning 13 September 1903. The London School of Tropical Medicine, under the direction of Manson, had first focused on the study of malaria in India, and then turned to sleeping sickness in Uganda and later other British colonies, including Northern Rhodesia and Nigeria.

In July 1903, upon his return to England from the Senegambia expedition, John Todd was amazed to find that what he and Dutton had considered to be 'their' parasite was being studied by so many other scientists. By that time, there was an air of urgency and competition.[19]

Politics and commerce in tropical medicine

From the beginning, the field of tropical medicine, called 'colonial medicine' on the Continent, involved questions both of commerce and of politics. The connection between medical science and economic development recurs in administrative documents in the Belgian Congo. As one researcher explained, 'the elucidation of [sleeping sickness] has a large bearing upon the development and prosperity of Africa'.[20] Ending such an epidemic disease would assure a fledgling colonial administration not only live labourers, but also international prestige.

Medical researchers were fully aware that 'the future of imperialism lay with the microscope'.[21] Later apologists for colonialism often pointed to the extension of Western medicine as being one of the most positive aspects of their administrations. And it was recognised as a powerful asset. In 1924, Todd explained that 'Medicine is now more than the healing of the sick and the protection of the well. Through its control of disease, medicine has come to be a world factor of limitless power.'[22] Good health alone allowed Europeans, unlike their forbears, to be permanent visitors to the tropics.

Scientists and governments were not alone in expressing an interest in tropical medicine. Alfred Lewis Jones, Chairman of the Elder Dempster Shipping Line of Liverpool, was the principal founder and first chairman of the board of the Liverpool School of Tropical Medicine from 1898 until his death in December 1909. Joseph Chamberlain, Secretary of State for the Colonies, made a plea on 25 May 1898, for the formation of schools in which to prepare colonial officers for the tropics. Jones was quick to respond and in November 1898 he offered the Royal Southern Hospital in Liverpool £350 per annum for three years to promote the special study of tropical disease. He said that 'money spent in our School of Tropical Medicine is an investment, and we expect dividends from it'.[23]

From its inception, the Liverpool School had very close relations with the city's commercial community which had, after all, played a central role in its formation. Jones was well acquainted with the Belgian king, Leopold II, whom he called 'Great Chief', and Jones' shipping line was a major transporter of Congo products. His company, Compagnie Belge du Congo, possessed the very profitable monopoly of the Congo–Antwerp trade. Chairman of the African section of the Liverpool Chamber of Commerce, Jones was also consul of the Congo Free State in Liverpool, and one of the leading defenders of the State during the great 'Red Rubber' scandal.[24] Edmund D. Morel, the founder and principal force behind the Congo Reform Association in England, said of Alfred Jones, 'Posterity will forget his attitude on the Congo and only remember that he was a powerful captain of industry, a man of great energy and the creator of the Liverpool School of Tropical Medicine.'[25]

The Uganda epidemic, 1899–1905

In the five years between the close of 1900 and the end of 1905, sleeping sickness killed over a quarter of a million Africans in the British Protectorate of Uganda. This tragedy sparked off one of the most dramatic chapters in the history of medicine. Near the end of 1900, Dr Albert R. Cook, and his brother, Dr Jack Howard Cook, missionary doctors at the Church Missionary Society's station in Mengo (Kampala), Uganda, observed the first victims of a 'fever' which they soon informed the Ugandan authorities was sleeping sickness: it was, they added, spreading rapidly. Southern Busoga was soon considered the chief focus of the disease, and by the spring of 1902, local African chiefs reported that nearly 14,000 people had died.[26]

News in April 1902 from the Medical Officer at Jinja, Dr A. D. P. Hodges, that 20,000 people had died in the epidemic, increased alarm. The British Foreign Office, urged by Patrick Manson, had already asked the Royal Society to send a special commission to the Protectorate to study the disease.[27] A three-man team composed of Aldo Castellani, George Carmichael Low and Cuthbert Christy arrived at Kisumu in July 1902. On 15 October, Low was able to write to Manson informing him that young Castellani had spotted a 'fish-like parasite darting about', and that he believed 'a streptococcus, or an organism resembling it, to be the cause of the disease'.[28]

Combined with Dutton's discovery of the first trypanosome in human blood in December 1901 during the Liverpool School's expedition to Gambia, Castellani's finding meant that the aetiology of human sleeping sickness was now understood for the first time. The British government took an early lead in sleeping sickness research, an understandable response to the potential threat to their human resources in Uganda. In fact, by 1902, sleeping sickness had become the most important administrative question in Uganda. Unaware at first of the complicated ecological nature of the disease, the British feared that it might spread along the Nile river, even to Suez. There were even fears that the disease might spread to India, with incalculable economic consequences.[29]

Over the next few decades, the Foreign Office, and later the Colonial Office, as well as both schools of tropical medicine, were engaged in research projects and special commissions related to sleeping sickness. Especially important was the establishment of the Sleeping Sickness Bureau in London which collected and published the latest research on the disease. International conferences were held in which Britain, Belgium, France, Portugal, Germany and Italy participated.[30] Both the Foreign Office and the Colonial Office sent questionnaires to a number of African territories in an effort to discover more about the disease.[31] In fact, it was the British Foreign Office from which the Congo Free State government requested information about the disease in late 1902.[32]

From Busoga the disease spread rapidly east and west, and by the end of 1903 there were over 90,000 deaths.[33] By November 1904, it was epidemic as far west as the shores of Lake Albert, which bordered the Congo Free State. Official calculations of mortality rates varied, but Bruce, a reliable witness, claimed that in Busoga, with a population of 300,000, as many as 200,000 had died! In 1905, one member of the Royal Society's commission estimated that in the past three years sleeping sickness had caused an annual mortality of 100,000 in Uganda.[34] Another reliable source, Brian Langlands, later asserted that in Uganda between 1900 and 1920, deaths from the disease numbered between 250,000 and 300,000. All the colonial powers in Africa took note of events in Uganda. We will never know the total mortality for certain, but it is obvious why administrators of all African territories were alarmed.[35]

At the turn of the century, most medical authorities held the view that epidemics of disease erupted under particular conditions; this was the notion of circumstantial epidemiology. Thus after the discovery of the aetiology of the disease in 1902, it was believed that a region containing people, *Gl. palpalis* and trypanosomes, was circumstantially ideal for the outbreak of sleeping sickness.

In 1908, Bruce was convinced that the spread of sleeping sickness in Uganda had been clearly the fault of the British. He asserted that he could positively demonstrate the manner in which the disease had been disseminated for the past twenty years by native movements in response to European demands for labour. 'Pax Britannica' had allowed freer travel throughout central Africa and was responsible for the spread of sleeping sickness.[36]

Most other researchers, however, tended to accept Sir Harry Johnston's view that the infection had travelled with Stanley's Emin Pasha relief expedition and had reached the Congo–Uganda border at Lake Albert in 1888–9. The men left behind by the Emin Pasha expedition, the so-called 'Soudanese' remnants, were blamed for later spreading the disease. The Soudanese were former troops under the command of Emin, who with their numerous kin, totalling 4,500 according to Gerald Portal, had been forced southwards from Equatoria (southern Sudan today) by Mahdist victories. Many of them chose not to make the long trek to the east coast in May 1889 with Stanley, but instead settled in what became the Uganda Protectorate. Over two years later, on 5 October 1891, Lugard began the exodus southwards of 8,000 so-called 'Soudanese' soldiers, wives, children and slaves whom he wished to settle elsewhere. They moved along the western side of Lake Albert to the Semliki river in eastern Congo where they survived in large part by raiding local peoples and causing them considerable hardship. In 1893 Portal, the commissioner of Uganda, recruited about 450 of the soldiers, who, with their very numerous entourages, were relocated in a scattering of posts around the northern shores of Lake Victoria. It was later argued by epidemiologists that these activities ensured the further spread of the disease.[37]

In part, this was accurate. At the same time, contemporary medical experts believed that for a given disease, there was a proper medical response. Disease was an invader, medicine was the vanquisher. Experts responded by seeking and then combating the 'germ' with an appropriate weapon in the form of chemotherapy, or medicine. Congo State administrators believed that some regions, like the Uele district in northern Congo, with their still uninfected populations, frequent

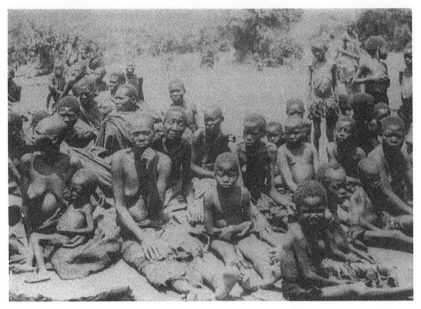

Plate 6. Sleeping sickness victims, Buvuma Island, Uganda, 1902.

movements and the presence of *Gl. palpalis*, were severely threatened and required prompt, preventive action. A disease which could annihilate such staggering numbers of people in Uganda evoked an impressive response.

Sleeping sickness and propaganda

But there were other powerful motives, besides the purely medical, behind the response of the colonial powers. King Leopold II of Belgium, probably the most ambitious imperialist in Africa, had more than one motive for protecting the human capital in his private state.[38] After all, the Congo was very much his creation. In late 1903, some eighteen years after Leopold had founded his empire, John Todd described the position thus:

The King of the Belgians is absolute sovereign here and this is not a Belgian colony in the proper sense of the word. The King of the Belgians made the state, and it is practically his. He must be a very smart man indeed to have made use of his position as a Ruler to so successfully exploit the country. He is boss of the state both as ruler and in the same way as some of the big mine owners out West are sovereigns of certain towns . . . [39]

At the invitation of Leopold, the Liverpool School sent an expedition to study sleeping sickness in the Congo Free State. This consisted of three experienced scientists, J. E. Dutton, J. L. Todd and Cuthbert Christy, who arrived at Boma in the autumn of 1903. Officially, the expedition remained eighteen months, although Christy left much earlier and Dutton died of fever in February 1905. In these months, the entire length of the Congo river and most of the Lualaba were examined for the disease while more general observations were made on the sanitation of the state posts. The researchers relied upon written and oral reports for vast regions of the state but in spite of these limitations their conclusions and advice to the Congo Free State authorities formed the basis of a public health programme for decades to come.[40]

Leopold established a precedent for later colonial administrations by insisting upon the importance of the new field of tropical medicine, medical provision and public health policy as essential features in the justification, sometimes rationalisation, of colonisation. His decision to invite British scientists to investigate sleeping sickness in his state becomes explicable in this context. So, while diseased and dead Africans were an economic loss to all involved in the Congo adventure, Leopold had a second powerful motive for his quick response to the discovery of sleeping sickness. He intended to make the most of this opportunity to combat the increasingly effective anti-Congo State propaganda campaign being waged in Britain. In March 1900, E. D. Morel, an Englishman who had worked for Jones' shipping line since 1891, wrote a series of articles exposing the scandal of 'red rubber' in the Congo Free State. He publicised the shocking mistreatment by state agents of Congolese men, women and children, who were driven without mercy to collect rubber. In 1902, Morel made a number of public speeches and published articles in Europe where his condemnation of the 'Leopoldian system' met enthusiastic response. His book, *Affairs of West Africa*, held Leopold personally responsible for these atrocities. On 20 May 1903, a debate in the British House of Commons on the 'Congo question' resulted in a resolution indicting the Congo Free State government. As a result, on 5 June 1903, the British consul at Boma, Roger Casement, began a tour of Upper Congo to investigate the situation.[41] The resulting 'Casement Report' was submitted to the Foreign Office in December 1903, and a heavily revised version was sent to the Congo State in early February 1904. In March 1904, the Congo Reform Association was officially established. An increasingly effective lobby, this group successfully pressured the 'Leopoldian regime' for many years.

The association was dissolved in June 1913, some five years after the Congo Free State had passed into the jurisdiction of the Belgian government as a colony.[42]

It is clear that Leopold's invitation to the Liverpool School to investigate sleeping sickness was related in part to his concern for his international image. It is also clear that he knew the potential propaganda value of attending benevolently to an epidemic of sleeping sickness. It was an opportunity not only to prevent dangers to his labour force, but also to take part in a prestigious, international quest. After a visit to Leopold in August 1906, John Todd made this revelation in a letter to his family:

After we'd finished telling the old man how to make the Congo healthy and promised to administer a lovely coat of whitewash to his character in the eyes of the English, he created Boyce, Ross and myself officers of his Order of Leopold II . . . We commenced yesterday what is intended to become quite a political move – an *entente cordiale* – a renewal of the intimacy of Belgium and England, which Congo jealousy has placed under a cloud.

This scientist had no doubts about the lively connection between health, economics and politics. He added: 'The anti-Congo papers will certainly say that they [funds allocated by Leopold to the Liverpool School] represent the bribe to the School (and myself in particular) for saying nothing concerning Congo atrocities and administering a lovely coat of whitewash to the Free State.'[43]

6

Discovery: Liverpool scientists in the Congo

The scientists

On 23 September 1903 the team of scientists from Liverpool arrived in the Congo Free State to begin assessing the public health situation, particularly with reference to sleeping sickness. The Twelfth Expedition of the Liverpool School of Tropical Medicine consisted of Doctors Joseph Everett Dutton, 28, John Lancelot Todd, 27, and Cuthbert Christy, 40, each of whom recently had taken part in previous trypano-somiasis research expeditions in Africa. Dutton had participated in the Third Expedition concerned with malaria in Nigeria in 1900 and in two expeditions dealing with trypanosomiasis, in 1901 and 1902, both to Senegambia. Cuthbert Christy, a most difficult and irascible man, had been briefly attached to the Royal Society's first sleeping sickness com-mission to Uganda in 1902. When they reached the Congo Free State, the British team was joined by Dr Inge-Valdemar Heiberg, a reserve captain in the Norwegian army, who was one of the many non-Belgian military doctors employed by the State. Heiberg's career of six terms spanned nearly twenty years. Beginning as a *médecin d'expedition* in the Lado enclave, he became director of the first sleeping sickness lazaret at Ibembo in 1907 and the first *médecin en chef* of the Congo on 28 January 1911. As an illustration of the small number of tropical health specialists at the time, Dutton and Todd were already acquainted with Heibert whom they had met in Liverpool where he had completed the new tropical medicine course in May 1903. Dutton explained, 'We were delighted when he told us that he was put at our disposition and was to act as a guide, aide-de-camp and everything else.'[1]

On 30 June 1904, after spending nine months in Lower Congo at Boma, Leopoldville, Matadi and the Cataract area, the researchers began to examine peoples and stations upstream along the Congo river where they visited state and mission posts as far as Kasongo. Everywhere the emphasis was on European centres, as the primary concern of the administration was European health. The expedition returned to Boma on 27 February 1905.

In spite of the great stretches of the country personally investigated by the researchers, they did not actually observe the vast majority of the territory of the Congo Free State.

Only a small part of our facts was obtained by personal observation. 23 months were spent in the Congo, and during that time we travelled some 2,000 miles . . . several short journeys of from 1 to 7 days' duration were made off the main line of travel. The conditions obtaining were carefully noted on each locality visited, and residents, missionaries, State officials and natives were thoroughly questioned.[2]

They did not travel along major tributaries of the Congo river such as the Ubangi, Itimbiri or Aruwimi rivers into the north-eastern portion of the Free State but relied upon secondary oral and written accounts from state agents, medical staff, commercial representatives, traders and African informants. A major source of information for areas not personally observed was the questionnaires distributed by the Free State on behalf of the researchers. In fact, the researchers' fieldwork in the north-east consisted of sixteen days near the river in the vicinity of Stanley Falls. Yet rather ironically it was the north-east which between 1905 and 1930 experienced the full brunt of the public health campaign suggested by the researchers.

There were only a few reports about the situation in the north-east and they were based upon the most unscientific evidence. For instance, the commandant of Stanley Falls reported that he had been as far north as Avakubi in 1896 and to Bafwaboli five years later and each time he had 'seen' no sleeping sickness. The researchers were informed of a few cases of the disease by a state doctor who had just finished his term of service in the Lado enclave, and while the doctor did not believe those cases to have been contracted in the enclave he did believe that the disease was present among natives around the important administrative post of Bambili in Uele district.[3]

The primary purpose of the Liverpool survey was first and foremost *scientific*. The motive of the scientists was analysis of the aetiology, pathology and epidemiology of the disease(s) caused by trypanosomes. Advice on the management of public health among African societies, so crucial in the history of the Belgian Congo, was of secondary importance to the researchers. The main point was quite clearly the solution to the intriguing puzzle of this exotic tropical disease.

Yet long before the researchers had completed their survey in February 1905, they had submitted a series of reports and advisory statements which resulted in public health measures with which the State hoped to control the spread of the disease. Their advice was much heeded by the Congo authorities, and as the Liverpool investigation was a crucial episode in the history of sleeping sickness and the evolution of the public health service in the Belgian Congo, we must examine its activities and conclusions in some detail, paying particular attention to the motivations and preconceptions of the participants.

The Liverpool scientists inaugurated some features of the routine later followed by the annual sleeping sickness survey teams which examined the populations in the colony after World War I. For many Africans, their experiences with the Liverpool researchers were, if not their first, then certainly among their most memorable encounters with the new European rulers. Those memories were not pleasant. The team of scientists – travelling with a large entourage and many loads of equipment and accompanied by government administrators and porters borrowed from the army, whose instructions were carried out by chiefs and headmen – most certainly represented the new, oppressive state no less than its directly employed functionaries. In addition, the scientists' rather rough handling of individuals during examinations doubtlessly added to the unpleasantness of memories of those initial encounters with European medicine. We must not forget that there was a vast gulf between African and European perceptions of what constituted disease and the two groups had different opinions of appropriate responses. The European scientists, with their unexamined attitudes of superiority, simply never considered that gulf to be of any significance.

Objectives

While officially the purpose of the expedition was two-fold, it was soon referred to simply as a 'trypanosomiasis mission'. The researchers had been instructed by Leopold to investigate and report upon the sanitation of the principal state posts in addition to continuing the 'School's work on human trypanosomiasis and its connection with the sleeping sickness in animals'.[4] It was still assumed by many in the scientific community that these were two distinct diseases. Dutton and Todd informed the chairman and committee of the school that 'it is most necessary to study the relation between trypanosomiasis and sleeping sickness, both of which are present there (in Congo). We wish to find the carrying agent of the human trypanosome and to make further observation on the relation of the tse-tse fly to trypanosomiasis.'[5]

Todd wrote to his brother, Bert, on 8 July 1903 before embarking for the Congo, that both he and Dutton were pleased at the opportunity of going,

because it gives us a chance to complete the work we commenced in the Gambia and especially since it will enable us to examine the probability of the hypothesis, which Colonel Bruce and other workers in Uganda have put forward concerning sleeping sickness. They say it is caused by trypanosomes. We do not believe it at present.[6]

On 29 July 1903 Dutton and Todd informed Sir Patrick Manson that they could still say nothing about the relation of trypanosomiasis and sleeping sickness. Of course, they knew that just recently David Bruce had shown that trypanosomes appeared in startling numbers with great frequency in those affected with sleeping sickness. If it really were the causal agent of sleeping sickness, 'it is a very important "bug" indeed. Privately I don't think that the particular variety of it which I know, is. We hope to prove its relation, or no, to sleeping sickness, while in the Congo, and also to find out how the parasite gets from individual to individual.'[7]

Sanitation

Leopold's other primary objective for the expedition was an inspection and report of the sanitation of state posts, but not a great deal seems to have been done because the scientists were frankly of the opinion that the study of sleeping sickness was of far greater importance. There are few references to sanitation in their reports, only one of which was published in the Liverpool School's *Memoir* series. In that era, 'sanitation' in the colonial setting meant action concerning conditions in which malaria flourished. This objective was referred to by Dutton in his long letter to Ross on 1 February 1904, some five months after the researchers had begun: 'We have delayed writing reports on the mosquito sanitary questions, though we have practically done all the inspections, as I think while we are here we should devote all our time to the sleeping sickness question. It appears to us of vital importance to the State; the mortality from this disease is distinctly great.'[8]

According to the researchers the population of the capital, Boma, consisted of some 400 to 450 Europeans and 3,000 to 4,000 Africans, and while there was no sewage system in the town, it compared most favourably with the towns they had previously visited in British West African territories. They were informed that excreta and rubbish were simply emptied from government wharfs into the river, which 'sometimes affects the water supply when the [tributary] river backs into the Congo'.[9]

Felix Fuchs, the governor-general of the Congo Free State was reported to be 'very wide awake' with respect to the researchers' sanitation advice and by 8 November 1903 he had already commenced on some of their recommended improvements such as swamp drainage and clearance of water grass along the water front. But in May 1905 upon his return to Leopoldville, Todd recorded that there were no public latrines, rubbish was dumped 'by order' in the middle of the town and the doctor told him that during his entire tour in Leopoldville the Conseil d'Hygiène had never once met.

Finally, besides dealing with the specific subjects of sanitation and sleeping sickness assigned to the researchers, the expedition made notes on other endemic and epidemic diseases and Dutton, in particular, paid some attention to African terminology and procedures in relation to disease and illness. Their notes contain observations relating also to socio-economic and political conditions.

Method and routine

The scientists used a number of techniques quite foreign to African experience. They examined people and corpses, blood and lymphatic fluid. Microscopy played a major role in the research and it should be pointed out that even many years later when it was routine, a microscopic study of one blood-slide for the presence of trypanosomes averaged twenty minutes! Todd explained that the microscopy involved 'no necessity to think of the work – it's done reflexly [sic] – and my mind is left free to all sorts of curious thoughts . . . '.[10] Blood samples were generally taken from a finger while lymph fluid came from the posterior cervical glands and from cerebral-spinal fluid drawn from the lower spine by means of a lumbar puncture, a most painful procedure even in clinical conditions. The cervical glands were aspirated with a syringe – yet another strange procedure for the people. Todd noted that it was 'only after passing Coquilhatville that gland palpation and puncture were employed . . . permitting us to form a really accurate idea of the percentage of natives infected with trypanosomes'.[11]

No time was wasted and work began almost the moment the

scientists arrived in the Congo Free State and their field diaries reflect long and busy days. The sheer number of tasks undertaken daily for the next two years are impressive by any standard. Within a week of arrival they were settled in and working at a hospital for Africans where they examined the first ten cases of sleeping sickness. They quickly fell into a routine of days spent at the hospital of working in their own quarters on specimens with microscopes. Variety was provided by numerous visits to nearby locales to examine Africans.

By April 1904, after five months in Leopoldville and 465 examinations, the researchers had identified 54 Africans infected with trypanosomes. In three other major centres, Boma, Matadi and the Cataract area, examinations of 707 people had revealed 49 infections. To give an idea of the rate of infection being discovered in the Congo State, in the Gambia the scientists had only been able to identify 6 cases of trypanosomiasis after 1,071 examinations of finger blood, while examinations by exactly the same method of 1,015 people in Lower Congo revealed 46 cases.

The six months spent at Matadi, Leopoldville and Boma were occupied with many experiments as well as the clinical observation of victims of the disease. Seeking the mode of transmission of the parasite, the scientists made many attempts to feed a fly on an infected rat or guinea pig and then successfully transmit the trypanosomes to an uninfected specimen. During this period, they performed many autopsies, a procedure which greatly alarmed local Africans and gave rise to disquieting rumours about the 'true purpose' of the scientists' work.

Physical examinations involved palpation of cervical glands at the back of the neck as well as careful scrutiny of individuals for tell-tale signs of the disease. Records were kept of temperatures, pulse rates, abscesses, bowel conditions and a wide range of accompanying symptoms and conditions. As far as possible, the scientists recorded patients' names, approximate ages, sex, home villages, length of stay in their present locale and length of present illness. Naturally, careful note was made of the presence of trypanosomes in all samples.

It was slow work. Dutton reported to Ross that the 'investigations here naturally progress slowly (1 tsetse fly takes a whole day to dissect)', but so exciting was this research that he and Todd made it quite clear that they did not want to leave Congo until they 'had something good' or were 'fagged out' and if the school could not afford to continue paying them, they were prepared to finance themselves.[12] They visited state officials and nearby religious missions. For instance, in October 1903 they visited the American Baptist Missionary Union station, Banza Mateke, and the Ecole Scolaire, where they took blood samples from fifty pupils. They also examined soldiers' children at a camp which contained, they were informed, about 250 men. In the same month, Dutton and Heiberg inspected the hotels of Boma and the prison where blood samples were taken from the prisoners. On 24 December 1903, Todd outlined a typical day's schedule:

6–6:30 a.m.	rise and work until 11
11:00	breakfast
11:30–2	writing and microscopy
2–6:30 or 7	work
7:00	bathe and dine

Often he worked again after dining or just fell asleep 'like a log'.[13]

The confusion over trypanosomiasis and sleeping sickness continued. Early in November 1903, Dutton and Christy spent several weeks inspecting Wathen mission station where sleeping sickness had been reported as endemic. Christy visited four villages where missionaries had reported much sleeping sickness, but he said he could find none. In other areas thought to be infected, African houses had been burnt with the result that Africans began to hide victims. But Christy was certain that there was no sleeping sickness around Wathen. His explanation for the non-existence of victims was that many cases purported to be sleeping sickness were in face trypanosomiasis cases![14] He wrote:

Although reports from Bentley and others to the Government and handed to us stated that whole villages were and had been decimated by sleeping sickness, what does it mean? Almost any case of illness of whatever sort is put down by the natives as sleeping sickness and the diagnosis seems to be infallibly accepted by the missionaries who of late have heard more of sleeping sickness than is good for them. Apart from the recent fuss made about sleeping sickness every missionary who comes to the Congo is primed before he starts from home with idears [sic] of the awful disease called Negro sickness of the Congo of which no exact symptoms have ever been published till recently.[15]

Christy's comments are a distant reminder of the impact on both African and European of the declaration of a frightening, and apparently new disease, like AIDS, attaining epidemic proportions.

Questionnaires

A questionnaire had been used with some success by the Royal Society's commission in Uganda in 1902, and in fact it was their set of nine questions which was first employed in the Congo. On 18 May 1903 the governor-general distributed the form to all territorial agents, missionaries, military camp commanders and state doctors and that October the Liverpool scientists requested that their own questionnaire be sent to all of the previous informants as well as to all commercial agents. Most of the responses, however, came from district administrators and Free State physicians.[16]

A wide range of issues was covered: did sleeping sickness exist in the district? When had it appeared? What was the population of the district and had there been any changes? Was the disease endemic or epidemic? Did it appear to have been introduced from elsewhere? Did the native recognise it? Did they have a name for it? Respondents were asked to comment on the contagiousness of the disease. Had a European ever contracted sleeping sickness?[17] There were further questions about the presence of tsetse and the disease in animals, commonly called by its Sotho name, *nagana*.[18]

The responses to the questionnaires varied in both length and quality. Some were only cursory while others were far more detailed. For instance, the Baptist missionary William Holman Bentley, stationed at Wathen in the Cataracts district, returned eleven pages of informative detail. He described the disease as a widespread disaster in his region with 'hardly a village escaping its ravages'. It was not a new disease as there had been occasional cases over twenty-five years previously. By 1886–7, the 'ravages were terrible at Manteke 180 kilometres southwest [*sic*] of here and it became epidemic in the district. I regard the disease as an endemic which became epidemic.' He then described the course of the symptoms, the ecology of his area, the labour patterns of the African populations, their diet, and he even suggested how the disease was transmitted by means of saliva.[19]

Responses to the questionnaire provided a variety of useful information. For example, the commandant of the military camp at Luki, in Lower Congo, supplied a list of all the victims of sleeping sickness in the camp since the time of their arrival in June 1903. Of fourteen people, two, both women, were from the Uele district in the north-east. There were 300 men and 100 women in the camp. Commandant Bouillot reported that Africans advised that the way to avoid contracting the disease was to avoid stepping on the spittle or urine of a victim. One informant reported that sleeping sickness was very frequent, although several years previously, he said, it had been unknown. He provided a recipe for a therapeutic remedy employed by his people.[20]

By February 1904 fifty administrators and physicians had replied to the questionnaire with ten replies coming from the north of the State. While the responses were instructive, many lacked precise details and Dutton explained that 'it will, therefore, scarcely be possible to make a comparison between the replies received to the two questionnaires for the purpose of extending in what directions and with what rapidity sleeping sickness is spreading. Neither will it be possible to form a very accurate idea of the localities in which tsetse flies and man-biting flies occur.'[21] Yet, it was based upon such imprecise information that the Liverpool scientists formulated their epidemiological maps which presented most of the north as an area free of sleeping sickness and an area which had, at all costs, to be protected from an invasion of the disease.

Physical examinations

It was the physical examinations which brought the scientists into their most intimate contact with Africans and in those encounters we can discern some of the attitudes which account for misunderstanding on both sides. The researchers were well-trained professional scientists of the highest calibre, and they attempted to carry out carefully controlled observation and analysis in order to test hypotheses in as objective a fashion as conditions would allow. However, the techniques involved in Western science, coupled with the new political and economic structures, caused considerable grief to many Africans. This was especially true when European medical measures directly conflicted with traditional beliefs and practices. The scientists employed 'invasive techniques', that is, their needles and knives punctured and cut the flesh, procedures with which even most Europeans were uncomfortable. At the same time, the intimate contact occasioned by physical examinations generally reinforced European assumptions of superiority and faith in the legitimacy of their colonial venture. In one of the approximately 200 letters addressed by Todd to his mother while in Congo, he mentioned the shock expressed by Dr Heiberg at some of the methods of the scientists. Todd described how casually and *swiftly* an African was stretched out on the ground and a lumbar puncture performed. Even in the best conditions, a lumbar puncture is a difficult and painful procedure. Another time, Todd explained how the researchers had 'rather horrified' some missionaries 'by the rapidity and indifference with which we lumbar-punctured. You should have seen his eyes bulge as the patients were put on the floor and "done" with no waste of time.'[22]

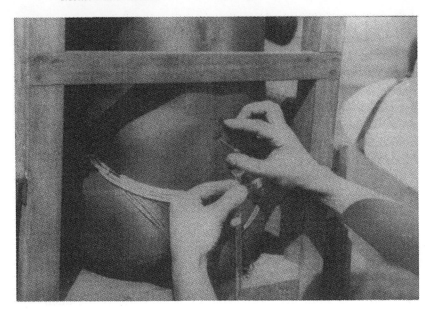

Plate 7. Lumbar puncture in field, 1935.

The researchers came into close contact with various categories of Africans. Speaking no African languages, however, they had to work through interpreters who were most often the local administrators with whom the recently conquered peoples could not have had very pleasant relations in the best of circumstances. For instance, near Bamania mission on 10 July 1904, Dobbelaere, the agent in charge of the agricultural plantation, acted as interpreter. The purpose of such plantations was the production of food for Africans compelled to labour for the state or for the production of cash crops. When the scientists arrived on the scene, we can assume that most Africans were not given even the most rudimentary explanations of what was happening but were, instead, simply ordered about.[23]

The vast majority of the Africans physically examined by the researchers were those already labouring and living within the new colonial state structure. In addition to their own personal staff and assistants, the *capitas* (headmen) and state-appointed chiefs, the Force Publique, labourers, porters and other auxiliaries were all examined. These included a few medical helpers; labourers in both the urban and rural sectors; and small numbers of students, mostly the sons of African chiefs at the colony's training school at Boma, the capital. Significant numbers of Africans had been drawn into the mission network, and so the researchers visited missions and their orphanages and schools. They also visited prisons, military training camps, administrative and military posts, wood-fuelling posts for riverboats, state agricultural plantations, hospitals – anywhere Africans had been drawn into the colonial structure and economy. Since August 1903, when sleeping sickness had been listed as a contagious disease, administrators had been instructed to isolate suspected victims; thus a number of such 'establishments' already existed by the time the Liverpool scientists arrived. Naturally, these Africans were also examined.

Whenever possible the researchers attempted to examine the wives and children of the auxiliaries. However, it was frequently difficult to examine the women, children and even the elderly. The attempts to examine Africans within their own 'traditional' settings away from European centres were few. For instance, during October 1904, Dutton and Heiberg made a short trip 'into the bush' up the Lowa river to observe the conditions of Africans in an area reportedly free of sleeping sickness and 'where the influence of the white man and traffic is not much felt'. They soon discovered that it was especially difficult to examine women who were outside direct contact with the state.

The majority of those examined were between the approximate ages of 14 and 30, as it was that age-range which was more commonly drawn into the colonial economy. The scientists estimated the age of Africans from their appearance so we must take age statistics as only a general impression.[24] Later, Todd reported that almost 90 percent of the total number of trypanosomiasis cases seen in the Congo had been young adults. He accounted for this in part as being due to the fact that 'the natives of the Congo were unaccustomed to Europeans, and the tendency was for women, children and the aged to hide from the members of the expedition'. In opening up the country, large numbers of young men, sometimes with their women, were drawn to the European settlements to act as labourers and soldiers, and Todd explained that such persons were easily examined. 'The cases of trypanosomiasis seen in European posts came almost entirely from among them.' Certain occupations, however, such as labouring on plantations, were to a large extent performed by women. Thus, younger children and older adults most often escaped examination. We must keep in mind the skewed sample examined by the scientists when considering their statistics and the conclusions based upon them. Not only were age and sex misrepresented in their survey but the fact that most Africans studied were those already within the state economy with its attendant stresses most certainly affected the infection rates calculated by the researchers.

Most often the researchers would simply arrive at a state post or mission, request those in authority to assemble likely candidates for examination for trypanosomes or sleeping sickness and set to work. In the case of those Africans already within the state sector this was fairly straightforward, but with those not directly involved with the state such as dependents and villagers there were often difficulties. Orders would be passed from either the scientists or higher authorities to the local administrator, who might prevail upon the local contingent of the Force Publique to assist in rounding up persons to examine. The local administrator would also inform the state-appointed chief and his *capitas*, or headmen, to cooperate in assembling people.[25] The scientists were very impressed by the efficiency of state operations and Todd openly praised the semi-military nature of government and its extremely detailed instructions to administrators.

A variety of means was employed to identify individuals who might be ill with trypanosomiasis or sleeping sickness. The Trappist monks at one mission used children to inform on the ill who were being hidden by their relatives from European eyes. The monks sent boys into the villages where they were to throw down sticks in front of the huts in which patients were being hidden. The scientists reported how the state administrator sent soldiers with canoes to surround one town so that the ill could not be whisked away by their kin into the surrounding brush before the team arrived.[26] One can only speculate on the terror which preceded the scientists during their tour of the Congo State.

All the time, the sick were 'weeded out' from settlements and in many cases transported by state agents to new sites which were most often located more conveniently for the state nearer main rivers or routes of communication. At another mission station the missionary's wife collected together some 200 people for examinations. Africans already established outside their own traditions and now living within European influence thus found it necessary to cooperate with the new authorities. In this case, it seems, army and state coercion were not necessary.[27]

Dutton has left us a vivid description of the expedition on the move which gives some idea of its impact. A variety of transport was used. For nearly two months a small steamer was put at the expedition's disposal for use as a floating laboratory and as transport between Leopoldville and Stanley Falls. At other times they travelled along the river by canoe. Along one stretch, each member of the expedition had a large canoe –

about 30 feet long – with twelve to fourteen paddlers. At each stop a drum summoned women who had to carry the scientists' *350 loads* of equipment and supplies to sheds for the night. Dutton explained that everything operated smoothly, with both women and paddlers 'willing and smiling'. He added: 'to a European mind it seems hard on the women to carry heavy boxes; but in reality it is not so, they are accustomed to hard work. It is a mistake in Africa to apply European ideas to the native.'[28] This important European misconception about the differences between themselves and the 'natives' is of great importance when considering the history of health, for it was assumptions like this which affected health policy and practice at every level of the colonial state.

Individual Africans do occasionally emerge in the records. Some of the researchers' case notes are available, and they contain names of individuals, ethnic identities, approximate ages, home regions, occupations and diagnoses, with additional notes in some cases. Attempts were sometimes made to follow up individual victims. For instance, a retrospective entry in one of Todd's notebooks reveals that all the sleeping sickness victims at one stop had ' . . . died soon after we left . . . the administrator . . . says they were quite uncared for'.[29] From Canada many years later, Todd tried, usually without success, to find out what had happened to several former victims. Only very occasionally could a state doctor report upon the outcome for an individual victim of the disease who had been personally observed or examined by the researchers as they had passed through his territory years before.[30]

Researchers' perceptions of Africans

These vignettes provide clues about the relationship between the medical doctor and the scientists with their quite different goals. They also demonstrate the more obvious relationship between the Europeans and the Africans telling us something about the unquestioned assumptions making up the late-Victorian view of Africans, who were, after all the subject of Todd's study. Africans, it was thought, while human were nevertheless of a lower order. Most European colonists in Africa wasted little rhetoric eulogising their newly-acquired subjects. In stark contrast to the eighteenth-century literary and artistic ideal of the 'noble savage', European imperialists of the early twentieth century generally possessed a quite different view of Africans, one which emphasised a *biological* as well as cultural inferiority.

The attitude of the Liverpool scientists towards the people whom they were examining in the course of their research was not so different from the prevailing attitudes of most Europeans in the Congo Free State. There were moments of sympathy and sensitivity for the hardships of the African situation, but most often observations of that nature were immediately followed with rationalisations for that situation. The scientists also implied strongly that such hardships were of a long-standing nature, and while some were imposed by the state, many would be ameliorated as the state developed.

Impressions of brutality and suffering alternate with expansive views of a dynamic, improving country in which fortunes could be made. Late-Victorian pride in well-rewarded labour alternates with Dickensian pathos over the African's plight. For example, in Matadi on 8 November 1903, Todd wrote to his mother that the

natives have been wonderfully squeezed by taxes and disease, so that the remnant are most miserable and quite unlike what one would imagine from Stanley's descriptions of a rich and populous country. Every steamer coming down the river is loaded with ivory and rubber. They are not adequate to transport the supply and we are told there are hundreds of bags waiting at various riverside posts to be shipped.[31]

In general, Dutton emerges through his letters and diaries as a more gentle, observant and perhaps humanitarian individual than Todd, whose writings convey a sharper cynicism and, some would say, realism. 'Life isn't worth much. I have seen more deaths since I have been here, than I ever saw in Montreal, during three years in hospitals.' Todd wrote this before he had been in the Congo Free State even one full year.[32]

African perceptions of the scientists

African perceptions of the scientific mission can only be inferred from their actions as reported by Europeans, and this perspective makes it extremely difficult to ascertain the subtleties of the situation. Generally, those who were able to do so ran away themselves or hid victims of sleeping sickness, or even all seriously ill patients, from the European authorities. This response was understandable since from August 1903, when sleeping sickness notification and isolation of victims were made obligatory, Africans had feared being taken far from their kin. Their own isolation practices generally removed victims to the edges of settlements but, more importantly, such decisions were taken by their own recognised authorities. Illness became yet one more area of life, like labour, which Europeans controlled and which often involved physical upheaval.

Not all Africans shunned the European scientists. For instance, at Kasongo, Africans pleaded with the researchers for assistance for sick kin. In April 1905 a girl, about 13, with sleeping sickness was brought by her relations to the researchers in the hope of assistance, but there was no space in which to keep her. 'It was most pathetic and very human to see their disappointment,' reported Todd, 'and the solicitude with which they persuaded the child to drink our hated – and useless – medicine.'[33] He also reported:

Some of the natives believe that we can cure sleeping sickness (we've never given them any hope) and more than once some poor wretch has come with his bed, a rolled up mat containing all his belongings, and said that he intended to follow us everywhere. I shall never forget the tears and absolutely hopeless forlornity of a boy at Leopoldville and of a woman recently, who tried to get on our steamer, were refused and left gazing on the beach.[34]

In addition to physical upheaval, we have already seen how European management of disease caused enormous psychic disturbance in African societies. There was much fear of the strange activities of the scientists. Not only could the Europeans force people to submit to physical examinations, they also could perform painful invasive procedures such as taking blood and lymph samples or spinal fluid by means of lumbar punctures in the roughshod manner referred to above. Rumours were rife about the fate of those unfortunate Africans identified as ill and isolated by the Europeans in places from which, most often, they never again reappeared. What happened to them? Todd explained to his mother: 'We are told that we are believed to eat parts of those on whom we do autopsies, and to preserve other portions for the purpose of making medicine. Hope the news doesn't spread. If it does, it will be awkward.' He also described the absolute apathy of Africans who had been sent to the state hospital for sleeping sickness in Leopoldville. The hospital was, in reality, a rough shed. After only a few days surrounded by dying people, the new victims quickly succumbed to overwhelming depression. His description of the filthy, vermin-filled hospital where people starved among the 'droning of flies' makes such depression entirely understandable.[35]

Liverpool conclusions and advice

The scientists from Liverpool shared with other European specialists basic assumptions about the nature of contagious disease, its transmission and control. They tended to rely upon knowledge derived from the metropole rather than to make the effort to understand the African socio-economic environment in which the epidemic was taking place. These assumptions, coupled with the conviction of their own superiority and the belief in their civilising mission prevented more open attitudes ón their part during the Congo survey. Their view that they, as scientists and specialists in the new field of tropical medicine, were the only ones qualified to seek solutions to problems of health in the Congo State blocked communication, and they tended, if not simply to over-look, to completely discount many opinions of people 'on the spot'.

Not all local views were ignored but conclusions based upon their own research were given priority. Only after the views of men on the spot appeared to be substantiated through their own research did the scientists seriously credit them. For instance, the view of some Africans that 'famine and hard times' were directly related to sleeping sickness was eventually accepted by Todd who said that such factors 'may decide a declaration of disease in persons already infected' as it did with animals. In 1904, missionaries at Lukolela reported that sleeping sickness had been long endemic in the region and this was corroborated by old chiefs of 70 who remembered its presence when they were boys. They then described how after a 'big' war eight years previously in the region of Irebu, sleeping sickness spread among the conquered people who had been forced to scatter, leaving their unharvested food crops behind. These missionaries were convinced that food shortages and famine were one of the major precipitating factors for sleeping sickness.[36] Further-more, some missionaries insisted that sleeping sickness epidemics had not been the *initial* cause of demographic decline but were in part a result of other socio-economic factors.[37]

Most African views on the subject of health, when rarely solicited, were considered more as items of curiosity than as relevant infor-mation. With such an approach, it would not be simple to transfer European ideas and techniques of epidemic disease management to the radically different circumstances in the Congo. And it was going to be an enormous task to impose health measures on confused, often hostile African societies. Most significantly, Europeans were generally ignorant about African societies, especially about their ideas and practices in relation to disease and misfortune. How could the Congo Free State convince African populations, their most precious resource, that draconian measures were being imposed for the benefit of the Africans when such benefits were not at all evident?

What did the Liverpool scientists learn from their long sojourn in the

Congo Free State? They discovered certain facts about trypanosomal infections, and they mapped the supposed epidemiology of sleeping sickness in the Congo State, labelling zones as endemic, epidemic or free from infection. The information about the disease was of considerable importance to the international scientific community and for their own reputations in the new field of tropical medicine. But the epidemiological mapping of sleeping sickness in the Congo State, coupled with the new knowledge of the aetiology of the disease, was a watershed in the country's history and shaped its public health policy for decades to come. At the outset of the research, Todd had described the two main objectives. How did the parasite get into people? Was it a fly as some thought or possibly a tick? And, did trypanosomes cause sleeping sickness as the Royal Society's commission in Uganda believed? If they could discover the insect vector of this disease, they could then work on prophylaxis along the same lines as malaria, e.g., eradication of the insect.

The Liverpool researchers came to several important conclusions regarding human trypanosomiasis. The expedition confirmed that *T. gambiense* was the pathogen responsible for the form of the disease prevalent in the Congo Free State. On 1 February 1904, Dutton had written to Major Ronald Ross that he had found *T. gambiense* in the stomach of a tsetse and he enclosed an example on a slide in his letter. He concluded under a heading ,'Trypanosomiasis in Congo in Relation to Sleeping Sickness', that[38]

(a) there was a low percentage of *T. gambiense* infection among the natives of the Lower Congo region;

(b) most cases were accompanied by symptoms, though not all, and there were three varieties of cases:
  (i)   trypanosomes with no symptoms;
  (ii) trypanosomes with slight symptoms; and
  (iii) trypanosomes with symptoms similar to those in animals with *nagana*; this form was what doctors had called 'the sleeping sickness';

(c) sleeping sickness in the Congo did not resemble the epidemic sleeping sickness of Uganda as the Congo variety showed none, few, or only occasional classic symptoms;

(d) death was inevitable among sleeping sickness victims; however, as secondary infections – septic pneumonia, pleurisy, dysenteric diarrhoea, meningitis, etc. – were common, it was difficult to ascertain those deaths caused specifically by sleeping sickness.

(e) parasites were found sporadically in blood and spinal fluid. The expedition advised that it was important to watch cases of trypanosomiasis very carefully in order to exclude secondary infections.

The researchers had demonstrated the phenomenon of symptomless carriers of the parasite, and this finding led to the expedition's recommendation of the feasibility of palpation of the cervical glands for purposes of diagnosis. This technique, it was maintained, was most suitable for mass surveys of the African populations. In effect, the expedition's conclusions in this regard formed the basis for the public health policy and measures of the Congo administration for decades. That policy was firmly grounded on the notion of a contagious disease which could be combated only through its identification and containment by means of isolation, as there was no available therapy. And long after late 1905 with the introduction of the drug atoxyl the basis of the public health programme with regard to sleeping sickness remained identification and isolation.[39]

Based upon their personal observations and information derived from questionnaires and other reports, the researchers published a map of the 'Distribution of Sleeping Sickness in the Congo Free State, 1905', which was most influential in policy decisions taken by the State administration (Map 5). The map indicated a huge area infected with the disease extending from the Lower Congo along the main river into the Ubangi region. Another large area where sleeping sickness was epidemic lay between Kasai district and northern Katanga, while four large areas in north-central, central and southern Congo were indicated as 'Areas not reported on'. That left a large, triangular-shaped portion of northern Congo which was shown as 'Non-infected' with the exception of six small, isolated foci which had been reported. The researchers had no first-hand knowledge of the situation in the north and nearly all of the very few reports they had received emanated from non-medical personnel.[40]

The *actual* epidemiology of sleeping sickness is a very contentious issue and for the purpose of this study it is not necessary to enter into the debate of when, where and how the disease spread. Of importance here are the responses of the colonial authorities to the scientists' *understanding* of the epidemiology of the disease. The fact that the Uele district contained very old foci of endemic sleeping sickness is not as important to the argument as is the Belgian belief that it was not only free of infection but that it was in dire danger of becoming contaminated.

It is important to remember that sleeping sickness was perceived, as

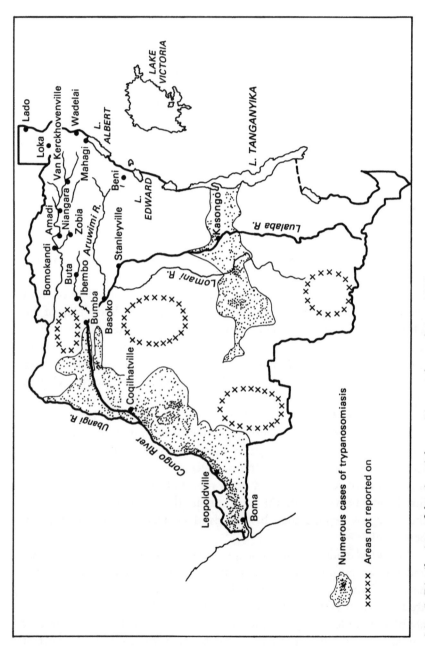

Map 5. Distribution of sleeping sickness, Liverpool expedition, 1905.

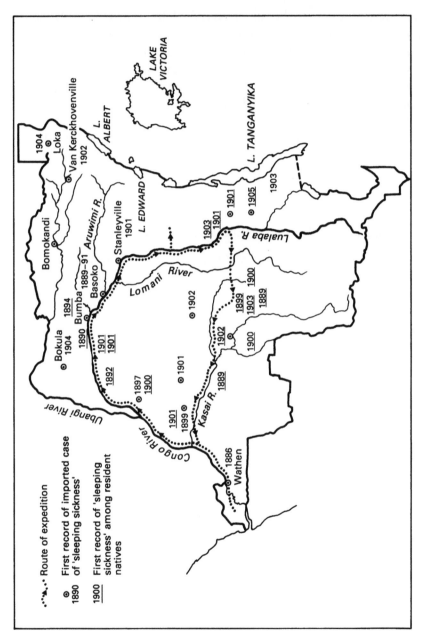

Map 6. Distribution of sleeping sickness, Liverpool expedition, 1906.

were most diseases, to be an 'invasion' of the 'enemy', pathogenic parasites, to be rooted out and prevented from entering populations and regions. The very language employed to discuss the disease reflected the view of disease as alien invader. 'Campaigns' were organised in the 'struggle' or 'fight' (*la lutte*) against sleeping sickness; and uninfected peoples and zones had to be 'defended' against invasion of the 'dreaded scourge'.

Before moving on to an examination of the advice of the Liverpool scientists, it will be helpful to quickly review their theory of the history of sleeping sickness in the Congo State. This theory reveals clearly their epidemiological assumptions.

Epidemiology of sleeping sickness in the Congo

Based on his researches, John Todd postulated the history of the spread of the disease in the Congo as follows. He explained that in 1884 Europeans had as yet no influence in the Congo basin and that the whole eastern province was controlled by 'Zanzibaris' and their allies, who ruled Central Africa exacting tribute from Avakubi to Cabinda.[41] Todd believed that these traders had never travelled much below Basoko on the Congo River where in 1888 the Free State forces had established a military post to stop them. He pointed out that none of the 'Arab' routes directly touched districts now discovered to be infected with sleeping sickness.

Todd described shorter-distance trade routes which he believed to be more 'purely' African and which he believed predated the East Coast traders' routes. For instance, Africans from between Tschumbiri and Nouvelle Anvers regularly took slaves from the Ubangi River to Leopoldville, where other middlemen African traders from the neighbourhood of Lutete (Wathen) bought the slaves and then later resold them at San Salvador in Lower Congo, in present-day Angola.

Todd believed that sleeping sickness had existed for probably *more than half a century*, in other words before the 1850s, at Wathen in Lower Congo, and it seemed probable that the constant stream of travellers may have carried sleeping sickness back up-river midway between Nouvelle Anvers and Upoto. Bumba was the highest point reported to have sleeping sickness *before* Europeans arrived. Todd then described the brisk inter-village commerce along the river in salt, fish, camwood powder, slaves and iron tools which, he said, explained the extension of sleeping sickness to Bumba.

He concluded from evidence of Europeans of long residence in the Congo and from African informants that sleeping sickness had not been known above Bumba in 1884 and he explained

No district in which sleeping sickness has once existed is known to have ever become entirely free from the disease. Cases may become more rare, but they do occur, and the natives always know and have a name for the disease. [But up-river] on Upper Congo, between Basoko and Kasongo, the disease is *quite* unknown and the natives either coin a new name to describe it, or use the Ki-Suaheli name.

He continued his history with the founding of the Free State in 1885, after which time steamers made transport on the great rivers rapid and easy. In 1888 the administration took its first step to 'suppress the slave trade'; and fortified camps were established at Basoko (1888) and Lusambo (1889). Expeditions were sent to all parts of the country, but it was in 1891–2 that war really commenced. He referred, of course, to the large military expedition of exploration and conquest begun by Commandant Van Kerckhoven in 1891 and discussed in chapter 2.[42]

Todd, the only member of the Liverpool research expedition to survive or remain the full period of the survey in the Congo Free State, concluded at the end of the tour that sleeping sickness was indeed epidemic. He believed, like so many of his contemporaries, that the disease, long endemic in the Lower Congo, had become epidemic and spread from west to east. The principal agents of that spread, he believed, were the numerous Africans who, because of the new colonial state, had been and were still moving about within the territory. Because of this focus upon the movements of populations as the major cause of the spread of the disease, Todd's advice to the authorities centred upon the necessity for state control of such movements.

Liverpool advice

The major element of the recommendations to the Congo State authorities on sleeping sickness management was the implementation of a cordon sanitaire. This was especially important in view of the fact that there was as yet no cure for the disease, but even long after 1905 with the introduction of the first drug, atoxyl, the cordon sanitaire remained the central feature of the sleeping sickness programme.

The scientists had not been the first to recommend isolation of sleeping sickness victims in the Congo State. In January 1903, when

Charles Liebrechts, the Secretary of State for the Interior, first requested advice from Liverpool about sleeping sickness, Professor Ronald Ross responded. (Ross was already well known for his research into malaria in India and identification of the insect vector, the *anopheles* mosquito.) Based upon the contagion theory, Ross had advised the immediate isolation of all cases of sleeping sickness, which he believed might possibly protect villages not yet infected with the disease. He believed that it could not be eradicated once it had manifested itself in a village, and he postulated that the disease was transmitted from person to person, most likely at night among persons sharing the same hut. He suggested that the authorities should instruct village headmen to construct isolation houses about half-a-mile from their villages and that they should make arrangements for sufficient food to be brought from the village to the patients in isolation. He further suggested that the Congo Free State should 'appoint several intelligent natives as inspectors with, perhaps, a European officer as director'. It is noteworthy that Ross's advice reveals the underlying assumption that the logical conclusions arising from European scientific research into the cause and possible prevention of a disease would be accepted and acted upon by very different societies. It did not seem to matter that, in addition to the tremendous differences in culture, the African societies had only recently been conquered or were still in the process of conquest.[43]

The Liverpool scientists recommended a policy of simple containment and prevention of the spread of sleeping sickness through the establishment of a cordon sanitaire. Their advice followed the general scientific consensus that sleeping sickness was a contagious and infectious disease, and that there were uninfected as opposed to infected zones within the Congo. It was particularly important, they said, to prevent infection from being imported by travellers and porters from neighbouring French Congo, Sudan and Uganda. They suggested that *all* Africans with swollen glands should be isolated and examined and they advised that victims' families should not be allowed to visit. Special efforts should be made to encourage chiefs to cooperate in the policy of 'search and isolate', and efforts should be made to inform African leaders of what was happening. Total isolation was not necessary for victims who were still physically able to work and, anticipating objections from European employers, the researchers pointed out that the *gambiense* variety of sleeping sickness is an exceedingly chronic disease and that infected people may remain in apparent health and be perfectly capable of steady work for several years. They assured employers that isolation 'will not mean the loss of a labourer, but only his transfer to an already infected district'.[44]

In agreement with Ross's earlier advice, the scientists urged the use of a medical passport system as a means of controlling the movements of people. At all costs, the uncontrolled movements of people must be halted. But African mobility was a vital factor in State development. Labour supply was a crucial and never-ending problem for the functioning of the army, transportation (which needed porters and paddlers), road and railway construction, agricultural production, mining enterprises and commerce (which needed porterage). The scientists stressed that Europeans should no longer be able to introduce large numbers of infected labourers and soldiers into uninfected districts as previously had been the practice. The scientists presented as an example the case of the first *noted* case of sleeping sickness in February 1901 in an African from Uele district in the north. The victim was an Uelian soldier who had taken part in a mobile military unit used to 'put down' a rebellion in 1896 around Kasongo, far to the south of Uele. No other victims were noticed among the local natives at that time. But, six years later, in November 1902, the military commandant of Stanley Falls again travelled upriver with 150 Uelian soldiers. This time, according to the military commandant, just after these men had passed through eastwards on their way to Kivu, an epidemic erupted.[45]

The scientists further advised that it was vital to supervise all river traffic in order to protect the north-east from contamination, and suggested that all transport along the Itimbiri and Aruwimi be checked at their confluences with the River Congo. In early 1903 they recommended that Africans be forbidden to travel on state steamers and that Ibembo post on the Itimbiri should become an observation post for all travellers entering or leaving the north-east. Monitoring the population in this manner would prevent European settlements from becoming new disease centres.[46]

Another very important aspect of the Liverpool scientists' advice to the Congo State administration concerned the development of the medical service. At that time all doctors were part of the state administration, and they were directly responsible to their local administrator. Thus, the medical service had no autonomy or centralisation, making it very difficult to coordinate an overall policy. Such an overall health policy was essential, according to the British scientists, for the control of a disease like sleeping sickness. Thus, they advised the establishment of a post of Principal Medical Officer who could supervise a medical service.

Furthermore, they advised that Congo Free State doctors, like the British, be required to follow a specialised course in the new field of tropical medicine before going out to the Congo State.[47]

Legacy of the Liverpool expedition

The Liverpool expedition to the Congo State has been discussed at some length because of the impact it had upon the history of public health and the African societies affected by it. While Belgian researchers were working at the same time on the problems of the mysterious disease, it was to the British specialists that Leopold turned for assistance and advice. As representatives of one of the first European schools of tropical medicine, and with several research expeditions already behind them, the opinions of the British scientists carried much weight. Their advice was quickly accepted and acted upon. Their epidemiological assumptions and their perceptions of sleeping sickness as a contagious and infectious disease formed the basis for their advice of a cordon sanitaire and its attendant features of population control. Those assumptions precluded the asking of important questions about the ways in which the disease manifests itself in societies. Although they were acutely aware of the hardships being experienced by Congolese who had been drawn into the networks of the state, they not only neglected to relate those hardships to the disease, but they even warned against the mistake of applying 'European ideas to the native'. Disease, like any enemy, had to be fought with all available weapons, and the erection of defences was vital. The socio-economic conditions in which people lived and laboured were not seriously considered as contributing factors in the incidence of disease. Thus the advice of the experts was directed at the enemy as they perceived it. It did not touch upon the deeper causes of disease which are to be located within the web of relationships, that is the ecology, in which it occurs.[48]

Perhaps most importantly, the Liverpool scientists' assumption, based upon the flimsiest evidence, that northern Congo Free State was free of sleeping sickness and constituted a great 'uninfected triangle', was to have the most profound effect upon that region. Coupled with their conviction that sleeping sickness was contagious, providing there were tsetse flies to transmit it, and that *anyone* could succumb, regardless of the particular circumstances of his physical and emotional state, their advice to cordon off the north and to erect defences for its protection completely overlooked important factors. While it is not wholly fair of the historian to condemn the actions of those who precede us, especially in light of the scientific knowledge now available, nevertheless it is relevant to draw the reader's attention not only to the important ecological nature of many diseases in general, but also to that of human trypanosomiasis in particular. The residents of northern Congo experienced major disruptions of their social ecology between 1891 and 1930, and while the region did *not* apparently experience epidemics of sleeping sickness of quite the severity of those in other parts of the colony, there were serious outbreaks. In addition, the north contained epidemic foci of the disease, such as that in the north-central region of Gwane, which can be connected to the serious upheavals of the region and the stresses that these caused to its inhabitants.

7

The campaign. Part one: Sleeping sickness and social medicine

The idea of social medicine in the Belgian Congo was born in the special campaign against sleeping sickness. In the words of one colonial doctor, sleeping sickness was a 'scourge which even an administration as unfeeling as the Congo Free State could not ignore' and by the mid-1930s most Belgian colonials tended to regard their medical and public health programmes as a form of compensation for the hardships caused by their colonisation of African peoples.[1] But for Congolese populations, the campaign against sleeping sickness had other important implications which affected their existence in ways far beyond the more traditional boundaries of public health. It became widely accepted that the special sleeping sickness campaign was the basis for both the colonial medical service and a public health programme since it was, as in several other African colonies, the first real effort made by the Europeans to deal with the health of Africans.[2] It was during this phase that the real 'medicalisation' of the Congolese began. People were systematically introduced to the idea that European doctors and their medications were the solutions to problems of ill health. The Belgian sleeping sickness campaign was elaborated and refined over time until by the 1930s it formed the core of the colonial public health programme. Yet the large-scale campaigns waged against one disease, sleeping sickness, often became so bureaucratised and routine that it was almost impossible to implement important changes in public health policy to deal with other health problems. 'The various colonial sleeping sickness campaigns became a kind of conditioned reflex . . . routine, even a fixation of ideas with the result that all epidemics were fought in stereotyped manner without asking if methods were best from region to region.'[3]

The strategy

The campaign operated on two fronts which the Belgians referred to as *médicamenteuse* and *biologique*. The former included all the more purely medical aspects such as development and the training of staff, European and African; the creation of the itinerant medical missions which by 1930 were examining nearly 3,000,000 people annually; the gradual evolution of a network of rural clinics, injection centres and hospitals, and research into the disease and possible cures. The second front, *biologique*, was primarily administrative and involved public health measures intended to control the incidence and spread of the disease. Many of these measures were in effect early attempts at 'social engineering'. Features of this front were the identification and mapping of infected and non-infected zones and the creation of cordons sanitaires to protect mainly non-infected regions such as large portions of the north-east; isolation of infected individuals in one of the special lazarets located on the fringes of uninfected zones; the regrouping and resiting of African populations as part of the overall programme with which the Belgians hoped simultaneously to solve public health, political and economic problems; and, finally, a score of administrative measures designed to regulate and control numerous African activities in order to control the epidemiology of sleeping sickness.[4]

Disease was regarded as an enemy agent against which the Belgian colonial administration fought on these two fronts.[5] The administration of the Congo Free State, which was only gradually altered after the *reprise* in 1908, quite naturally conceptualised the battle against sleeping sickness as a 'struggle', which would require all the logistics and strategy of a military campaign. Sleeping sickness, the foe, had to be isolated – cordoned off, contained and eliminated. After 1903–4 when the aetiology of the disease was first understood, the enemy became more clearly identified and those factors believed by the Europeans to cause the disease – trypanosomes and tsetse flies – could be targeted for the attack. Supported by the assumption that superior European science with its technology and medicine would succeed where primitive African societies simply floundered, the colonial authorities had no doubts about their methods. After all, 'we know how primitive and futile was the knowledge of the natives in matters of hygiene', said a medical administrator in 1943.[6]

Disease, like recalcitrant Africans, would be forced into submission. The new colonial authorities attempted total control of future labourers and taxpayers. This would require systematic and total protection from infection as well. The major feature of the early campaign against sleeping sickness, the cordon sanitaire, reflected the paternalistic nature of Belgian colonial policy in which health priorities formed a part of the justification for the methods of the social engineer. African societies, like the labouring classes in Europe, had to be controlled for their own protection. There was a crucial difference, however, in the scope of measures possible in the colonial setting, where social engineering could sometimes be exercised to an extent unimaginable in the metropole.

A profusion of legislation from both Brussels and Boma was increasingly sanctioned by the judiciary and enforced by the military and the police (see appendix A). At the same time, an evolving medical infrastructure of personnel, facilities and procedures was directed at locating, isolating and dealing with all those infected with the parasite. As we saw in chapter 4, the Belgians, like the French but unlike the British, focused primarily on one factor in the epidemiological web, man. Thus, from 1906, when the first drug became available, they concentrated increasingly on 'sterilising' the human reservoir of infection, thereby preventing the circulation of the parasites to uninfected people.[7] Victims in the first stage of the disease when the parasites frequent the peripheral circulatory system are particularly infectious as the vector flies can then transmit to new victims. Clearing a victim's blood of the parasites is referred to as 'sterilisation'. While British policies for sleeping sickness inconvenienced specific groups of people considered to be at risk (for instance, in Northern Rhodesia), their public health policy never had the overall impact on the total population as did the Belgian campaign. From the early decades of this century, prolific regulations and prohibitions combined with the mass medical surveys affected the lives of immense numbers of Congolese. The legislation and many of the policies were increasingly aimed at monitoring a wide range of social and economic activities by strictly controlling the location and movements of population.[8]

The cordon sanitaire affected the people in many ways: people's freedom of movement was subject to strict controls which included surveillance and a system of compulsory medical passports; homesteads and villages were reorganised into larger groups and forced to move to new locations; and there were increasing attempts to regulate many areas of African social and economic life which affected, for instance, kin relations and marriage. The sleeping sickness regulations affected nearly every aspect of life from taxation, trade and transport to fishing and the production of one of life's necessities, salt. The volume of legislation and instructions produced between 1903 and 1930 to combat sleeping sickness is striking indeed.

Proliferation of health services

By 1930 there was a great deal of confusion among those involved in health care in the Belgian Congo. Within the state sector, it came about because from 1903, concurrent with the development of a colonial medical service, a special sleeping sickness service evolved and much overlap developed between the two. Then, in the 1920s, the colonial administration took steps to establish a separate public health service which would take on many of the 'preventive' functions pioneered by the sleeping sickness service. In addition to health provisions made directly by the state, other agencies in the Congo played a quite significant role in medicine and public health and they were especially important in their roles in the sleeping sickness campaign. From the beginning both Catholic and Protestant missions had involved themselves to varying degrees in 'health ministry', with the minority Protestants taking a striking lead until the 1930s. In 1910 the colonial administration had officially enlisted all religious missions in the sleeping sickness campaign, and some missions established their own lazarets, which usually functioned as general clinics as well.

The mix of agencies involved in health care created new problems. The colonial medical service, the special sleeping sickness service and the religious missions each took part in the sleeping sickness campaign, and while all efforts were desperately needed in the huge task at hand, the lack of coordination among health workers often resulted in inefficient use of extremely limited resources. Furthermore, tensions among the European sectors sometimes dissipated energies which would have better benefited Africans afflicted with sleeping sickness. For instance, the vast majority of the religious missions in the Belgian Congo were Catholic, the official religion, which often meant that Protestant missionaries were at a disadvantage in relation to the administration.

The unclear status of colonial doctors was another area of strain which in turn weakened the campaign. Between 1885 and 1908, during the period of the Congo Free State, doctors formed a part of the military and were under the command of the officers who administered Leopold's state.[9] Soon after the transition to a colony in November 1908, a medical department was created within the Belgian colonial ministry; nevertheless, colonial doctors still remained under the direct authority of the various provincial and district administrations. Pressure from within the ranks of the medical staff for an autonomous medical department increased, but it was not until after World War I, in the early 1920s, that such a service was finally created. From 1903 most of the research and medical staff who concerned themselves with African health had concentrated on sleeping sickness, but the absence of an autonomous medical administration crippled any attempts to develop a unified policy to combat the sleeping sickness epidemics.

It is possible, however, to identify four phases of the sleeping sickness campaign in northern Congo between 1903 and 1930: (1) 1903–9, when most efforts were concentrated on implementing a cordon sanitaire; (2) 1910–14, during which major reforms were introduced to the sleeping sickness programme and a colonial medical department began to take shape; (3) World War I (1914–18), when a first survey of sleeping sickness was completed in Uele district and local administration in the Congo, considerably isolated from the metropolitan government (based in London during the war), stressed control of population movements; and (4) 1920–30, when an autonomous medical service and separate sleeping sickness missions were created with the eventual result of much overlap and blurring of responsibilities between the two services. In the remainder of this chapter, I will discuss the first two phases of the campaign. The period 1914 to 1930 will be discussed in the next chapter.

First phase, 1903–1909: cordon sanitaire and isolation

No sacrifice . . . appears to me too great in order to safeguard the . . . intelligent population of Uele.   Commissaire General Bertrand.[10]

The first official legislation of the campaign was a circular distributed by Vice Governor-General Felix Fuchs, on 5 May 1903. In this, Fuchs was responding to the advice of Dr Broden, director of the Bacteriological Laboratory at Leopoldville who, in agreement with Ross at Liverpool, had advised in April that soldiers and labourers with sleeping sickness should no longer be allowed to retire to their home regions but should be, instead, isolated in lazarets at state posts. Fuchs in his circular thus averred that isolation of victims was the 'principal precaution to take in order to check the spread of the disease'. On 26 August sleeping sickness was added to the list of contagious and epidemic diseases subject to the decree of 20 October 1888 which required that all suspects be isolated and the authorities notified.[11]

The tactic of a cordon sanitaire with isolation of suspected victims of contagious and epidemic diseases was already widely subscribed to by most authorities, whether they were medical, administrative or non-governmental. In fact, many local administrators on their own initiative had implemented that practice earlier, as the Liverpool researchers discovered during their survey. But medical men generally were doubtful about the efficacy of complete isolation. In 1902, Dr Rossignon, a state doctor at Boma, had advised that long and strict isolation would be difficult especially as it would necessarily separate victims from their families. He therefore suggested shorter-term isolation with some visiting allowed, since sleeping sickness was not as 'immediately contagious as a disease like typhoid'.[12] Broden raised the 'delicate question' of what to do about victims' families. Should they also be isolated? In April 1903 he wondered if these same measures should be applied 'chez natives'? But, added Broden, considering the 'insouciance and negligence of hygiene of the Africans', how could such surveillance be achieved? He reminded the governor-general that during the cholera and plague epidemics in Asia Minor and Arabia more than one port in the Mediterranean had become infected in spite of the cordon sanitaire. He feared that the Congolese manifested the same 'hatred of all hygiene measures conceived of by Western civilisation' as did the oriental populations, and that would preclude a successful cordon. Nevertheless, the Congo State could but attempt to protect uninfected regions.[13]

But Fuchs stressed the need for complete isolation, which as much as possible should be on islands in the rivers, and that access to such islands should be absolutely forbidden to non-infected people. It would be fatal, he continued in his circular of May 1903, to return victims to their home villages, because they would spread the disease. If islands were not available, then victims must be isolated at least two to three kilometres from the posts. He also formally forbade riverboat transport to all victims. It seems that Dr Broden's musings only one month before on the 'delicate question' of family relations were to be overlooked. Relatives must not visit isolated members; therefore it would be important to make the people understand that these measures were being taken in their own interests. Territorial administrators, as well as all religious and philanthropic bodies in the State, were instructed to investigate villages and alert the chiefs of the measures they were to take which included, naturally, isolation of victims a certain distance from the village, burning of their huts and, upon death, burning of all their clothing and daily utensils. There were no instructions on how these aims were to be achieved even when suitable language translators were available, and there was no discussion of the relevance of possible cultural differences among African societies, especially in the areas of disease management.[14]

December 1905 instructions

In December 1905, the year the Liverpool researchers had completed their survey, the campaign was further systematised and formal instructions were issued to all colonial agents. Infected individuals were absolutely forbidden to travel, *except* to lazarets on instructions of a doctor. Anyone could easily recognise enlarged glands, particularly the cervical glands at the back of the neck which were then considered to be the major symptom of infection.[15] Furthermore, any intelligent individual was capable of palpating those glands to detect enlargement, a technique, incidentally, which had been used for decades. Agents were instructed to send suspected victims immediately to the nearest medical post which housed a microscope so that lymph fluid and blood could be examined for trypanosomes. However, under *no* circumstances was a suspect to be sent to an uncontaminated region. All suspected victims were to be sent to special isolation centres, or lazarets, which would be constructed at least two kilometres from the post and villages. If victims had to use river transport to reach a lazaret, 'they were placed in movable cages surrounded on all sides by fine wire net'. It was particularly important to supervise all river transport, and doctors had the legal right to board all craft for examinations. In addition to the above instructions aimed at all agents, doctors were to keep careful registers of examinations, examine the gland fluid of all suspects, send all victims to lazarets and oversee the clearance of brush for 200–300 metres around posts, along river banks and a crossing and watering points. The doctors posted in the northern centres of Libenge, Lisala, Buta, Basoko and Stanleyville were to be especially strict in following these instructions in order to prevent the spread of contamination.[16]

With no cure possible, there were no significant policy changes between 1903 and mid-1906, and as sleeping sickness was always fatal, the only feasible measure had been the total isolation of all suspected victims. But with the development of a new drug, atoxyl, the situation was greatly changed. In December 1906 new regulations were issued as a result of this development. An arsenical compound, atoxyl was valuable for victims in the first stage of the disease while parasites were present in the peripheral circulatory system. It was mistakenly believed that it could effect a cure in four to six weeks, thus *regular screening* for victims made sense. For instance, the eminent scientists, Patrick Manson and Robert Koch, believed that atoxyl would be for sleeping sickness what quinine was for malaria. Understandably, the scientific community was euphoric over this discovery. Excited at the prospect of fame for the Liverpool School, Ronald Ross wrote to Todd in April 1906, 'Now this is the biggest thing our School has ever done . . . our School will reach greater fame than ever!' Illustrative of the international and political nature of the early course of tropical medicine, Alfred Jones, Chairman of the Elder Dempster Shipping Line of Liverpool and close personal friend of King Leopold, offered to pay £1,000 for research on atoxyl in the Congo Free State if the 'Great Chief' would match the sum.[17] Not everyone was as euphoric. Some doctors were reluctant to use atoxyl which they considered to be dangerous even in the hands of specialists.[18]

Surveillance and search

Nevertheless, from 1906 the emphasis was on the use of the new drug. 'Incessant surveillance' with the full cooperation of *all* Europeans was henceforth the battle-cry of the sleeping sickness campaign. Identifying victims in the advanced stages of the disease was not as difficult as finding those in the early stages of infection. The latter were both more contagious and, it was believed, more curable. All territorial agents were instructed to palpate their personnel and their families and to send suspects to the doctors for blood and lymph examinations. Europeans, as well as Africans, with suspect glands were to undergo examinations. In regions designated as free of infection, suspects were to be sent immediately to lazarets or observation posts located in contaminated areas and note of the diagnosis was to be made on their travel papers. Daily injections of 5 cc of atoxyl in a five per cent solution were given for about three days.

Legal sanctions accompanied the new December 1906 measures, and Europeans who were negligent in carrying out these instructions were warned that they were subject to disciplinary measures. All doctors in the Congo Free State were legally *obliged* to assist in the campaign by searching for victims and they were to be especially strict in the uncontaminated regions. From the beginning of the sleeping sickness campaign, the central government continually stressed the importance of gaining the cooperation of African chiefs and authority figures. Thus, territorial administrators were to teach native chiefs how to look for suspect glands and African authorities were to report suspects immediately. It was imperative that Africans understood the role of the tsetse fly, so administrators were to demonstrate the flies and to convince the chiefs of the importance of clearing away from their villages all tsetse-sheltering brush.[19]

Some state doctors questioned the policy of isolation as a blanket measure. For instance, in 1905 Dr Zerbini informed the governor-general that he could not approve such a radical measure. It was his opinion that there were so many Africans with enlarged glands that isolation of all would be impossible because of the lack of personnel; such a measure would also paralyse commerce. Furthermore, he said that 'one could not sequester people without clinical symptoms' other than enlarged glands. Finally, he had doubts about the ethic of imposing upon individual liberty such a sweeping policy. After all, he pointed out, in Europe, individuals with infectious tuberculosis were allowed to retain their liberty even when the public at large was at risk of infection.[20]

Some doctors also were concerned about the legality of treating patients against their wills. Responding to the queries of a state doctor in 1907, the Director of Justice, de Meulemeester, put the state firmly behind forced treatment, although with some reservations. He declared that the state had not only the right, but the obligation, to take necessary measures in order to prevent the spread of a contagious and infectious disease. He admitted that it was necessary to recognise individual liberty as much as possible, but it was the state, not private individuals, which took decisions on the best means to fight an epidemic. This was true *even* in constitutional countries where the individual was sacrificed to matters of public security or public hygiene. He did admit some doubts about the classification of sleeping sickness as a contagious disease. Diseases such as plague and cholera with their rapid spread and conclusion in either death or cure clearly justified severe measures on the part of the state. On the other hand, since sleeping sickness in the Belgian Congo appeared to be a slowly evolving disease with a long period of incubation, the issue of isolation of victims was *exceptionally* grave. On the question of the right of the state to impose a treatment which sometimes resulted in blindness, the director of justice believed that such a medication would be inhumane and its administration to unwilling victims would be contrary to elementary principles of 'natural law'. If blinding resulted for all those who received the treatment, then it could be used *only* with the consent of the victim, who would have to be forewarned of its danger.[21]

The cordoned triangle

Perhaps the most significant feature of the act of 5 December 1906 was the cordon sanitaire it placed around Uele district. This was achieved by means of a series of lazarets located on the periphery of the district. Between 1907 and 1910 key lazarets and observation posts were established at the state posts of Ibembo, Barumbu, Stanleyville, Aba and Yakoma. A glance at the map of the district with its cordon of lazarets, each of which also served the important function of observation post, or screening point, reveals their strategic locations. Ibembo was on the Itimbiri river, the major communication route for most traffic in and out of the north-east and the Sudan. Barumbu was situated on the Congo river near the major military training camp for the region. Stanleyville was the provincial capital, while Aba at the frontier with Sudan lay on a principal route used by the numerous trading caravans from Uganda; and, finally, Yakoma guarded the confluence of the Ubangi and Bomu rivers, the latter forming the boundary between French and Belgian territories. Later, an important observation post and lazaret was established at Ango on the Uere river in the heart of a seriously epidemic region. These then were the major sleeping sickness lazarets for the north-east, and for the period of this study they served as focal points in the strategy of the sleeping sickness campaign. By 1912, there were fourteen observation posts in the colony and the epidemic areas were designated as the Semliki basin, Kivu, the Kwilu basin, and Kwango.[22]

Lazarets shared certain common attributes. Most were in part served by Catholic nuns, often employed by the state for that purpose. Each state lazaret was allocated a specific number of labourers who were employed in a variety of ways. For instance, each lazaret was generally assigned individual hunters whose duty it was to supply the patients with meat. Lazaret directors were expected to secure provisions such as cereals and vegetables by purchasing them from local markets. The fact that markets did not exist in all regions of the Congo did not seem to matter and this is another example of the ways in which Europeans often neglected to base their policies upon the realities of African social and economic organisation, basing them instead upon European assumptions. Lazaret directors were responsible for plantations attached to the lazarets where the inmates were expected to grow some of their own food. Directors were also expected to maintain liaison with the local territorial administration at all levels – *chefs de poste, chefs de district, administrateurs territorials*, legal officers and the Force Publique. The latter obligation proved for many lazaret directors and staff to be an almost intractable problem during the first decade because most of the early territorial administrators were not at all interested in the public health programme and neglected the prescribed measures for sleeping sickness.[23]

Other features common to most lazarets included chronic shortages of staff, supplies (including medicines) and funding. While these problems were in part ameliorated by the reforms of 1910 and the real insistence from 1912 onward that *only* the very advanced, insane and recalcitrant victims be isolated, there was still the enormous number of patients to be managed by the out-patient clinics, and the ongoing tours of the surrounding district, surveying and searching for new victims.

Ibembo lazaret

Ibembo lazaret, at the 'gateway' to the north-east and opened in May 1907, was considered by the administration as the most important element in the cordon sanitaire of that region. Since 1889, Ibembo post had been the major staging point for military expeditions into Uele, and by 1907 it was also an important military training camp.[24] The Liverpool researchers, assuming that most of the Uele district was free of sleeping sickness, had suggested that a major observation post and isolation lazaret be established at the state post of Ibembo on the Itimbiri river in order to supervise the major communication route to the north-east. All boats, canoes and caravans travelling north were required to stop at the observation post, and *no one* was to travel on until examined by the doctor. African travel documents had to bear a record of all physical examinations, and everyone, African or European, was obliged to submit to examination for sleeping sickness before entering non-contaminated regions.[25] It was not until the end of 1908 that a large palisaded *zeriba* (an enclosure with one solid, locked and guarded gate) had been erected and it was not until August 1909 that a 'lock-up', or an inner *zeriba*, was ready for the advanced, or 'mad' cases. The original idea had been to house a maximum of 250 patients, but the number increased rapidly even before the site was prepared.[26]

The main principles of the lazaret system were described in the vivid reports of the first director of Ibembo lazaret, Inge Heibert, who had different ideas on the purpose of this institution from those held by the government.[27] He advised that camps should be located at the limits of contaminated areas, rather than inside them, and he stressed that the increased traffic caused by labour recruitment from infected areas was highly instrumental in the spread of the disease. He suggested that all recruitment be accompanied by thorough medical examinations which should be repeated along the transit routes and, in effect, constitute a *passage au tamis*, or sieve, to catch sleeping sickness victims. But the main responsibility would rest with the doctor at the gateway to uninfected regions, i.e., Ibembo for the north-east. Examinations should, whenever possible, include the native population, especially along major communication routes. 'In cases where a part of a village is found infected, the most energetic measures should be taken. One should decide for each case if infected individuals should be sent . . . outside the territory or if they should be interned in the lazarets.' Heiberg also described how a search tour should be conducted to trap all suspects. The doctor should begin at a point the farthest from the centre of the area and in that way 'brush ahead of him like the hunter' all suspects and expel them through the observation post, or 'key' to the district.

Once inside the lazaret, victims would receive atoxyl injections and periodic examinations which were carefully recorded in registers. They were kept in varying degrees of isolation, from complete 'lock-up' to relatively unrestrained surveillance. According to Heiberg, prison-style confinement was administratively preferable for both Europeans and Africans. The boundaries and tasks were clear and public order was not disrupted, 'except, perhaps, at the moment of internment of a sleeping sickness victim'. No meeting could occur between victims and African soldiers or natives and, more significantly, no arms would find their way inside the lazaret. 'After all', the doctor added, 'it is isolation which makes a lazaret.' There were, however, disadvantages with the prison-style system, which required 'energetic and firm surveillance' and other stringent measures. The major problem was the ever-present threat of rebellion, and the doctor consequently favoured more liberal and open lazarets, keeping strict isolation for the really difficult or advanced cases.

Those Africans not in state employment were the responsibility of either their employers or their own chiefs, but in either case the chiefs were expected to contribute towards the provisioning of the lazarets. When questioned about this in June 1908, the Secretary of State in Brussels repeated that the state 'had entirely fulfilled its obligation by putting people into lazarets and providing free medical care', although he had previously admitted, 'These people are unwillingly held and prevented from earning their livings.'[28] All able-bodied victims were required to work without salary on the construction and maintenance of the lazaret facilities, as well as on the cultivation of their own food. In March 1909 the Ibembo director requested permission to give small daily salaries as 'one could then ask them to do slight work . . . We cannot without injustice not give them fifteen centimes a day.' He suggested that the funds could be raised through a supplementary tax in Uele district, as after all it was only fair the Uele population should pay. The vice governor-general did not agree.[29]

The 1906 regulations indicated that government supplies would be sent for the care of the patients, but three-and-a-half years later, in June 1910, the lazaret director Dr Bottalico reported that patients lacked both food and covers. 'We have had no meat or fish, as what should go to the patients has been taken for the labourers and soldiers. I cannot obtain rice or salt . . . people who are here only under observation often stay months and receive no salt or oil and are forced to roam about haggling'.[30]

Patients' families were not officially allowed to visit them in the lazarets, but kin often accompanied victims. The conflict which arose from the Belgians' misunderstanding and ignorance of this widespread African practice in relation to disease management provides a rich area of enquiry for the historian.[31] In the early Congo, administrators all too frequently revealed their ignorance of African social and medical practices. But sometimes humanitarian concern broke through, as in August 1907 when an unusually sensitive zone administrator addressed the governor-general: 'I want to know if the families of the patients can live at the post and if they can be rationed by the State, as often, if one member is hospitalized, the others in the family do not want to leave. It would be cruel to send them away . . . '.[32]

The problem of accompanying kin also illuminates the Belgians' extremely legalistic approach to native affairs. For instance, the doctor at Stanleyville lazaret in 1907 asked if he should return the *legitimate* wives of victims to their home villages, pointing out that this would be done only after ascertaining the legitimacy of marriages, and only one wife would be considered. He was instructed that he should keep the wives at Stanleyville and give them state rations until their husbands either died or departed.[33]

Heiberg warned that it was of paramount importance to treat the patients with kindness, goodwill and indulgence. They must be carefully nourished and understand that they came first where food was concerned. He advised that it was best to allow people to live in culturally similar, small groups – 'village style' – with a former sergeant or corporal or the Force Publique appointed as the headman. Doctors and administrators should enter as little as possible into the people's internal disputes. In September 1910, the district commissioner reported seeing small groups of individuals from different, often mutually hostile tribes apparently content with life in the lazaret.[34]

Labour supply for Ibembo, as well as for the other lazarets, was a constant problem. In May 1907 the ministry in Brussels informed the governor-general that each zone with up to 100 sleeping sickness victims would have three African *infirmiers*, a category of medical auxiliary loosely comparable to nursing aides. In August 1910, the minister authorised funding for a European assistant, or *agent sanitaire*, at each principal lazaret and an African clerk at each of the twenty-six lazarets; but in December 1910 the vice governor-general announced that he had only been able to appoint one African clerk and no nursing aides, and he was in urgent need of twenty-six clerks! His problem was that literate and trained Africans leaving the colonial school at Boma were in great demand and were assigned to the military and economic sectors.[35]

The shortage of labour meant more work for the interned victims, who generally performed their tasks most unwillingly and only under constant threat of punishment. A sad irony was the use of former internees of the lazarets as labourers in and around those establishments, as was the case at Stanleyville in 1911. One doctor suggested a tax exemption for those victims not in strict isolation inside the lazarets who contributed labour. This idea was apparently not approved by the administration which a number of times emphasised its view that Africans must continue to contribute to the *mise en valeur* of the colony. The state had fulfilled its obligation by providing lazarets and doctors. Africans were obliged, therefore, to provide the supplies and their labour.[36]

Other lazarets

Stanleyville

There were other lazarets around the periphery of the great triangle of the north-east: Stanleyville, Barumbu, Aba and Yakoma completed the circle. Stanleyville lazaret, directed by Dr Trolli, was opened in 1907 for people from Aruwimi district and for victims discovered aboard passing rivercraft. By the end of 1908, 345 people had been hospitalised and the mortality rate was a staggering 27.7 per cent. In December 1908, it was

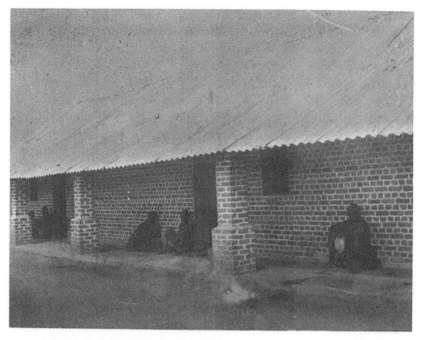

Plate 8. Stanleyville lazaret, 1912.

reported that victims at Stanleyville lazaret refused to cooperate; and while the vice governor-general had recently stopped the use of the army in implementing the sleeping sickness policy and delegated this duty to the police, it was now agreed that it might be necessary to establish an army post near the lazaret to enforce measures. By 1910, the average number of patients isolated in the lazaret at any one time was about 150.[37]

Barumbu

Barumbu lazaret in Aruwimi district near Baroko on the Congo river lay directly south of Ibembo. Its declared purpose was the isolation of Africans still outside the state sector, that is, 'natives'.[38] Thus, we see that at this time it was implicitly understood that most of the sleeping sickness measures and programme were aimed at those Africans who lived in some contact with the colonial state while the mass of people outside such contact were not much affected by the public health programme.

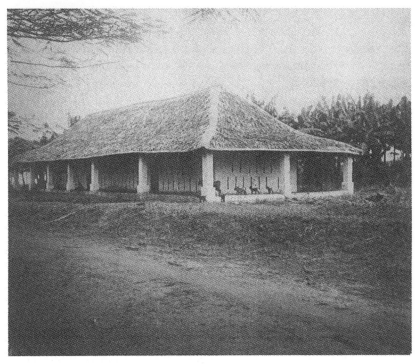

Plate 9. Barumbu lazaret, 1910.

Opened in June 1909, Barumbu soon proved extremely unpopular with Africans. It was almost empty when the vice governor-general visited it in January 1910, as most of the 'natives' had run away, leaving only state employees. He explained that coercion could not be considered as it would seriously affect the credibility of the whole sleeping sickness campaign in the eyes of the natives. But when the vice governor-general again visited the lazaret in September he was astounded to find more than 200 'natives' in residence. It seemed that following the apparently successful treatment of an important chief and his son, word spread quickly among the people and there had been an enormous change of attitude toward the lazaret.[39] Dr Van Goidtsnoven, the physician at Barumbu, had further dispelled African fears of the lazaret by repeated demonstrations of the gland puncture which he performed on himself. By March 1911 there were 209 Africans isolated at Barumbu and by July, 263. Of the 209 in March, only 20 were soldiers and former labourers.[40]

Aba

Aba was located in the Yei river region close to the Lado enclave. In January 1909 the colonial minister, Jules Renkin informed the governor-general that he had decided to establish a lazaret inside the Lado enclave where sleeping sickness was increasingly reported, with the idea that a lazaret established near the frontier would serve as a screening post to catch infected porters from Uganda, a matter of great concern because of the large number of Ugandans crossing into the Congo. However, by March 1909, with the impending transfer of the enclave to the British, there were doubts about locating a lazaret in the far north-east. Thus, plans were deferred although it was agreed that in any case there would be a frontier observation post. Eventually a lazaret was established at Aba.[41]

Dr Errera, stationed at Aba in early 1909, considered the entire Yei river region to be infected with trypanosomiasis, adding that he had first heard of infections among the natives in early 1907. In his report of December 1909 he said that 3.4 per cent of the caravan porters who had been examined at Lado were infected. Since there were some 2,000 Ugandan porters annually travelling through Uele district, he calculated that some 68 persons would be spreading sleeping sickness.[42] However, in his report for the second quarter of 1910, Dr Errera listed only twenty-seven victims, of whom just two were local 'natives'. At that time he also explained that while the 15 April 1910 instruction had been to limit inmates to only those in very bad condition, he preferred to intern victims who were still reasonably mobile so as to dispel the image of 'death and desolation' which tended to surround the lazaret.[43] His successor, Dr Vincent Rosas, reported in May 1911 that victims at the lazaret came from Aba, Faradje and Dungu and that by June of 1911 not one of the 136 inmates was a 'native'. They were all instead Africans with some connection with the European colonists. For instance, many were Ugandan porters whom the doctor, like his predecessor, was convinced had introduced the disease into the area.[44] Some idea of the numbers of people screened for sleeping sickness at this frontier post can be gained from the reports of Rosas who examined 3,323 people between April and December 1910 and issued 725 medical passports. In addition to these numbers, he had examined the residents of eight villages.[45]

Yakoma

In 1909 a lazaret was established at Yakoma. Dr Rodhain had surveyed the region of Upper Ubangi in 1905 for sleeping sickness, which he believed to have been a recent introduction. He attributed the spread of the disease into the region to the increased canoe traffic which served to provision state posts along the river between Libenge and Yakoma, which was located at the confluence of the Ubangi and Bomu rivers. He reported endemic sleeping sickness on the Belgian side, having noted forty-five cases during his survey. The spread of the disease from neighbouring French Congo was especially to be feared as it had been present in epidemic form across the river for some time.[46]

The authorities thus decided to establish an observation post and lazaret at Yakoma. But when the first director, Dr Arthur Zerbini, arrived there on 14 November 1909, he found that nothing had been done to construct such a facility. He was told by the post administrator that there was no available African labour to construct the lazaret, but it was Zerbini's opinion, like that of so many other doctors, that the territorial administration was not in the least concerned to cooperate with public health works. Zerbini immediately complained that since he did not know the local African language, he needed the assistance of a clerk and an *infirmier*. Finally, in February 1912, the colonial minister wrote to say that a European assistant was on his way to Yakoma.[47]

A year after Zerbini had first arrived at Yakoma, he was able to report in a quite different vein. There now existed a lazaret-village built in accordance with the recent reforms, with eighteen huts, *en pisé*, suitable for four to six persons each, and located some two kilometres from the post. The region was 'filled with trypanosomiasis cases'; and from all sides 'they come to enter the lazaret to receive care'. The doctor was puzzled by such an extraordinary response. 'Perhaps', he thought, 'it was due to the decent, clean houses, blankets and weekly food rations' which were provided by the state for the victims.[48] Not only were Africans freely coming to the lazaret from the Belgian Congo, but many from French territory crossed the boundary Bomu river to seek medical attention at the lazaret.[49] Between November 1910 and August 1911, more than 200 victims of sleeping sickness had been buried at Yakoma more than doubling the size of the post's cemetery but no one knew how many 'natives' had died of the disease.[50]

One of the most interesting aspects of Yakoma lazaret in the early days was a surprisingly perceptive observation made by its director. Astonishing in light of the prevailing theories of epidemiology, Zerbini observed that in addition to the 'germ' of the disease, other crucial factors were the geographical and social conditions. He noted that among the Azande, those of the ruling or aristocratic class, or the chiefs and notables, rarely succumbed to sleeping sickness while those of 'lower social orders', those with no rights (as he described them) were often terribly afflicted with the disease. Zerbini concluded that sufficient diet and good living conditions rendered people like the Azande chiefs and notables more resistant to the disease. Thus, he advised, the state should not direct all of its efforts only to the campaign against the tsetse fly, but it should also aim to 'ameliorate the situation of the natives'. A contemporary marginal note added in Brussels to Zerbini's report ran: 'I think this is one of the best remedies.' Early this century, there were signs that a few individuals in the metropole and the colony propounded a more 'holistic' approach to the management of public health.[51]

Lazarets in trouble

By 1910 the prison-style, total isolation system was clearly in difficulties. Serious problems had arisen almost immediately with the initial policy of 1905–6. Lazaret doctors had realised very soon that, in contrast to earlier hopes, atoxyl cured only very few patients in the early stages of the disease – and there were some relapses – while it had no effect on those in the advanced stages. Africans were very quick to observe the poor results. The mortality rates were appalling – at Ibembo lazaret by 1911, nearly one-third of those admitted had died. Furthermore, there was a dreadful side-effect with atoxyl injections – up to 30 per cent of those treated became blind as the drug atrophied the optic nerve.[52] People were terrified of the campaign and the lazarets became popularly known as 'death camps'. Wild rumours circulated that the colonial officials were not only causing the disease, but were rounding up people in order to eat them. A missionary's advice of 1902 that the state should establish 'colonies of incurables' had been made a reality.[53]

Heiberg vividly described the problems of placing in total isolation an already hospitalised victim. Such transfers were 'probably not without force and probably not without fighting and bloodflow'. The garrison at Ibembo post was insufficient for such transfers without violence. It took 'at least 150 soldiers with three Europeans to effect a quiet entry into a lazaret', and after their isolation, the patients required constant, firm surveillance with a double guard at the entry of the *zeriba* and two ordinary guards at two corners of the post. In all, it required thirty-six men, four non-commissioned officers and one European to effect surveillance.

Heiberg did not delude himself that the patients would be content and not attempt to flee. Although such a mass attempt had not been yet made, Heibert still believed that each indulgence, amelioration or favour on his part was seen by the Africans as weakness and, in fact, only increased their irascibility. He argued that he required 'at least a serious number of guards for proper surveillance' instead of the spectacle of five, unarmed soldiers sent from the post. When the victims saw a large, irresistible force, he declared, they would resignedly enter the isolation, but, he continued, 'if on the other hand, one appears with a handful of soldiers, the patients mock them'.[54] In addition, it was necessary to have a cleared no-man's zone around the entire lazaret. That was especially important to prevent the patients' friends and kin throwing arms to them. It was vital to regularly search *everyone* who entered the lazaret.

Heiberg had found that sleeping sickness victims were nearly all in a constant state of 'hyper-irritability' and that in almost 13 per cent of the cases, they were mad and would manifest that in maniacal outbursts. The least spark sufficed to cause chaos – a malcontent, a punishment, less food than a comrade, a woman problem – all could lead to a riot 'as we have seen several times'. Heiberg had experience working in European asylums for the insane which makes it most relevant to note his views on the difference between an insane European and an African sleeping sickness patient. According to him, nearly all European patients in an asylum would have their own *particular* delusions. That made a *coordinated* riot in a hospital an unknown, even impossible, event. But in the Congo, thought Heiberg, sleeping sickness victims had a different kind of 'insanity'. Their disease reduced, but did not destroy, their power to reason. Sleeping sickness victims were obsessive – they had fixed ideas such as 'the injustice of their imprisonment'. One hundred sleeping sickness victims with the identical 'obsessive' idea comprised a formidable threat. When the local administrator visited the lazaret in September 1910, he was repeatedly approached by patients with the same complaint that they were being prevented from 'seeing home'.[55]

Heibert's views on the insane and 'irrational' behaviour are of interest in that they reveal contemporary European attitudes about the insane as obsessive people who have fixed ideas and who act individually, not in groups. Among Africans, however, Heiberg proposed a different kind of insanity, that of a group of people *sharing* an obsessive and irrational idea.

Furthermore, he could only view the Africans' desire to escape his Western biomedicine in order to return to their own people and ways of dealing with misfortune as totally irrational, or insane, behaviour.[56]

All along, some victims managed to escape into the surrounding areas, but the growing frustration and hostility of victims isolated at Ibembo was given expression in two serious riots in 1909 and 1910 confirming Heiberg's fears. The Ibembo riots signalled the need for reform. As Heiberg said of the lazaret in 1910, 'Strictly speaking, it was a permanent prison and should bear the inscription, "Abandon all hope, ye who enter here."'[57]

The sleeping sickness campaign, like other Belgian colonial policies, was highly centralised with most instructions issued directly from Brussels. There was no colonial medical department as such until 4 December 1922. A medical service had functioned in Brussels since 1 December 1909, but doctors in the colony remained under the authority of their local territorial administrators. Instructions concerning the campaign were passed along a rigid line of authority from the minister of colonies, to the governor-general, provincial vice governors-general, district commissioners, *chefs de zones* and *chefs de postes*. Doctors usually received their instructions from the district commissioners who were, in turn, advised by a 'chief' doctor for the province. Doctors were very much a part of the territorial administration.

Before the *arrêté* of December 1910 which established the first medical department for the Congo, there was no true 'medical authority who made sanitation regulations'. All such regulations were issued by civil and military authorities. Thus measures such as medical passports and epidemiological maps upon which the cordon sanitaire was based had emanated from non-medical administrators. Ordinances controlling African life – village siting, fishing, salt production, travel, kin relations – were all drafted by non-medical staff.

At the same time, doctors who were instructed to carry out the sleeping sickness measures often found themselves in the impossible situation of having to request assistance from the local territorial administrator. And, very often, the administrator was reluctant to support the doctors' requests. The main reason for the lack of cooperation was the local administrator's wish to retain a modicum of tolerance from his African subjects. Implementing public health measures made the territorial administrator more unpopular than he already was among the people. Pressed to achieve certain political and economic goals, namely the recruitment of labour and collection of tax, the territorial administrators

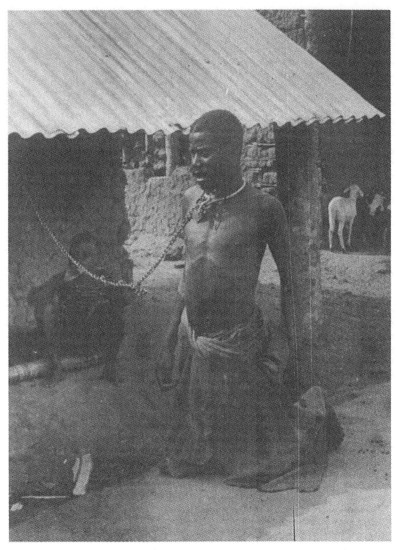

Plate 10. 'Un fou' (in an advanced stage of sleeping sickness), Stanleyville lazaret, 1912.

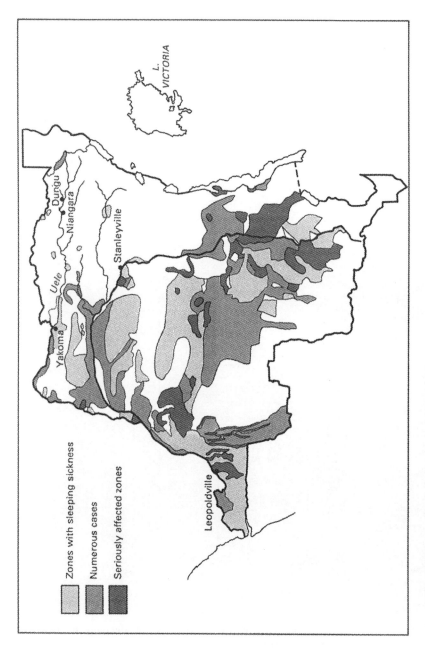

Map 7. Distribution of sleeping sickness, March 1910.

Zones with sleeping sickness

Numerous cases

Seriously affected zones

L. VICTORIA

Dungu

Niangara

Uele

Stanleyville

Yakoma

Leopoldville

would often ignore medical and public health measures as much as they could.

As of 1909 the major features of the campaign were the cordon sanitaire and isolation in lazarets. One doctor recalled these two features as 'the great panacea for public health in the Congo'. Combined with the ineffective, even dangerous, chemotherapy, the campaign evoked intense distrust from the people. Furthermore, this doctor said, the sporadic surveys for victims in African villages were viewed as 'little more than manhunts' and the result was that 'people fled the doctors more quickly than they did the tax collectors!'[58] We have already seen how the army was required to assist doctors to examine Africans and then to effect their isolation, and how in 1909 and 1910 serious riots erupted in Ibembo lazaret requiring the army to regain control. Clearly, the combination of a complicated and blundering bureaucracy with an isolation system from which the only exit was death or escape and in which one-third of those treated became blind was a failure.

African responses to the first phase of the campaign made it apparent to the colonial administration that no public health programme could be really effective unless everyone involved, African and European, cooperated. Slowly, the realisation dawned that medical and administrative staff would have to cooperate in order to effect sleeping sickness measures. There had been calls before for the understanding and cooperation of African authorities in the campaign to examine all of the people and to isolate infected individuals but by late 1909 it had become clear that the understanding and cooperation of *all* Africans affected by the campaign would be necessary. The responses of the people to the Belgian sleeping sickness campaign were indeed a significant factor which shaped the future development of public health in the colony. Many of those responses will be discussed in chapters 9 and 10.

Second phase: 1910–1914

The second phase of the campaign can be located in the period from 1910 to 1914, the years following the transition of the Congo Free State to the Belgian Congo. During this period, immediately preceding World War I, there were significant reforms in both health policy and the colonial medical service. The shift began in 1910 when a series of reforms were introduced. The major shift in policy, following the recommendations of Drs Broden and Rodhain of the Leopoldville laboratory, was that lazarets were to be more open; they were to become 'village-lazarets' in which only the very advanced or difficult patients would stay.[59] Unlike the prison-like atmosphere of the earlier lazarets, the new institutions would accommodate members of the victims' immediate families. All other victims of the disease would be treated as out-patients and attend injection clinics which would be conveniently located near their own regions (only inside infected zones). These patients were known as 'ambulatory'. Thus victims would be able to continue labouring or producing food.[60]

The reforms reflected administrative concerns as well as purely medical ones, and several issues were involved. First, there was the serious matter of the notorious reputation of the Leopoldian adminis-tration of the Congo Free State which the Belgian government wished to dispel. Then, too, the Belgians were still very much in the process of establishing state hegemony in several parts of the Congo including the north-east. Thus, while still engaged in the process of conquest, the administration of the new colony *had* to appear to be more humane in order to avoid further condemnation by the Great Powers.

While it is important to see events during this phase in the context of the broader political policy of improving the image of the adminis-tration, it must be pointed out that medical personnel in the Congo had been lobbying for some time for the creation of a separate administrative department which would permit the rationalisation of both the health service and public health policy. Following a tour of a district much infected with sleeping sickness, the governor-general in 1910 proposed a structured campaign to combat the disease throughout the colony. The combination of pressure from colonial doctors for a medical department and the apparently increasing epidemicity of sleeping sickness had already resulted in the creation of such a department at the end of 1909, although the special sleeping sickness programme was not put into effect until 1918.[61] The new medical department, like other areas of colonial administration, was based in Brussels where it remained so firmly centralised that one contemporary commented that the Belgian campaign against sleeping sickness was fought from offices in Brussels, not Africa.[62]

Sleeping sickness and administrative control

Sleeping sickness policy was intertwined with broader issues of territorial administration, and this linkage began to surface clearly during the second phase of the campaign. For instance there was the issue of

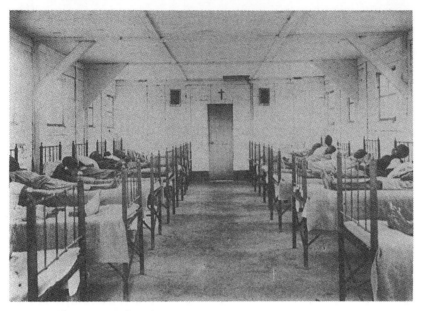

Plate 11. Kinshasa lazaret, 1914.

controlling movements of people both within the colony and across its international frontiers. North-eastern Congo, as we saw in chapter 2, bordered three other colonial territories all of which contained areas of seriously epidemic sleeping sickness by 1910. The movements of people in and out of the Congo was therefore a major concern for the administration. There were a number of reasons for such movements. The major ones included normal kin relations, particularly among the very numerous Azande who found themselves divided by three colonial frontiers. Other causes for African movements were trade, both local and long-distance; the disruptions of conquest and colonisation, especially from war, labour recruitment and tax requirements; and, finally, sleeping sickness.

Several of the social and economic reasons for population movements are discussed at greater length in chapter 10 but it is important to be aware of their existence while examining the evolution of public health policy. There was significant interplay between sleeping sickness measures, particularly those concerning the cordon sanitaire, and the broader economic and social concerns of territorial administration. It would be far-fetched to impute Machiavellian motives to those who made public health policy and to the territorial staff who implemented measures. Nevertheless, sleeping sickness measures formed part of the system of control used by the new Belgian rulers. Remember the director of the Nigerian medical service who toured several colonies during 1929 in order to compare their sleeping sickness programmes. He observed the startling absence of African travellers in the Congo compared to Nigeria.[63]

Medical passports

The crucial element in the reform of sleeping sickness policy was the introduction on 30 April 1910, of mandatory medical passports.[64] Formerly, all Africans travelling beyond their home regions had been required to obtain a travel document, a *feuille de route*, and as we have seen, doctors were obliged to record on them details of all medical examinations (see appendix B). From April 1910 the new medical passports superseded the less specific travel documents in the ever-increasing attempt to control every movement of Africans. All Africans – porters, couriers, soldiers, employees of the colony as well as natives in the service of private agents – had to carry medical passports. In addition, 'those who travelled freely' were to possess them. For this last category it was necessary to gain the cooperation of the African chiefs, now themselves 'legitimate' representatives of the colonial administration. This measure was especially important, in the view of the colonial authorities, near international boundaries where the spread of sleeping sickness was particularly threatening, for, as mentioned above, by 1910–12, it was obvious that both Sudan and French Equatorial Africa had active foci of sleeping sickness. Eventually, there was some cross-border cooperation among colonial administrations but it was never possible to eradicate old patterns of African social and economic interaction. This was especially true in those areas where colonial boundaries intersected ethnic entities such as the Azande. The 1910 decree also granted doctors the powers to coerce and punish recalcitrant people as well as to delimit the zones in which travel permits would be mandatory.

There was one large gap in the rigorousness of this control. A decree of 17 August 1910 greatly limited the degree of control exercised by state administrators in granting travel visas to those Africans recruited by European firms or the Force Publique. In the event, administrators were nearly always forced to comply with such requests for visas.

An important element of the revisions of public health policy was the standardisation of observation posts. These were strategically located surveillance and screening stations at which a medic, ideally a European *agent sanitaire*, but very often a lone African *infirmier*, was based with a microscope. It was his duty to screen all travellers, being especially alert to those coming from regions known to be infected with the disease. A major function of the observation post was the issuing of medical passports in the attempt to further control movements of people.[65]

It has been said that, considering the large numbers of victims and restricted resources and personnel, much of the voluminous legislation was 'of academic interest' only or a 'paper war'. While it is true that many of the instructions could not be successfully implemented because of the lack of resources, mainly personnel, it would be a mistake to dismiss the early sleeping sickness policy as *merely* a paper war. Many state officials ignored the regulations, but others made considerable efforts to enforce them.[66]

1910 reforms: missionaries and sleeping sickness

The second phase of the campaign brought about the standardisation of missionary participation. Before 1910, some mission societies in Congo had involved themselves with medical work, and several specifically assisted victims of sleeping sickness.[67] In 1906, with the opening of the School of Tropical Medicine in Brussels, mission societies had been encouraged to send representatives along for elementary training. In January 1910, however, Jules Renkin, the colonial minister, formally instructed nine Protestant and thirteen Catholic mission societies to take part in the campaign against sleeping sickness. In future, mission representatives were required to complete a theoretical course at a school of tropical medicine as well as a course of 'practical' work in a laboratory specialising in sleeping sickness. Renkin proposed that the 1911 colonial budget cover the cost of such a course for missionaries at the Leopold-ville laboratory. He believed they could help with patients in the second stage of the disease and could be authorised to use atoxyl. Missions without doctors could isolate patients in the advanced stages of the disease. There would be two kinds of mission lazaret: medical and non-medical. The state would supply missions with necessary equipment and medicines and it would pay the salaries of nursing sisters from religious orders.[68]

The Uele survey and the Gwane epidemic

The first organised survey of sleeping sickness in northern Congo took place in Uele district in the period of the second phase of the campaign. Between 1907 and 1910 the director of Ibembo lazaret had made repeated proposals for an organised sleeping sickness programme focusing upon what was believed to be the 'great uninfected triangle' of Uele. His proposal in 1912 included a request for 600,000 francs with which to create an effective cordon sanitaire. He suggested that special sanitary brigades, teams of thirty-six men, could isolate the infected areas by clearing the brush along porterage routes and at major river crossings, thereby creating natural zones.[69] In response, King Albert allocated 1,250,000 francs for a concerted campaign and plans were begun.[70] The outbreak of war in 1914 postponed the full implementation of campaign plans for five years, however, and it was not until 1919 that the first permanent sleeping sickness team, or mission, began in Kwango.

In the meantime, in 1913–14, a first widescale survey for sleeping sickness was made in Uele district as an immediate consequence of the Belgian military campaign against the powerful Azande ruler, Sasa. From the time of the Liverpool study until 1912, it had been believed that there was no real problem with the disease in the district except at a few isolated foci – along the Itimbiri river as far as Ibembo, in the extreme north-east of the territory, and immediately around Aba near the Sudan frontier. But that complacency was shaken during the campaign, which the Belgians launched in 1912 to finally crush their long-term foe, Sasa. Sleeping sickness was for the first time found to be present to an alarming degree in northern Uele district.

On 30 May 1912, the state doctor accompanying the military expedition, Grenade, reported seeing victims of the disease in a village twenty kilometres north of the Uere river. Very soon after, the administration ordered the immediate and 'quiet' evacuation of the troops who had been used in the war against Sasa.[71] Then on 27 June Gemio, a soldier at Sasa post, died of sleeping sickness. By 24 July, the zone chief had ordered that the passes of 150 of the soldiers who had sojourned in the region of the battle with Sasa should be specially marked with the message: 'these soldiers have stayed in a region suspected of sleeping sickness and should be examined as soon as possible by a doctor'.[72] Two weeks later, on 4 August, the region north of the Uere river was declared by the provincial government, as advised by Drs Grenade and Russo, to

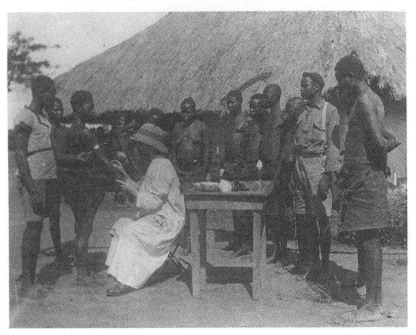

Plate 12. R. P. de Graer injecting victims, 1924.

be 'contaminated'. The director of Ibembo lazaret, Dr Boigelet, added the region between the Bili and Bomu rivers to the area now to be cordoned off, and control measures were applied. And in Brussels at the end of the year a report to the central government from the Department of Hygiene included an official declaration of an 'infected zone' along the Gwane river in north-central Uele district.[73]

The governor-general was informed that the health of both European and African troops involved in the operations against Sasa had deteriorated because of the privations and overwork they had suffered. He was also told that sleeping sickness was now 'ravaging' the populations between the Gwane and Bomu and that yet another contaminated zone existed at the confluence of the Uele and Bomu rivers.[74]

By mid-1912, then, it was well established that sleeping sickness was not only present, but present in serious proportion, in northern Uele district, and it was presumed to be spreading along both the Uele and Aruwimi rivers. Arrangements were made, therefore, for Dr Jerome Rodhain to survey the district for the disease. Between May 1913 and December 1914, Rodhain personally examined *83,000* Africans for sleeping sickness in the course of five separate trips along the major

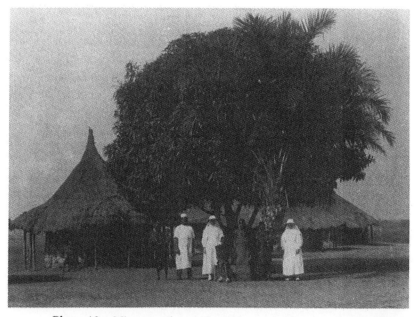

Plate 13. Niangara hospital, Uele and Sisters of Fichermont, *c.* 1930.

commercial and official communications routes in the district. In all, a total of 200,000 people were examined during the survey.

It must be recalled that Uele district had been scheduled to be opened to free trade in July 1912, so the administration felt it was imperative to discover the extent of epidemic sleeping sickness. 'Opening' Uele meant essentially that there would be an influx of mineral prospectors as well as numerous traders and their agents and porters, and that meant greatly increased movements among many resident Africans as well.

Between 21 July and 2 November 1913, Rodhain examined the territory of Uere-Bili. The doctor was accompanied by an administrative representative, A. de Calonne-Beaufaict, a practice which would continue with future medical surveys and which would understandably lead Africans to equate the public health campaign with other aspects of state hegemony such as tax. Calonne-Beaufaict left a report of his tour from which we learn that although more than 1,100 people were examined, 'they were, of course, the least timid ones' and he complained, ' . . . what singular mistrust! . . . They only knew us as conquerors and not as organisers.'[75] Since the first report of the disease, during the campaign against Sasa, no doctor had visited the region. The Belgians had ruled the

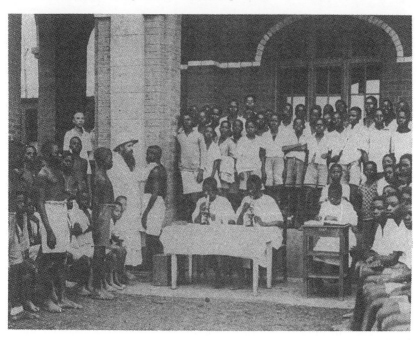

Plate 14. Tumba post: sleeping sickness survey at a mission school, *c.* 1930.

territory of Uere-Bili indirectly through the powerful Azande chiefs, Sasa and Mopoie, and thus no state troops had occupied the region before 1909–10. Rodhain believed that situation explained why no cases of sleeping sickness had been officially noted. He discovered the basins of both the Gwane and Asa rivers to be infected with the disease, and Africans told him of the deaths of many people.

When Rodhain left Uele district in December 1914, he hoped it would be possible to confer the sleeping sickness survey upon a successor, but the war and consequent reductions in medical staff prevented that. In his report of the survey, he emphasised the danger that sleeping sickness would be spread by the constantly increasing movements of peoples throughout the region, much of it occasioned by administrative policy. He stressed the importance of the cordon sanitaire. All river traffic should be 'limited to that strictly necessary'.[76] His survey revealed the presence of several epidemic foci in Uele district. Like the survey conducted a decade earlier by the Liverpool researchers, the advice emanating from the 1913–14 survey had considerable impact on the development of policies for the control of this disease. Of particular importance was Rodhain's emphasis upon mobility of African populations as a danger leading to the spread of the disease.[77]

The Uelian outbreak, referred to here as the 'Gwane epidemic', increased and spread for many years. But in spite of repeated warnings and pleas from local administrators and the few medical personnel in the region, it was not until 1923 that the central government finally began to respond. The long delay raises a number of questions about the disparity between declared policy and practice in public health and gives cause for the perception that, perhaps, public health policy was not always really motivated by the desire to protect Africans from sleeping sickness.

Agglomeration and consolidation of Africans

Another significant feature of the second phase of the campaign was the emergence of a discernible policy regarding the organisation and structure of African societies. Restructuring African societies would remain for decades an important and troublesome issue for the colonial authorities. It became a particular problem when public health authorities came into conflict with territorial administrators, for the two departments had quite different motives for wishing to reorganise Africans. When the two were in agreement over the reorganisation and resiting of a group of people, there was less conflict, although increasingly, territorial administrators were loathe to involve themselves in this particular form of administration which was so unpopular with the people.[78]

From very early in the campaign against sleeping sickness, the regroupment and relocation of African populations had been a much-used tactic. Ostensibly to protect people from the danger of infection through proximity to the infected tsetse flies, the regroupment and relocation of entire populations served other requirements of the territorial administration, especially during the early colonial period when the hegemony of the state was still very much under threat. Territorial administrators preferred their subjects to be conveniently sited for ease of administration even though many agents on the scene were extremely reluctant to tamper with this aspect of African life for fear of increased hostility and resistance. This tactic was important in labour recruitment and tax collection. It was simply easier to deal with groups of people conveniently located near communication routes or state centres than it was to 'chase up' scattered individuals far from routes used by the colonials. With people like the Azande and many Babua whose normal settlement pattern was dispersed family clusters separated by stretches of forest or savannah, the policy of regroupment was especially controversial.

Missionaries were another colonial sector much concerned to 'agglomerate Christians'. As the Dominican Vicar-Apostolic of Niangara complained in 1927, the Africans in his diocese tended to settle in 'scattered fashion' averaging five or six people per square kilometre north of the Uele river and that it was very difficult for missionaries to 'agglomerate' them.[79]

During this early period of the campaign, it was quite unrealistic to think of major restructuring of African societies, if for no other reason than the lack of staff and resources to enforce such a policy. Nevertheless, it was often mentioned, and it was an important feature of sleeping sickness policy. The topography of most of northern Congo made it infeasible to attempt to relocate Africans away from tsetse areas, and when such moves were executed, people simply returned to their rivers to fish and to their plantations to cultivate.[80]

By 1910, doctors had been delegated considerable powers by the central government to request the reorganisation and relocation of Africans within their districts. Also by 1910, doctors had the right to request assistance from the army – the Force Publique – as well as the cooperation of the territorial administration, in their attempts to implement the public health policy. Thus it was not uncommon for the doctor to arrive in an area accompanied by armed soldiers and an administrator, and then to begin a systematic examination of the people, who were obliged by this show of force to present themselves regardless of activities they may have been engaged in at the time. The doctor was also entitled to the cooperation of the local *capitas*, or village headmen appointed by the state, as well as that of the *chef médaillé*, also a colonial appointment. But these were not the only authority figures available to implement the programme. From 1912 most posts had, in addition to their contingent of the Force Publique, other law enforcement agents in the form of police who might be territorial or local. Finally, by 1912, the central government had made it quite clear that *every* European in the district was obliged to participate in the campaign against sleeping sickness and, while it was certainly not the case everywhere, there were many examples, as we shall see, of individuals fulfilling that task by examining their own employees.[81]

Summary

Thus, during the second phase of the campaign, 1910–14, a series of public health policy reforms was undertaken which was linked to the wider changes occurring in the administration of the new colony. The sleeping sickness campaign was increasingly standardised and missionaries were required, in principle, to participate. The strict isolation policy was 'humanised' by the introduction of village-style lazarets. But liberalisation of the policy of isolation of patients was coupled with ever-increasing controls over African lives in the form of regulations on their movements, their residential patterns, and so forth. Sleeping sickness regulations flowed from Brussels to Boma and thence to the local administrators, who found themselves responsible for a bewildering array of rules.

By the outbreak of World War I, there was both confusion over the regulations regarding sleeping sickness and at the same time irregular and varying enforcement of them. The public prosecutor at Bambili complained on one occasion that 'the texts regulating sleeping sickness being so numerous, incomplete and unclear', he could not unravel a particular infraction. Again, on 9 June 1914, another public prosecutor, this time at Buta, asked the district commissioner to supply him with a complete set of all sleeping sickness regulations. It may have been a 'paper war' in the sense that limited resources and staff precluded thorough application of the sleeping sickness rules, but these requests from legal officers demonstrate that there was some attempt to follow 'the letter of the law'.[82]

8

The campaign. Part two: the surveys and tensions

Third phase: World War I

The period of the First World War can be considered as the third phase in the campaign against sleeping sickness in the Belgian Congo. Unfortunately, the war began just at the time when the colonial administration was in the process of addressing the problem of a medical service and public health policy in the Congo. An outstanding feature of the period of the war was the manner in which the colonial administration contradicted its own public health policy and, in fact, aggravated human sleeping sickness in northern Congo. The reprise of the Congo in 1908 had not been widely popular amongst Belgians at home but the war revealed, for perhaps the first time, the fact that their government *needed* the labour and resources available in its colony. Evacuated to Britain because of German occupation, the Belgian government looked to its African colony for material assistance in the war effort. North-eastern Congo was suddenly of great importance for three reasons: gold, rubber and labour. We can get some idea of the effect of the war by examining the figures for gold production in northern Congo during the war. In 1913, the total sales from Kilo-Moto amounted to 4,676,852 francs, but by 1918, the sales were 12,394,256 francs and in 1919, 19,796,000 francs. In six years, the sales had quadrupled.[1]

But the constantly increasing demands for gold, rubber and men forced the colonial administration to contradict much of its own recent public health policy in the north-east.[2] The labour demands required an intensification of the movement of population throughout the north-east, and that meant that the recently imposed cordon sanitaire became a hindrance to the war effort. Until the early 1920s both rubber and gold production remained particularly labour-intensive activities which required substantial production forces as well as numerous porters (see chapter 3). The latter transported the gold and rubber as well as the

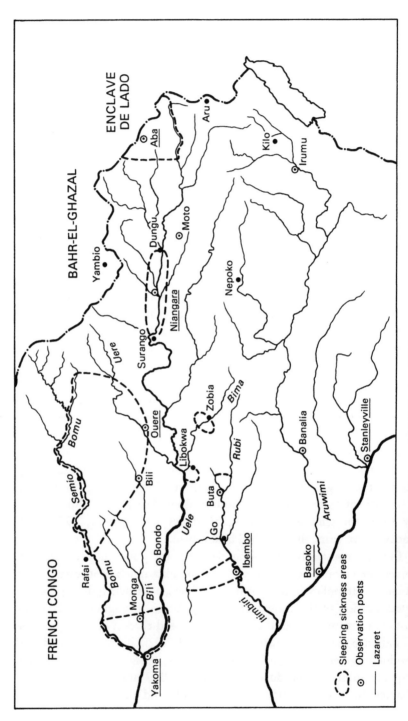

Map 8. Distribution of sleeping sickness, Uele District, 1914.

supplies and food provisions for the mines. Thus, during World War I, Uele district was particularly pressured to produce workers, principally porters for the Kivu region, mine workers and soldiers. In 1915 the district of Lower Uele furnished 600 recruits for the Force Publique, 800 for the gold mines of Moto, 120 for the eastern frontier plus an *unspecified* number for palm-oil companies, trading concerns, religious missions, road construction and state posts. The district commissioner commented in his report that there had been 'grave difficulties' obtaining these labourers and that nothing was as helpful 'as a show of force'.[3] There were endless requests for porters for the war effort in Kivu where, in October 1915, the district commissioner was informed that the number of porters required was 'unlimited'. Single *chefferies* had to provide convoys *en bloc*, a terrible strain on local manpower.[4]

A further difficulty for colonial policy in the north-east was the loss of territorial and medical personnel, transferred elsewhere during the war. These transfers seriously threatened the public health policy as well as the political administration of the region. At the beginning of 1915, Dr S'Heeren, a major figure in the Uele sleeping sickness campaign, left for the European front. The doctor at Niangara went to Europe leaving in his place a pharmacist to continue with the sleeping sickness campaign in the region, and there was concern that Dr Olivier, director of the Ibembo lazaret, might also leave for Europe. Another problem was that a large proportion of doctors in the Belgian colonial medical service were Italians who were now called away. That came about as it had not been possible in the early years of the service to recruit sufficient numbers of Belgians.[5] On 30 June 1915, *all* Italian officers under the age of 39, were summoned for military service by the Italian government and the Belgian Congo lost at a stroke a significant proportion of its doctors who in 1914 had numbered eighty-one. There is an interesting footnote to this event. The *adjoint supérieur* of Uele asked the district commissioner to withhold information of the call-up from the Italians because he was afraid they would leave their posts before replacements were made.[6] However, an Italian agent at Niangara learned by radio of the call-up and he notified his compatriots who then prepared to leave.[7]

It is clear from the evidence that, at the local level, administrators in northern Congo were genuinely concerned to continue the sleeping sickness campaign. The provincial administration, too, was aware of the problem and throughout the war issued its own instructions for the protection of the district. It continued to urge the maintenance of vigilant observation posts for the cordon sanitaire. In July 1915, for example, instructions were issued that the observation post of Ango must continue its vigilance by examining all Africans passing from infected into non-infected regions, and all territorial agents were warned that infractions would be punished.

At the same time the added pressures for rubber production intensified conflict between the central and provincial administrations with regard to sleeping sickness policy. In spite of evidence that there were foci of epidemic sleeping sickness such as those discovered during the military campaign against the Azande ruler, Sasa, the central administration had always been reluctant to sanction local government's declarations that such regions were epidemic, because it wished to avoid the self-imposed restrictions of a cordon sanitaire. The war further exacerbated such differences of opinion. In August 1915 the district commissioner of Uele reported that the situation *vis-à-vis* sleeping sickness had worsened in the areas already afflicted by the Gwane epidemic. Rubber collection was widespread and now was carried out *exclusively* in tsetse-infested gallery forests. In addition, he reported, there were very many traders and *capitas* travelling throughout the territory spreading the disease. It was quite clear, complained the district commissioner, that for reasons of a political and economic nature, the central government simply refused to officially recognise as epidemic the region in north-central Uele district bordered by the posts of Titule, Bili, Semio, Lebo and Bondo. Such recognition was required before a cordon sanitaire could be legally enforced. The important observation post at Bili did not even have a European agent. Would it not be possible, he asked, to recruit military *infirmiers*, or even soldiers, who might have received training on sleeping sickness at the school of tropical medicine?[8] But five months later, in January 1916, Bili was still without even an *infirmier*, let alone a European agent.[9] A shuffling of the limited number of medical personnel took place. At Ango, for example, an African *infirmier* had to be left entirely on his own to run the post, with authority to issue medical passports, and Bili lacked even an *infirmier*. Nevertheless, a slow-down, almost cessation, of the campaign to control sleeping sickness in northern Belgian Congo took place. In May 1916 the district commissioner of Lower Uele lamented that since Dr Rodhain had departed in December 1914 there had been 'no real sleeping sickness campaign' in spite of the vivid evidence of an epidemic between the Bomu and Uere rivers.[10]

A major consequence of the war for Uelians was the increase and spread of epidemic sleeping sickness.[11] In the territories of Gwane, Bili and Dakwa where the disease was already serious, sleeping sickness now became intensely epidemic with entire *chefferies* afflicted. The increased demands for both labour and rubber meant that the region was subjected to more stress than ever, while the decrease in medical attention meant less was being done about it than before. The region would have to wait until 1918 and the end of the war before the first really effective steps were taken to cope with the increase and spread of the disease – the first effective steps, that is, from the point of view of the 'medicalisation' of the region.

Fourth phase: *missions maladie du sommeil*

The most highly organised attempts to deal with the problems of endemic disease were the mobile services set up in Africa to combat human trypano-somiasis and on to these were later grafted field units with wider terms of reference, whose diagnostic and treatment facilities were directed at a number of different endemic disease problems.[12]

The decade 1920–30 during which the special sleeping sickness missions were launched and developed can be considered a fourth phase of the public health programme for sleeping sickness. The policies of this period were taking shape as early as 1917 and became effective in 1919, but their full impact was only experienced by the Congolese from 1920 onward. The heart of the programme in this phase was the *missions maladie du sommeil*, the special teams which were to systematically survey certain regions of the colony in order to identify and treat victims in their own villages. The cardinal features of the teams were their mobility and their attempts to examine the entire African population of the colony. New staff were recruited specifically for this ambitious campaign, and the hope of the governor-general, who first enunciated the programme in August 1917, was that the colonial medical service would be able to recruit medical staff in Europe when military troops began demobilising following the end of the war. This was to be no ordinary public health programme. It was important, stressed the governor-general, 'that the agents who lead brigades into villages be "men of heart" with generous altruism and that they be conscious of the grand nature of the task'.[13]

The first sleeping sickness mission, or team, in the Belgian Congo began functioning in south-western Kwango district in 1919, followed by the second team in Uele in 1920. Within four years three more sleeping sickness teams were established in Bangala, Stanleyville and Mayumbe districts. So well did this policy take hold that by 1932 there

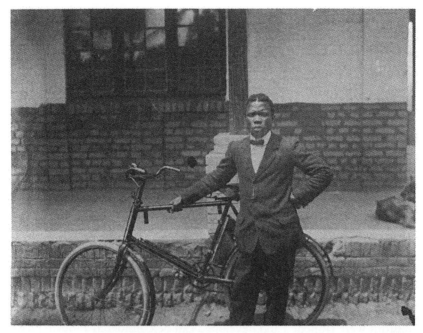

Plate 15. An *infirmier*, 1914.

were at least five such teams operating in the north-east alone, in the regions of Uele, Semliki, Stanleyville, Basoko, Kivu and Maniema.

In his report to the League of Nations in 1922, Dr Emile Van Campenhout sketched out his ideal of how a sleeping sickness team should operate. It would consist of five medical officers. Each of them, along with a European sanitary agent and twelve literate native injectors, would enter a sector of territory and install himself in a village which would form the centre of a group of about ten similar teams. Examinations would begin using the method of gland palpation, and careful records would be kept. One of the African assistants would be posted in that village, and the European sanitary agent would remain for one week supervising and getting the operation set up and underway, so that the African assistant could carry on the work thereafter. Meanwhile, the medical officer would move to a second village to be followed one week later by the European sanitary agent. The process would be repeated until all twelve injectors were posted, a task which would require three months. The medical officer would then commence a tour of inspection of the twelve injection stations, continuing for three months to supervise

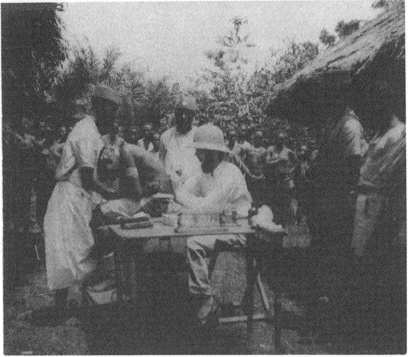

Plate 16. Lumbar puncture at Gemena, *c.* 1935.

treatments, search out new cases, resite villages, and supervise brush clearances. 'The region thus treated during six months would then be left alone for the next six months.'[14]

For many reasons, the reality of the missions was often far from the ideal envisaged by Van Campenhout. First of all, the frequent transfers and shortages of staff made difficult any continuity of a given project. For example, during 1931 a total of six doctors and eleven *agents sanitaires* had taken part in the team surveying Uele. Of those seventeen Europeans, only four had remained with the survey throughout the entire year. Even the direction of the team had been shared by two different doctors. All the other staff had been posted in the north-east between one and eight months with the average stay being six months. At the time of his report in February 1932, Dr Marone had at his disposal one doctor and five *agents sanitaires*, but he felt that five doctors and fourteen *agents sanitaires* were necessary in order to adequately conduct the mission. Furthermore, he said that he needed 260 African auxiliaries – *infirmiers, aides infirmiers,* microscopists and orderlies – in place of the 128 at his disposal. After all, it was the African auxiliaries who did most of the actual work of the team. Thus, understaffing and frequent transfers meant that the sleeping sickness teams could not fulfil the roles envisaged by Van Campenhout.[15]

Other difficulties became apparent during the fourth phase of the campaign. The different goals of colonial departments sometimes resulted in impasses over implementation of the public health measures. Doctors increasingly found themselves confronted with local administrators who were loathe to enforce public health policies and recommendations. In addition, increasingly through this decade, the special sleeping sickness teams overlapped with the colonial medical service until it became very difficult to perceive clear-cut roles for these two services.

1921 Uele survey

The reports of the missions at the beginning and end of the decade reveal the emergence of an institutionalisation of the surveys and some of their problems. Because of the intervening European war, Dr S'Heeren's survey of Uele in 1920–1 was the first since Dr Rodhain's extended tour of June 1913 to December 1914. Belgian medical staff at that time reasoned that demands for rubber and gold from the northern Congo during the war had meant greatly increased movements of people which, in turn, had spread the disease. They continued to believe that sleeping sickness, like plague, was a contagious disease spread primarily by the movements of infected people. As usual, the social and economic conditions obtaining among African peoples were not seen as contributing causes to increased incidence of disease.

Uele district had been a single administrative unit when Rodhain examined its western portion, but by the time of S'Heeren's survey the district had been divided into two sections, Lower, or western, and Upper, or eastern, Uele. In 1920–1, the sleeping sickness team surveyed only Lower Uele, a region of some 130,900 square kilometres. It was much the same area earlier examined by Rodhain. Based upon Jamot's model, S'Heeren devised a grid system, which he referred to as a 'chequerboard', whereby he divided Lower Uele district into ten medical sectors. This echoed the earlier idea suggested by Dutton and Todd of dividing the Congo Free State into a grid of infected and non-infected zones. S'Heeren stressed the importance of examining *every* single individual in the district. To do that, the teams would have systematically to visit each territory and *chefferie* and even each *capita*'s residence. Serious study of the maps of the region as well as the territorial census was vital.

The 1920–1 survey team for Lower Uele consisted of four doctors, three *agents sanitaires*, one European *infirmière*, and an unspecified number of African assistants. Among the latter would have been *infirmiers*, microscopists and, perhaps, some trained injectors although this was not made clear in the report. S'Heeren's method was first to inform a chief about the impending survey. Next, two *infirmiers* were sent to that *chefferie* where people were examined for swollen glands. The *infirmiers* also completed a medical census at that time. They then accompanied the suspected victims to the base of operations for that sector. It was very useful for the *infirmiers* to be accompanied by the local *capita* who was familiar with the territory and who could locate the isolated settlements. It was also useful to have along police agents who could assist with the 'recalcitrants' and those people who attempted to flee.

At the base for the sector, suspected victims' blood and cerebral-spinal fluid were examined by *infirmiers* trained to use the microscope. It was necessary to have at least two men for this purpose as there were twenty-five to thirty examinations per day. All adult males in the *chefferies* possessed identity cards which also displayed the names of any wives and children, and the sleeping sickness team were to make up dated medical visas with details of their examinations. It was necessary to complete the specimen examinations of all the people brought into the headquarters each day as they could not be expected to return the next day if not seen. The most important individual who helped with the survey, according to S'Heeren, was the chief, and if he happened to be cooperative the number of daily examinations was always much increased. For instance, when the people were working in their fields, they were most reluctant to break off to attend medical examinations and were only brought with great difficulty. But, added S'Heeren, the Azande *always* hid their women from the team, making this category of individuals 'la plus rebelle'.

S'Heeren believed that one could 'sterilise a region by repeated ambulatory atoxylisation'. Upon diagnosis, victims were immediately treated with injections of atoxyl alone, or in combination with other drugs such as scamin, émetique or diaxyl. The schedule of injections used by this survey had been developed at the Leopoldville laboratory by Dr Van den Branden, and it apparently quickly cleared a victim's circulatory system of trypanosomes thus making him non-infective for 'weeks, months and perhaps, years', according to S'Heeren. Van den Branden's formula for chemotherapy was as follows:

Day 1: 0.5 g atoxyl or scamin;

Day 2: 0.1 g émetique;

Day 3: 1.0 g atoxyl or scamin.

Most patients were instructed to attend 'ambulatory', or walk-in clinics fortnightly for further injections.

Victims sent to lazarets were given a different course of treatment which consisted of:

Day 1:   1.0 g atoxyl;

Days 2–9:   1.0 g atoxyl plus 0.1 g émetique;

Day 10:   lumbar puncture

If no parasites were present, the victim was kept in the lazaret for a further three months without medication. At the end of that period, a second lumbar puncture was performed and if the fluid was still free of trypanosomes, he still remained inside the lazaret for a *year*. Following that time, a third lumbar puncture was performed and if there were still no parasites, the patient could be considered, at long last, fully cured and he was released. They were the lucky patients. The unfortunate ones whose punctures revealed trypanosomes were considered to be chronic cases and were administered fortnightly injections of atoxyl. S'Heeren pointed out that these were the ideal treatment patterns. The reality was something else. Although ambulatory patients were *supposed* to present themselves for fortnightly injections, it was 'extremely rare' for patients to appear fortnightly or even monthly. S'Heeren voiced the ceaseless complaint of the coloniser, 'We do not know how to change African thinking . . . '.

The 1920–1 survey of the ten sectors of Lower Uele identified 1,445 victims of sleeping sickness after examining 160,000 people over a six-month period. The most heavily infected sector was Gwane where 1,014 victims were discovered among 10,813 examinations. Next worst was Bili with 102 victims found among 17,325 examinations. The lazarets isolated 236 patients (Ango, 68; Ibembo, 168) while the remainder were treated at the injection clinics.

Perhaps the most significant finding of the 1921 mission was its recognition of the long-standing and alarming epidemic in north-central Uele district. We have seen that there were over the years repeated reports of an increasingly serious and ignored epidemic in the region of Gwane, Bili and Dakwa. By 1918 the epidemic was reported to be 'ravaging' and, in 1922, 'decimating' Africans in the region.[16] S'Heeren reported that all along both the Gwane and Asa rivers sleeping sickness was very serious and that in the region of the Bomu river, many people had 'disappeared'. He considered the region to be a 'very dangerous focus of sleeping sickness'. One *chefferie* alone, Tuka, had 224 victims while another, Tupkwo, had 154.

'Mesures médico-administratives'

S'Heeren devoted five pages of his report to a series of complaints and suggestions. The other section of the report consisted of a two-page discussion of the main shortcoming of the survey – its lack of personnel. It is not surprising that, during the first organised survey for sleeping sickness in Uele since the war, the doctor was so critical.

S'Heeren was disturbed by the almost total disregard of the sleeping sickness regulations on the part of most residents in the district he examined. He was also very concerned about the need to resite specific populations he considered to be at risk. He reported that moving people was really executed only along the Itimbiri river because there whole villages were already established along the banks; thus they could be easily located and forced to move. But the doctor thought it 'nearly impossible to move the hundreds of tiny Azande groups far from the little rivers'. Water supply was the major problem in moving people, S'Heeren found, as 'well-digging was not only unknown, but unacceptable to the Africans'. He advised that the Belgians should follow the example of the British who had moved entire populations to totally new regions. As for clearing brush along major communication routes, S'Heeren admitted it would be a 'Titan's task' and enormously expensive.[17]

S'Heeren's most emphatic and radical suggestion touched upon the fields of economic and political administration. He suggested that the territories of Gwane and Bili should be totally closed for two years. He advised the administration to immediately put a stop to all trade, elephant-hunting and rubber collection in these heavily infected territories. Furthermore, he suggested that either the people in the region should be exempted from tax or it should be greatly reduced. In order to carry out these measures, senior doctors in charge of surveys and lazarets should be granted powers to enforce all public health regulations so that it would no longer be necessary to depend upon the territorial administrator, police and army to implement necessary public health measures. In other words, S'Heeren stressed the importance of restructuring

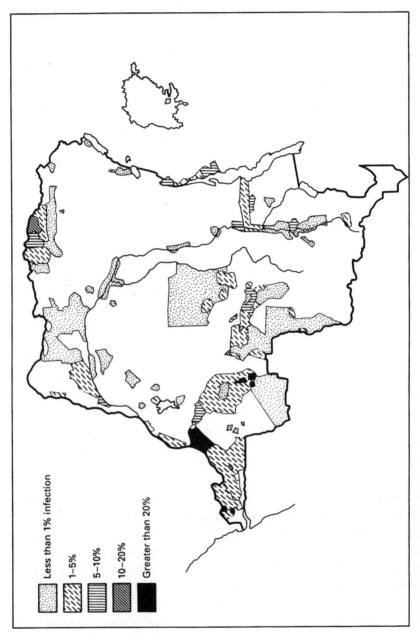

Less than 1% infection

1–5%

5–10%

10–20%

Greater than 20%

Map 9. Distribution of sleeping sickness, 1928.

African societies he considered to be at risk, and much of his complaint centred on the conservative nature of people, whom he saw as slow to adopt the colonial, Western form of medical response to epidemic disease.

1931 Uele survey

By the time of the survey of Uele a decade later, in 1931, the region had been redivided into three districts: Uele-Itimbiri, Uele-Nepoko and Ituri and contained nineteen administrative territories. This much-enlarged survey thus included all the region formerly examined by S'Heeren's team in 1921 plus an extensive area in the north-east of the colony bounded by the posts of Faradje, Aru and Watsa. It is interesting to compare S'Heeren's findings and scope with those of the report of the 1931 survey.

The first striking feature of the 1931 survey was the composition of its staff. In spite of the much greater territory and more numerous population, the numbers of European members on the team remained very small, averaging at any one time three doctors and five *agents sanitaires*. The real difference was in the number of African assistants. In 1931, there were 128 African assistants, a staggering increase over the 1920–1 survey. None the less Marone, head of the survey, insisted that he needed at least 260 African assistants in order to adequately survey the region. S'Heeren had not specified the exact number of Africans involved, but he had stated that it was advisable to have two *infirmiers* in each of the ten sectors. With its more numerous African assistants, the 1931 team examined many more people. In fact, Marone boasted that the 1931 medical census not only rivalled, but surpassed, the census made by the territorial administration for purposes of tax and labour.

Marone's fifty-one-page typed report provides interesting insights into developments over the decade. One area of development was in the chemotherapy of sleeping sickness. During the whole period of this study, there were few drugs available for treatment of the Gambian form of human sleeping sickness.[18] The major drugs used by the Belgians between 1906 and 1930 were, in order of appearance: atoxyl and a number of compounds based upon atoxyl in combination with other drugs like émetique, orpiment, etc.; soamine; salvarsan or '606'; neosalvarsan; suramin or Bayer 205; tryparsamide and its Belgian version, tryponarsyl; pentamidine; and melarsoprol. But atoxyl, a highly toxic arsenical compound composed of 37.69 per cent arsenic which caused

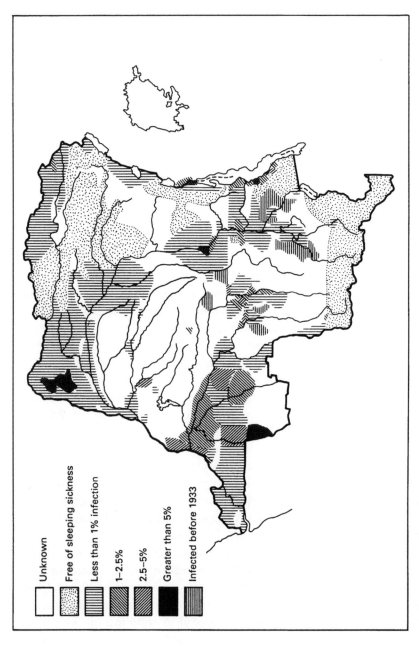

Map 10. Distribution of sleeping sickness, 1933.

Unknown

Free of sleeping sickness

Less than 1% infection

1–2.5%

2.5–5%

Greater than 5%

Infected before 1933

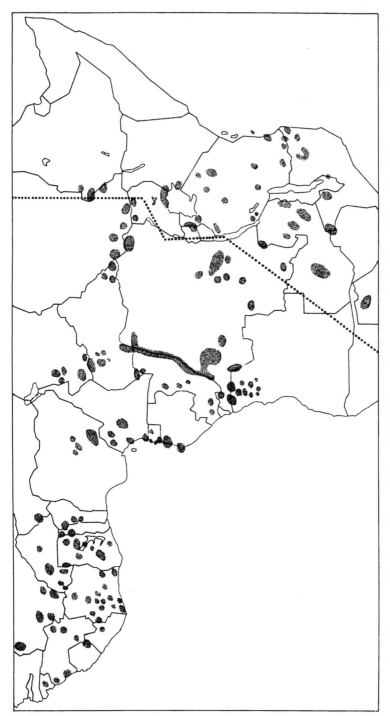

Map 11. Distribution of sleeping sickness, Africa, 1986. *T. b. gambiense* areas to left of dotted line; *T.b. rhodesiense* to right of line.

atrophy of the optic nerve and blinding, remained the main drug employed by the Belgians from 1906 until 1920.[19] Soamine was introduced in 1912, but it also blinded patients. In 1913, Dr Mouchet reported that the drug salvarsan and the combination of atoxyl and émetique could sterilise a victim of trypanosomes for periods of two to four months. Salvarsan, '606', had been developed by Paul Ehrlich and first used for syphilis in 1911, but he later introduced a better version of this drug, neosalvarsan.[20]

Suramin, or Bayer 205, was developed between 1916 and 1920, while tryparsamide was developed between 1919 and 1925. The latter drug was much experimented with and later used in the Belgian Congo where Dr Louise Pearce of the Rockefeller Institute made extensive clinical trials from 1920. Dr C. C. Chesterman, whose Baptist Missionary Society hospital and sleeping sickness work at Yakusu, near Stanleyville, was famous, also conducted trials of drugs, including tryparsamide. He suggested that 'it is probable . . . that visual trouble must be expected to occur in at least thirty per cent of second stage cases . . . With due care, however, this should not proceed to permanent amblyopia [blindness].'

The Belgians introduced their own version of tryparsamide in 1925, naming it tryponarsyl. Dr A. Broden of the Leopoldville laboratory found it less toxic than atoxyl with its dangerous toxicity and lack of stability in the tropics. The chief medical officer, Rodhain, announced in June 1924 that 'we will be able, no doubt, towards the end of the year to improve our therapy and substitute atoxyl with tryparsamide and Bayer 205'.[21] So, by 1931, the drugs for use with sleeping sickness, while far from ideal, were nevertheless a great improvement over the crude arsenical, atoxyl. Marone's routine for treatment was 2.0 g of tryponarsyl injected daily for forty days, followed by a lumbar puncture. If there were no trypanosomes, he considered the victim to be 'apparently' cured for the next six months, when there was another lumbar puncture. This action was repeated a total of four times at six-monthly intervals. Finally, if there were still no parasites in either the blood or spinal fluid, the patient was declared to be 'definitely' cured.

While chemotherapy had improved, the course of treatment, inconvenience and discomfort for victims of the disease remained considerable. By 1931, a series of injection centres had been established at carefully selected sites placed in the centre of infected zones. An *infirmier* was permanently posted at each centre where victims were expected to attend for injections. According to Marone, in areas where it was not possible to place an injection centre near the victims, the

Table 3. *Sleeping sickness in Uele district, 1931*

Sector	Victims 31 Dec. 30	New 1931	Died	Vanish	Lumbars
Gwane	428	16	31	3	300
Bili	42	3	1	0	61
Dakwa	346	56	7	1	n.a.
Doruma[a]	2,178	92	46	440	2,311
Faradje–Aba	624	274	22	4	622
Niangara	1,381	284	36	29	n.a.
Dungu	137	83	5	4	75

Note:
[a] Doruma also had a lazaret managed by Catholic missionaries and during 1931 it housed 154 victims.[22]

infirmier would go to the village of a chief or sub-chief and administer injections to the patients, who would have been summoned there. Most Africans, in Marone's experience, had been cooperative about attending for injections.

In 1931, the sleeping sickness team examined 306,277 people, almost twice the number seen a decade earlier. Previously identified, or 'old' patients numbered 5,136 while there were 809 newly discovered victims. Marone reported that of the total victims in 1931, 481 'disappeared', 148 died, and 4,305 remained in treatment. The statistics reported by Marone are given in Table 3.

Gwane territory in 1931

Sleeping sickness was apparently no longer so serious in Gwane territory, which now had been completely surveyed. Marone reported small foyers of infection, and only 16 new cases were diagnosed, bringing the total number of cases in Gwane to 478. This figure stood in sharp contrast to the 1,014 victims reported in 1920–1. In Bili territory, only one *chefferie* had been examined, and among its 2,079 people, only 3 new cases were diagnosed, for a total of 42 victims. Dakwa territory produced 56 new cases among 10,445 examinations, while the total number of cases was 346. Sleeping sickness appeared to the Belgians to have 'moved' eastward afflicting the territories of Doruma with 92 new cases among 57,257 examinations (2,178 total); Niangara with 284 new cases among 58,500 examinations (1,381 total); and Faradje with 274 new cases among 6,497 examinations (624 total). Dr Marone surmised that the Gwane–Bili–Dakwa epidemic had decreased whereas the eastern portion of Uele now seemed to be an epidemic region. It was the view of the chief medical officer for the province, Dr L. Fontana, that the reason for the diminished epidemic of sleeping sickness in certain areas, like Gwane, was 'medical action'. In other words, he stressed the role of medicine in victory over disease, overlooking the important role of economic and political factors in relation to disease. What was also not mentioned in the 1931 report was the fact that the earlier surveys had examined *only* the western portion of the district.[23]

The statistics produced by the sleeping sickness teams between 1921 and 1933 can be gleaned from their reports and from reports published by the provincial medical service (Table 4).[24] From 1922 the figures for both halves of Uele district were combined, making it difficult to ascertain how many applied to the Upper, or eastern, half. However, the total numbers examined only gradually increased until 1929 or 1930, and thus it may be that most of the people actually examined by the survey teams up to 1930 were still those resident in Lower, or western, Uele district. In fact, a later director of the colonial medical service informs us that it was only *towards 1930* that the 'methods of the sleeping sickness teams became good enough to produce reliable statistics'.[25] Consequently, Dr Marone's conclusion in 1931 that the epidemic of sleeping sickness had *moved* eastward may, in fact, only reveal the Belgians' own recent move eastward with their survey. We cannot overlook the possibility that sleeping sickness may have been present in eastern Uele district to a greater degree than was long thought to be the case.

Settlement pattern

By 1931 the sleeping sickness campaign reflected both major strands of Belgian public health – *prophylaxie médicale* and *prophylaxie biologique*. It was in the latter, the realm of 'social engineering', that colonial doctors were most often frustrated, especially as they increasingly found themselves in the awkward situation of making demands which conflicted with the goals of other sectors of the colonial administration. Marone, like S'Heeren ten years before him, discussed in his own report the two fronts of the sleeping sickness campaign, '*prophylaxie médicale* and *biologique*', but he complained that most of the reports from members of the 1931 survey 'were silent' on the latter. Only the report from the sector of Faradje-Aba included comment on this aspect of the campaign.

Table 4. *Sleeping sickness in Belgian Congo, 1921–1938*[26]

	Area	Exams	Total	New	Old
Surveys of Uele District					
1921	Bas-Uele	157,826	1,631	—	—
1922[a]	Uele	110,548	3,620	—	—
1923	Uele	157,843	3,208	608	2,600
1924	Uele	189,262	4,871	—	600
1925	Uele	155,928	5,182	956	4,226
1926	Uele	199,061	4,114	540	3,574
1927	Uele	200,642	4,429	—	—
1928	Uele	163,422	4,484	269	4,215
1929	Uele	276,412	5,485	862	4,623
1930	Uele	346,305	6,501	1,142	5,359
1931	Uele	306,277	6,056	839	5,217
1932[b]	Uele	260,554	5,671	954	4,717
1933	Uele	323,972	5,182	645	4,537
Surveys of Province Orientale and Stanleyville Province					
1930	P.O.	632,749	12,183	3,341	8,842
1931	P.O.	670,557	13,916	2,688	11,228
1932	P.O.	718,014	11,364	2,775	8,589
1933	St. Prov.	652,148	8,588	1,020	7,568
Surveys of the entire colony					
1923		about 1,000,000	44,891	19,709	—
1924		1,300,000	—	—	—
1925		1,500,000	98,512	—	—
1926		2,145,177	—	—	—
1927		1,704,477	—	16,260	—
1928		2,126,356	70,812	24,440	46,372
1929		—	—	—	—
1930		2,779,448	103,985	33,562	70,423
1931		1,959,604	87,577	19,248	68,329
1932		2,832,083	98,614	21,346	77,268
1933		3,572,423	121,893	27,939	93,954
1938		5,034,351	59,239	13,454	45,785

Notes:
[a] The 1922 survey revealed 1,549 victims in Doruma territory; 188 in Niangara; and a 'very bad' situation in Gwane–Bili.
[b] In 1932, Bili territory was not surveyed.

Marone's view was that *prophylaxie médicale* had benefited certain areas, like Gwane. Unfortunately, the administration had 'always demonstrated an aversion' to regrouping people upon medical advice, and the resulting lack of *prophylaxie biologique* meant that the disease, in fact, had spread into neighbouring territories (east to Dungu and Faradje). One advantage, in Marone's view, would be to have 'formed a collectivity of natives where only before had existed a unit' which would always be able to clear brush around residences. Furthermore, the little paths formerly connecting scattered homesteads would be unnecessary and would disappear giving way to main roads connecting villages. He admitted that it would take a long time to regroup all Africans along the newly made motor routes, but the regrouping of people into villages as described above would be an important first step in the direction of the full policy.

Another advantage of grouping Africans in villages would be the increased ease and efficiency of locating victims of sleeping sickness. As it was, it was very difficult to locate all victims, since many individual Africans were unwilling to come forward for examinations, while many African authorities refused to make their people attend the examinations. On the other hand, pointed out Marone, many miserable victims of the disease could not manage to get themselves to the sleeping sickness team for help either because they had been abandoned by their kin or because they had been hidden away from the medical authorities by the kin. Such things could not happen after people were forced to live in villages in which the sleeping sickness mission could move from hut to hut methodically examining each resident.

Tensions

Marone paid special attention to the serious lack of cooperation, even conflict, among various administrative departments in the colony and urged that doctors be granted sanctions to arm them in their attempts to effect *prophylaxie biologique*. This, for Marone, was *the* greatest problem facing the sleeping sickness campaign. He devoted fifteen pages of his 1931 report to a discussion of the one issue of regroupment and resiting of Africans. Since clearing all of the brush along important rivers was impossible, it was particularly important, he felt, to reorganise people into villages which should be placed at locations 'chosen by the medical service' in accord with the territorial administration. He added, however, that he, himself, had never 'had the honour of discussing this subject with a representative of the administration'. 'Comme on le voit, après le regroupement indigène, toute autre proposition faite en vue de faciliter le recensement des indigènes au point de vue maladie du sommeil est rejetée part Messieurs les Administrateurs.' As things were, he said, doctors could attempt only medical prophylaxis, while biological prophylaxis, the 'social engineering', was up to the territorial administration. Clearly severe tensions had developed between medical staff, who pressed increasingly for preventive measures, and territorial staff, who saw the function of medicine as curative and not administrative.

Marone's lengthy articulation of the frustration experienced by doctors in their attempts to advise and implement public health measures designed to prevent the spread of the disease, reveals the extent of this problem by 1930. From 1920, doctors had implored territorial administrators to heed certain measures which, they believed, would decrease the incidence of sleeping sickness. The measures focused on several main areas of African life including movements of population due to travel, labour recruitment, kin relations and trade. Doctors were concerned about African movements induced by their search for rubber and, increasingly, medical authorities made suggestions directed at state policies of taxation. They offered advice on policies concerning African economic activities such as fishing and trade. They advised the 'sealing off' of certain badly afflicted regions, asking that outsiders be prevented entry even when seeking their mandatory rubber tax. Medical advice related to sleeping sickness touched upon state policies concerning the growing of cash crops (such as cotton), and those concerning porterage and road construction were directly affected by the acceptance of such medical advice. By 1930 the issue of regrouping people into larger villages and resiting villages in areas considered safer from infection of sleeping sickness had become a major problem for medical staff and territorial administration alike.

Medical service and sleeping sickness missions

From the mid-1920s, demands by some doctors for increasing autonomy for the special sleeping sickness teams conflicted with the demands of others who recommended unification of the two increasingly separate services. Discrete sleeping sickness teams functioned alongside an evolving colonial medical service, but there was considerable confusion as the two services often competed for the same limited funds and personnel. Resources were shunted between the two services, often producing confusion over which staff or facilities belonged to which service and which functions were to be performed by each.

The relation of the sleeping sickness missions to the medical service became more, rather than less, unclear over time. S'Heeren, in 1921, had requested administrative independence with regard to the personnel attached to his mission. He had asked that his staff be engaged exclusively in the campaign against sleeping sickness, promising that they would work in 'perfect accord' with the local territorial administration. He had even suggested that the sleeping sickness team be financially independent, following the example of the one in Kwango district. Rodhain, who had been appointed chief of the colonial medical service the previous year, agreed with S'Heeren. But in 1924 Dr Van Campenhout, by now the director of the Service de l'Hygiène at the Colonial Ministry in Brussels and a man who just two years earlier had so solidly supported the special sleeping sickness team concept, suggested that the autonomous sleeping sickness teams be discontinued. He felt that one single, unified colonial medical service could better manage the sleeping sickness campaign.[27]

Metropolitan versus colonial view

The two contrasting views of Rodhain and Van Campenhout exemplify the differing perspectives from the metropole and the colony. Jerome Rodhain spent nearly a quarter of a century in the Congo (1903–25), where he began his career as a doctor in a military training camp. He soon took up duties researching sleeping sickness in the laboratory at Leopoldville, only leaving in the period 1910–12 to direct a scientific mission to the southern province of Katanga. Then between 1913 and 1915 he conducted the first survey of sleeping sickness in Uele district. Named chief of the colonial medical service in 1920, he remained in the Congo until 1925 when he returned to Belgium to take up a post at the School of Tropical Medicine. He became director of the school in 1929 and stayed until 1933 when he became director of the Prince Leopold Institute of Tropical Medicine.[28]

Emile Van Campenhout spent ten years in Africa, most of the time acting as a military administrator rather than a medic. He had taken part in the Van Kerckhoven expedition, but his duties involved very little medicine because of the dearth of administrative staff. Instead, he was a *chef de zone* and a *chef de poste*; between 1894 and 1897 in Bangala district

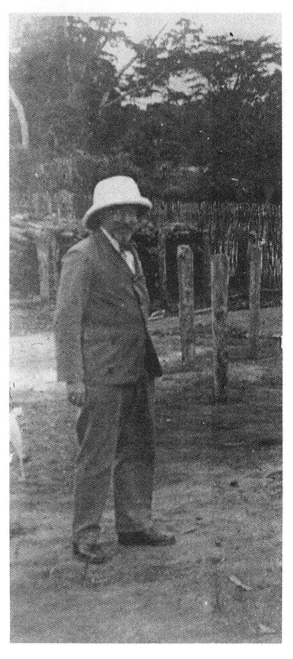

he spent much of his time administering the post of Nouvelle Anvers and commanding 'police operations' (a euphemism for enforcing rubber collection) in nearby districts. In May 1899, after seven years of active military service, he founded the research laboratory at Leopoldville where he began looking into sleeping sickness, which was then apparently epidemic in Lower Congo. In November 1900 he returned permanently to Brussels where, from its foundation in 1906, he managed the School of Tropical Medicine, teaching 'colonial hygiene'. He did not resign from the army medical corps until 1908, when he joined the newly established Service de l'Hygiène in the colonial ministry. He became *chef de division* in the service in 1910 and then, in 1918, its director. In 1924 he was named *inspecteur général*, which post he held until 1930. It was said that the Service de l'Hygiène in Brussels was the 'motor' of the colonial medical service and that Van Campenhout was at its centre.[29]

Rodhain, the head of the medical service in the colony, and Van Campenhout, the head of the hygiene department in the Colonial Ministry, had quite different views concerning the relationship of the sleeping sickness teams to the medical service. Not surprisingly, the Colonial Ministry favoured more centralisation while those in the colony favoured local autonomy. Some years before, in 1909, Rodhain had complained bitterly about this problem. Dr Van Campenhout, who was the director of the tropical medicine school and the main advisor to the government on colonial health matters, had left Africa nine years previously. In Rodhain's view, it was vital for one in such a position to have closer personal experience in the colony. He suggested therefore that for important posts in Belgium, the government should employ doctors who were at present working in the colony gaining first-hand knowledge of tropical health.[30] It was a tension between the centre and periphery which appeared in many areas of the Congo administration.

But the problem of redundancy and overlap between the two services was a real one. In the view of the *médecin en chef*, Trolli, in 1928 the sleeping sickness mission had 'lost sight of its principal aim', which was the survey of the district for all victims of the disease; and instead it had become 'bogged down' in the treatment of victims. Dr Schwetz, the *médecin provincial* for Province Orientale, thought that the same goals could be attained with half the staff if redundancies were eliminated: 'I have not been able to find a clear line of demarcation between the work of the regular Medical Service and the Sleeping Sickness Mission of Uele. The latter spends a great deal of its effort on "general medicine".'

At Buta the doctor was 'too busy with private patients'. In the Uele-Nepoko district, the situation was even more confused. Dispensaries directed by the district medical services were next door to dispensaries and, in one case, even a hospital directed by the chief of the sleeping sickness team. Throughout the decade the confusion increased between the roles of the sleeping sickness missions and those of the medical service until by the end of the twenties the medical tactics, too, were being challenged with explicit complaints about the 'creaking bureaucracy' of the system.[31]

By 1930, the sleeping sickness programme reached into every area of life for both coloniser and colonised in northern Congo, and it became inextricably entangled with other sectors of colonial administration. Measures advised by medical authorities to avoid the spread of sleeping sickness unavoidably affected areas of colonial policy such as transport, road construction and villagisation. At the same time, African life was markedly affected by public health measures.

Summary

Events in northern Congo between 1903 and 1930 are illustrative of the ways in which disease, especially when epidemic, can both illuminate social relations and affect the course of history. We have seen how sleeping sickness incidence and intensity increased in northern Congo as a result of the severe disruptions of the colonial imposition. After the 'discovery' of epidemic sleeping sickness in large regions of the colony, government responses were at first predominantly legislative, while the colonial medical service and a sleeping sickness campaign only gradually took shape. The highly bureaucratic nature of Belgian colonial policy was exemplified in the areas of public health and medicine. Local administrators were inundated with instructions, ordinances and decrees concerning sleeping sickness policies. By their very complexity, these policies led to confusion in carrying out the medical policy and often to administrative non-attention to medical requirements which conflicted with the political and economic demands on colonial officialdom. Perhaps more significantly, the policies touched upon myriad aspects of African life. The next chapter will examine African perceptions of the disease, the cure and the evolving public health programme.

9

The African response

SLEEPING SICKNESS AND AFRICAN SOCIETIES

Chapters 7 and 8, in discussing at length the main features of the Belgian sleeping sickness campaign until 1930, stressed the proliferation of legislation and directives. The colonial authorities hoped to control the spread of the disease through administration; in the early decades with no cure, the emphasis was very much upon *prophylaxie biologique*. As early as 1904, a state doctor had claimed that 'to stop the propagation and diffusion of disease is no longer a scientific problem but simply an administrative problem'.[1]

There is ample evidence with which to piece together the history of Belgian colonial medicine, the history of Europeans in Africa. But what about Zairean history? For instance, how did Zaireans perceive the enormous upheavals between 1891 and 1930? There can be no doubt that for many Africans populations, a significant feature of Belgian conquest and colonisation was increased incidence of illness and death. The ensuing brutal exploitation of the land and people meant that sleeping sickness, previously endemic in regions of the territory, sometimes spread and became epidemic. We can begin to understand the African point of view, firstly, by outlining the major cultural and social factors moulding their perceptions and, secondly, by examining their responses to sleeping sickness and the colonial public health programme. It must be stated at the outset that the major sources for this section are European; nevertheless, as will be demonstrated, a careful reading of the reports and accounts of independent travellers, missionaries, state agents and medical staff reveals much in the search for the African view.

Humans are key factors in the total ecological setting and it is through the relationships to their environments developed over very long periods that human societies in Africa have managed to survive. I have focused upon three representative societies of northern Congo, Azande, Babua and Mangbetu, in order to reveal some of the variety of responses to both outbreaks of sleeping sickness and the colonial medical service. In this way, I hope to dispel the simplistic dichotomy of 'the African' versus 'the European' and to demonstrate instead the subtleties of the historical past. There exists a popular image of helpless, backward Africans in the nineteenth century suffering a multitude of tropical diseases until they were 'saved' by European colonisation and its gift of medicine.[2] The truth is somewhat different as we shall see. Africans were no more passive or static in relation to the difficulties of their environments than they were later to be to the imposition of colonial rule.

African societies possessed social mechanisms and specialist knowledge developed over centuries which aided them in their difficult struggle to survive and multiply. In some regions across a wide swath of sub-Saharan Africa, ecological relationships had evolved which allowed survival in the face of the almost omnipresent threat of human sleeping sickness. However, it is important to note that generalisations about 'African' methods of coping with health problems can be misleading, if not incorrect. This means that some acquaintance with social and cultural factors of the African societies involved in this study is crucial to our understanding of events surrounding outbreaks of sleeping sickness. For example, the spatial patterns of settlements as well as attitudes concerning disease, epidemics, medicine and practitioners are vital if we want to comprehend African responses to colonial medicine.

The many and diverse populations of northern Zaire have been described as a 'mosaic' of peoples most of whom derive from three major linguistic families: Adamawa-Ubangian, Central Sudanic and Bantu. The term 'mosaic' is unsatisfactory insofar as it conveys a picture of ethnic fracture and opposition, an image which can hinder an attempt to understand the social history of the overall region. While use of the image has some basis in the linguistic diversity, its development during the colonial period was very much enhanced by administrative policy. Between 1906 and 1933 it was the policy of the Congo authorities to administer their new African subjects through so-called 'traditional' or 'customary' social and political structures. To that end, Belgian colonial administrators were instructed to research each African society which resulted in numerous ethnographic studies.[3]

These studies, taken together, enabled the Belgians to map the colony into distinct socio-political units or tribes. Tribes were perceived as discrete entities, the 'building blocks' with which to construct the new state; and, like blocks, entire groups of people could be shifted for administrative purposes or subjected to regulations *en masse*. This perception was clearly demonstrated in much of the public health legislation and policy. But the habit of perceiving African peoples as discrete tribes caused the Belgians to make an important error. They failed to understand the rich complexity of interactions among peoples which was responsible for a fluidity of ethnic relations and for the changing nature of social relations in different eras.

'Building blocks' and social engineering

The decree of 2 May 1910 regarding the appointment of official chiefs (*chef médaillé*) formed the basis of Belgian colonial administrative policy for nearly three decades. Each ethnographic unit was a *chefferie indigène* over which the local administrator was required to designate a 'legitimate' authority, or chief. Societies in which no such figure could be identified were either provided with a state-appointed chief or were amalgamated into another group. It was recognised to be a 'delicate task' and, as late as 1930, the official handbook for territorial administrators warned that the period of reorganisation would be an occasion for the 'discontented or ambitious to intrigue against the chief's position or to even overthrow customary organisation'.

The initial result of the typical literal interpretations of oral traditions collected by colonial administrators from the various peoples was a picture of an ecologically attractive region, Uele, experiencing 'waves' of invasion by outsiders converging from different directions. Invaders, the Belgians thought, had pushed into and displaced earlier non-food-producing inhabitants, namely hunter-gatherers. Such literal acceptance of the traditions resulted in the popular view that Bantu-speaking peoples had invaded from the south-west. Central-Sudanic-speaking peoples swept from the north-east, and later, Azande hordes had descended from the north-west displacing the two earlier groups. Based upon personal testimonies, memories and traditions, most of the early attempts to describe and explain the mosaic-like ethnography of the region include minutely detailed accounts of the order, or succession, of the invasions.[4] Early colonists in the region firmly believed that, had it not been for their own entry into the situation, the war-like Azande in a short time would have overwhelmed the entire region. The new colonisers saw themselves as 'rescuers', even saviours, of smaller African societies unable to effectively oppose the powerful Azande 'waves'.

Some notion of the time and effort expended by the Belgian administrators on 'sorting out' tribes, and their preconceptions and conclusions about the peoples involved, is relevant to an understanding of colonial responses to the problem of sleeping sickness. Very early on, administrators began categorising African groups, ascribing to them stereotypic attitudes and responses which later affected the formulation and implementation of public health policy. The categorising resulted in part from the ethnographic reports, in part from experience, and very much from a growing mythology. For example, it was widely believed that the Azande, in general, were secretive, wily and often non-cooperative; the Babua were fierce, rebellious and anarchic; the Mangbetu were 'cultured', cooperative and progressive. Such views often determined not only the formulation and implementation of public health policies but European expectations regarding them.

By 1914 the colony had been extensively divided into administrative units. There were, for instance, 183 *territoires* and by early 1917, western Uele district alone had 256 *chefferies*. In 1922 there were nearly 2,500 *chefferies* in Province Orientale alone while in 1928 Stanleyville district contained 840 *chefferies* and 170 *sous-chefferies* each averaging 150 adult males.[5] Already in 1914 a premature note of satisfaction had crept into the documentation regarding the 're-organisation' of African societies into so-called 'traditional' units.[6]

The new African representative of the state, the *chefs médaillés*, were in the very awkward position of having to assert themselves over peoples who often did not recognise any such authority. The colonial administration kept close watch over the chiefs' abilities to fulfil their roles as intermediaries for the state. When chiefs failed to implement state policies, their authority could be revoked; often they were imprisoned and they were always replaced. When chiefs, for example, were unable to enforce sleeping sickness regulations and make their subjects attend the obligatory physical examinations, they were removed from office and imprisoned. Uncooperative chiefs could be exiled far from their regions.[7] For years, European administrators complained that many Africans simply did not understand the new regime. According to a 1914 report, ' . . . chiefs are beginning to comprehend a little better their roles [but] . . . it is necessary to continually have a European present among them'.[8] In reality, the 're-organised' peoples rarely acquiesced as easily as Belgians had hoped they would.

African views of disease and medicine

I have already mentioned that in order to make sense of Congolese responses to sleeping sickness and the Belgian medical campaigns, we must first know something about their own ideas concerning disease and medicine. Such knowledge will allow us to discern more clearly the underlying explanations for what might otherwise appear to be the purely irrational behaviour of Africans, a widespread assumption on the part of the colonial administrators and medics. The need to understand the 'other' point of view has been recently addressed by international aid and health agencies involved in improving the health of underdeveloped regions of the world. These organisations now stress the real need to understand the social and cultural context of disease and health in order to realistically hope to bring about change for improvement. A good example of this more enlightened approach is the present international campaign against AIDS which stresses the need for sociological, anthropological and historical studies as a means of revealing the whole context of disease.

During the period covered by this study, most of the people in northern Congo did not make clear distinctions among sleeping sickness, the colonial medical service or public health measures, and the overall military conquest and political reorganisation of their lives. As mentioned in the first chapter, many Africans considered the increased levels of disease around the turn of the century to be the 'conscious work of Europeans – a kind of biological warfare'.[9]

If a medical historian were to explain events early this century in northern Congo with particular reference to sleeping sickness, he would probably describe the gradual spread of an epidemic disease and hopeful indications by 1930 of an ultimate medical victory. Statistics would illustrate the increase and subsequent decrease of infection rates, which the medical historian would present as proof of yet another victory for Western biomedicine. Western medical techniques, therapies and drugs would be credited for the abatement of the disease. This version of the history of sleeping sickness in northern Congo would contain elements of truth.

However, an account of the same events given by an African would differ considerably from the version of the Western medical historian. This account would certainly emphasise the dramatic increase in stress and turmoil experienced by peoples in the region. The African would explain that one major consequence of the disruptions experienced by the people and their environment was a marked increase of misfortunes, one of which was disease, and he would describe the different ways in which people responded in their attempts to regain control over their lives. The African version of the history of the region would contain elements of truth as well. The African might explain that some outbreaks of disease were caused by man while others were caused by ancestral spirits or God. For societies such as the Azande, diseases caused by man (witchcraft) included slow, chronic conditions, typical of endemic *gambiense* trypanosomiasis. For such a misfortune, certain measures were required to combat the ultimate cause which was most often disturbed social relations. Therefore, the African version of the history of sleeping sickness in northern Congo would focus on the response of entire social groups to increased tension, stress and disaster. The Western medical historian would focus on the appropriate response from within his cultural parameters which in the case of the cure and control of disease means a set of materials and techniques – medicine and medical practice. The African explanation of the same objective events – stress, disease and antidotes, or 'cures', for these misfortunes – would focus on the steps taken by the group to combat what was seen as the *true* cause behind the disease. As one scholar has expressed it, 'western medicine focuses on the individual patient and leaves the social context of his illness in pathological chaos'.[10]

There is a large and expanding literature on the subject of African 'traditional' medicine which goes far beyond the scope of this study. But several points are highly relevant in any discussion of African responses to sleeping sickness and colonial medicine. Robin Horton observed that Africans perceived 'a causal link between disturbed social relations and disease or misfortune' while Victor Turner's view of divination as a form of 'social analysis' is an elaboration of this idea. Another scholar, A. B. Chilivumbu, explained that 'most social investigators writing about African society agree that belief systems as part of the structural components are causally related to illnesses'. This means that the primary objective regarding a sick person is his reintegration into the 'social fabric'. There is, then, an intimate relationship between the illness of an individual and his social structure. John Janzen in his study of therapy among the Bakongo investigated that relationship and demonstrated the vital role played by the patient's kin. Kin were the 'therapy-managing group', crucial in the process of reintegration of the individual. Janzen discusses the inevitable conflict between colonial medical practice and the African necessity for group involvement in individual cure. The historian Randall Packard suggests that in order to begin to understand changes over time in African concepts such as witchcraft, the study must include examination of the ways that social and economic changes interact and affect conceptual shifts. We must be aware of the enormous complexity of a people's concepts of what constitutes disease and effects cure.[11]

This awareness means that to understand African responses to sleeping sickness during the early colonial period, we must distinguish as much as possible between reactions to the disease and reactions to the 'cures'. It is useful to make a further distinction by separating out those reactions specifically provoked by preventive measures taken by the colonial authorities. Preventive measures formed the basis of the public health programme; they were, in effect, administrative measures which were at the same time early attempts at social engineering and were, therefore, the aspect of the sleeping sickness campaign which most affected the largest number of northern Congolese. A final note: it must be stressed that African responses to European concepts of disease and medical practices naturally changed over time. Responses also varied to some degree among societies and among social groups making up those societies. It would be a mistake to assume an 'African response' common to all societies or which remained static over time but a few generalisations concerning African ideas of 'health', 'disease' and 'misfortune' can help us to understand what might otherwise appear to be irrational behaviour.

Misfortunes and their cure

Traditional medicine is a complete medical system with joint global concepts of health that includes at once somatic, psychologic, and social aspects. The herbalists approach sickness in a manner similar to doctors and nurses in Western medicine, whereas the other healers [are] more like psychotherapists or sociologists.[12]

So concludes a group of researchers who have examined 'traditional' medicine in Zaire in response to the World Health Organisation initiative of 1977. While the current policy of the World Health Organisation which encourages the incorporation and utilisation of so-called 'traditional' medicine by many countries is not approved by all, many Western medical experts, just as did many early colonial medical personnel, find it easier to recognise and accept the merits of the 'herbalist' than they do the diviner or prophet. When these functions are neatly separated in the form of discrete practitioners, there is less of a problem in assimilating the role of the herbalist. However, when herbalist and diviner functions intermingle in the form of a single practitioner, there is and was a serious problem for the European biomedical expert – how to separate the 'voodoo' from the efficacious herbal cures?

The Azande

In this section the reader is introduced to some of the major concepts and practices related to misfortune which would have pertained among Azande, Babua and Mangbetu peoples during the period of the study. In sketching these views, I realise the risk of imposing an 'ethnographic present' upon the cultural and social features of societies which, in reality, had evolved over centuries and naturally continued to change over time. With this warning in mind, let us turn to a review of Azande ideas on the subject.

These people make a sensible beginning for there is a rich literature on Azande-speaking peoples who today stretch across international boundaries and live in three countries: the Central African Republic, southern Sudan and northern Zaire.[13]

Misfortune, or kpele

For the Azande, and here there is great similarity with the ideas of both the Babua and Mangbetu, disease was only one manifestation of *kpele*, or misfortune, of which there were many forms. The most common response to the occurrence of death or disease was to enquire not only why it had occurred, but *who* had caused it since the vast majority of deaths and diseases were believed to be caused by humans employing either witchcraft, *mangu*, or magic, *ngwa*, the concept closest to the Western idea of medicine.[14] They realised, naturally, that cold temperatures could lead to pneumonia, for instance, or that syphilis could result from contact with a syphilitic person. But at the same time they believed a person would not have suffered the effects of either the cold or the syphilitic contact if, in the first place, the witchcraft or bad medicine had not been employed. They viewed death (*kpiyo, kurugbwe*) and most disease (*kaza, wokote*) as unnatural except in a few specific circumstances such as death of the very elderly. Methods used to discover the identity of the person responsible for a misfortune included oracles (*soroka*), divination (*pa ngwa*), and medicine (*ngwa*).[15]

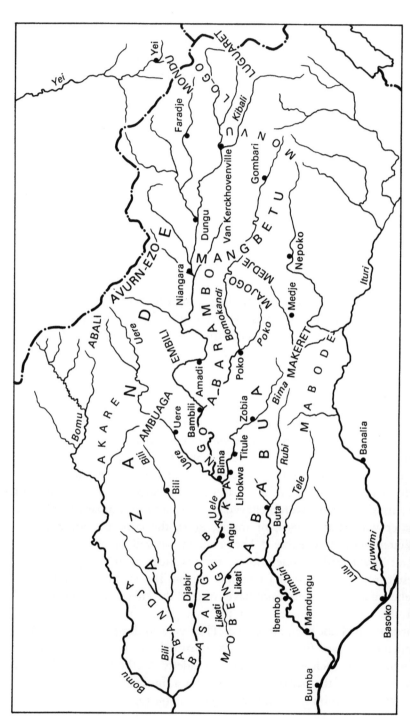

Map 12. Peoples of northern Congo.

The separate concepts, *mangu* and *ngwa* must not be confused. Most of the slower or chronic physical ailments, especially those without violent symptoms, were ascribed to witchcraft which meant that no antidotes, or 'medicines', were possible. This would have included many of the earlier stages of the slowly progressing *gambiense* form of sleeping sickness. However, sudden or acute maladies were often diagnosed as bad magic, or sorcery, which most often meant that somewhere there existed an antidote, or medicine.

Witchcraft, or *mangu*, which included both the material substance in which it resides and its mystical powers, was believed to be hereditary and could be found in the stomach or visceral area of a witch, who was called *ira mangu*, possessor of *mangu*. Being physiological, witchcraft required no use of magical materials or medicinal substances, spells and rites. Witchcraft was much dreaded by all Azande, but at the same time its existence provided the important opportunity for individuals and society to reduce, even dissolve, destructive tensions occasioned by otherwise incomprehensible misfortunes.

Magic, or *ngwa*, however, was characterised by spell, rite and condition of the performer, and particular emphasis was placed on the material element, or 'medicine', involved. *Ngwa* could be either good or bad. Evans-Pritchard described *ngwa*, medicine, as any object, usually of vegetable nature, 'in which mystical power [*mbismo ngwa*] resides and which is used in magic rites.[16]

Azande possessed an impressive pharmacopoeia of more than 400 therapeutic materials for treating over 100 specific maladies. Evans-Pritchard explained that in their naming and differentiation of diseases, Azande had shown a great amount of empirical knowledge. He reasoned that the proliferation of therapies for each malady, on the other hand, showed their ineffectiveness. Thus, they were often quite skilled at noting the early symptoms of some diseases: some European doctors believed that Azande were rarely incorrect in their diagnosis of leprosy, for example. They were also aware of the normal course of a disease once its symptoms had been noted. 'They provide an etiology and although it is often far from objective reality, it reveals a power of observation and logic.'[17] Therapies included careful washing of wounds and sores with hot water. Protection from the air was provided by leaves, wood-dust, bast and animal fur. Nicotine applied to sores acted as an antiseptic. A special clan of bone-setters, *amozungu*, possessed considerable knowledge and skill about broken and dislocated bones. They utilised splints and massage and people came from afar to these renowned experts. The *amozungu* remain influential today throughout the northern region of Zaire and southern Sudan with people often travelling quite long distances to visit them.[18]

By the 1920s throughout much of colonial Africa, European administrations were encouraging the investigation of African traditional medicine and the Belgians were no exception. 'Medicine' in the sense of Western biomedicine found its nearest equivalent in most African societies in the botanical substances employed as healing agents. The practices involved in their application as well as the entire structure of beliefs about the amelioration or removal (i.e. the cure) of both symptoms and causes of disease of the Africans were, however, resoundingly different to those of the Europeans and were most often the cause of very serious misunderstanding and even outright collision. Europeans were interested only in the material aspects of African therapy; very often, they attempted to suppress all manifestations of the deeper beliefs about the causes of the illnesses. In general, there was an enormous gulf between African and European ideas of the causes and appropriate therapies for diseases.

For a member of Azande society, 'medicine', or *ngwa*, was far more than a physical substance used in the treatment of disease in the European sense.[19] 'Medicine' also incorporated the notion of the manipulation of the inner life force, or power, which resides in most natural phenomena, animals, plants, elements of climate, etc. In 1913, A. J. Rodhain, the state doctor engaged in an inspection for sleeping sickness in Uele, explained that he had accidentally 'enhanced' the power of his Western biomedicines when it became known by the local people that he had in his possession a specimen of a rare animal, the tree hyrax, which the Azande believed possessed important mystical powers.[20] There were specific medicines for hunting, fishing, wife-finding, agriculture, fertility, illnesses and so on. There were good medicines, *wene ngwa*, and bad or evil medicines, *gbegbere* or *gbigbita ngwa*. *Ngwa* often included knowledge of a particular practice, or ritual, in association with possession of a particular substance or object. It might include one or both of these aspects. Most importantly, medicines helped people to cope with other kinds of misfortunes than just diseases. Azande possessed many medicines or substances used in magical rites. For instance, the *fili* or magic whistle, reputedly adopted from the neighbouring Mangbetu, was used to cure many diseases and it was an essential medicine for curing diseases used by members of *nebeli*, one of several secret societies in the region.[21]

An interesting example of the wide reputation of Azande medicines is provided by the British consul at Stanleyville in June 1907. The Belgian administrator at the post of Bafwasende on the Lindi river nearly 300 kilometres south of the Uele river, noticed an unusual amount of goat-selling taking place at the local market. He discovered that the local people, Mobali, were selling their goats in order to purchase a 'medicine' from the 'Azande sorcerers'. This medicine would 'supposedly turn bullets of the white men into water, and he reported that the Mobali, who were generally rather timid had become much bolder'.[22]

'Medicine' in many cases was the special or secret provenance of particular individuals, acknowledged authorities who could act as intermediaries. Among the Azande, these individuals were the *binza* or *ira avule*. One individual acted as both *binza* and *avule*. The former can be thought of generally as a herbalist or, according to Evans-Pritchard, one who practised 'leechcraft', while the latter functioned as a diviner, which according to Evans-Pritchard was the more frequent role. The diviner exposed witches while the *binza* thwarted them.

The *binza* manipulated his own special medicines, *ngwa*, to both divine or ascertain and combat the ultimate cause of misfortune which was believed to be *mangu*. He could determine if the agent was a living sorcerer or an ancestor spirit, an *atolo*. The Dominican missionary, A. M. de Graer, who made an invaluable study of Azande therapies, related that only a very poor individual approached European medical services; this was when he could not afford the fees for his own more trusted, therefore more efficacious, therapies. Furthermore, the power of the *binza*, and thus his prestige compared with European doctors, lay in his ability to cause as well as cure illness. Dr Graer pointed out that while Azande practitioners were generally most reluctant to discuss their knowledge with Europeans, some were willing to reveal powerful remedies 'convinced that we did not know how to use them because we had not been initiated in our youth into the art of healing by the absorption of the secret drugs that only they knew'.

The *binza* was never a member of the ruling clan, the Avongara, and while women were as eligible as men for training, most sources report male *binza*. The *binza* enjoyed no particular prestige and was not held in awe like his counterparts in Mangbetu and Buan society. His statements had no legal value, and while *binza* played important roles in Azande life, more frequently individuals would 'administer' a 'medicine' to themselves.

Widespread endemic conditions, or diseases which were slow to heal were usually believed by Azande to be ultimately caused by human agency. They believed such diseases to result from social conflict. At the other extreme, awesome epidemic diseases were often thought to be caused by God, *mboli* or *mbori*. Other Africans, like the Bakongo of western Zaire, make a similar distinction between an 'illness of God' and an 'illness of man'.[23] Only a few categories of misfortune were specifically ascribed to the realm of *mboli*; they included, for instance, locust swarms and leprosy.[24]

Mboli was associated with public ceremonial during times of drought or severe epidemic disease and Evans-Pritchard once observed part of such a ceremony during a severe outbreak of cerebro-spinal meningitis. *Mboli* could also be publicly called upon by an Azande individual when declaring himself innocent of having caused a specific misfortune. For example, an Azande 'blew water' (expelled a mouthful of water in a fine spray) and formally pronounced his innocence in front of a sick person saying 'Oh Mboli, this man who is sick, if it is I who am killing him with my witchcraft, let him recover.' Such declarations were customarily made as it was believed that one could be totally unaware of one's responsibility for another's misfortune; in other words, one could unwittingly harbour the power to perform witchcraft.[25]

Misfortunes ascribed to *mboli* allowed the Azande some recourse to social mechanisms with which to soothe societal tensions. In contrast, during severe epidemics, the only options were flight or the isolation or afflicted persons. Generally, people with epidemic diseases were isolated in little huts some distance from the homesteads. One state administrator in Uele district observed in 1912 that the 'Azande transport sick people to a gallery near a river where they construct a habitation and the relatives care for them'. Such individuals were in quarantine (*ledudu, kuboni*), or exile in the forest. It is significant to note that isolation often meant relegation to the very ecological niche most likely to harbour *Gl. palpalis*. Occasionally, victims were sent to a maternal uncle's homestead for protection from witchcraft, a practice which reportedly remains widespread throughout Uele.[26]

Azande regarded *binza* divination as less reliable than the oracles, *benge* or *dakpwa*, although divination by the *binza* was considered as equivalent to another oracle, the *iwa*. The *benge* oracle was a major feature of Azande culture during the period of this study but as recently as 1983 a documentary film reported the contemporary function of the *benge* oracle among the Azande of the southern Sudan.[27] *Benge* is the name both of the poisonous root (*Erythrophloeum guineense*) used in a ritual and of the ritual itself, which lies at the heart of what is in effect a judicial system. *Benge* both identifies and sanctions the legal process.[28] This oracle had become a primary method of dealing with misfortune and uncertainty among the Azande well before the twentieth century. In his now classic study, *Witchcraft, Oracles and Magic Among the Azande*, Evans-Pritchard investigated this subject in detail. It has recently been argued that the *benge* oracle was monopolised and manipulated by the Avongara ruling clan, and that it was far less accessible to commoner Azande. In the 1920s one missionary learned from Azande that, formerly, *benge* had only been used by Avongara themselves. It has been suggested that the desire to keep commoners away from easy access to *benge* might help to explain the lack of Avongara hegemony south of the Uele where the vine is prolific.[29]

The root which is the source of *benge* was obtained more frequently in Belgian territory, south of the British Sudan, in the great gallery forests near the Bomokandi and Bima rivers, both affluents of the Uele river. In this way, a prominent ecological setting for the transmission of sleeping sickness played a crucial role in African life. Azande of both Sudan and northern Congo were often faced with the difficult, sometimes danger-ous, journey south into *auro*, or foreign, territories. The journey was made doubly difficult after the British and Belgians began attempting to prevent movements of peoples across their colonial frontiers. Through-out the colonial period, the Belgian administration was confronted with the widespread practice of the *benge* oracle, and medical as well as territorial administrators commented upon it. Ironically, perhaps, the Belgians did not turn their attention to the potential hazard of sleeping sickness faced by the people who were forced into the very eco-system which harboured the disease-causing tsetse flies.

Concepts of the causation of misfortune and the appropriate responses were thoroughly interwoven into Azande social and political structure and formed, in fact, an important part of the base of political power and judicial sanction. Understandably the Avongara rulers often manifested great resistance to changes which would affect basic cultural values, especially those concerning medical practice. Evans-Pritchard reported, for example, that the powerful Azande ruler, Gbudwe, had been a 'stickler' for tradition. He found any form of magic intolerable unless it had been known by his father. While he approved of *binza* and other diviners, such as *aboro atoro*, he was very hostile to the introduction into his kingdom of new 'medicines', especially new ones from the territories south of his jurisdiction, i.e. from Congo. He is reported to have asked why a man should wish to have recourse to a new medicine for protection in the form of a magical whistle, the *zelengbongo*, when he, Gbudwe, gave all the protection against injury that a man could desire.[30] Another important ruler, Sasa, had ordered the execution of his own sons for the crime of daring to deviate from custom. This conservatism is especially important in understanding the confrontation and deep misunderstanding which arose between the Europeans and Africans, who held such different ideas of the aetiologies and acceptable therapies for the misfortune of illness. It manifested itself in Azande responses to new medicine whether African or European.[31]

The Babua

Like the Azande, the Babua nearly always attributed death and serious illnesses to witchcraft or sorcery.[32] Evans-Pritchard's distinction between sorcery as intentional bad magic utilising substances (medicines) and rituals, and witchcraft as either intentional or unintentional employment of *inherent* power for harm apply equally to the Babua view. There is evidence that when witchcraft was suspected, the Babua turned to their witchcraft experts, or 'specialists of *liendu*', so-called because of the ritual employed to locate the human agency which possessed *elimba*, or the ultimate cause of the misfortune. Autopsies were performed to look for tangible proof of *elimba*; abnormal development of the gall-bladder, it appears, may have been taken as an indication of *elimba*. The *benge* poison oracle, as among the Azande, was used to ascertain the guilt or innocence of those accused of witchcraft, and it was the only poison-oracle permissible for that purpose.[33]

   The Babua word translated as 'medicine' denotes *both* the principle and the material substance as does the equivalent Azande term. People as well as technological processes possessed their own dynamism – activating force – or 'medicine'. Thus the blacksmith, for instance, knew the 'medicine' of iron while the potter knew the 'medicine' of pottery. Natural phenomena possessed their own 'medicine' – the light of the new moon was considered a potent one. There were also individually named medicines for specific events. Calonne-Beaufaict explained that the Babua, like most of the Uelian peoples, thought of the 'force', or strength and power (the dynamism) of someone or something as residing in the skin or covering. Thus, the skins of certain trees, fish or animals were valued as important medicines in themselves. A Babua individual would typically describe his feeling of general malaise as 'feeling ill in all his skin'.[34]

Medicines acted upon man, animals and most natural resources. Man could also absorb medicine through either direct contact or from distant influences – the new moon was one such distant source. An example of medicine was *elanga*, a vegetable prepared in pumpkin oil which was considered a '*dawa* (medicine) of knives' or assurance of a successful business transaction. For physical disorders – what Europeans called diseases – there was a wide range of 'medicines'. Many of the remedies of botanical origin were considered to be efficacious by some of the colonial medical staff. Even when not proved effective, familiar forms of medicines such as a number of infusions prepared with specific vegetable items were utilised for conditions such as yaws, syphilis, and gonorrhoea, diseases which were considered inoffensive. With both yaws and syphilis, immediate isolation outside the village was also practised. One method of applying medicine was by means of small incisions through which the substances could be inoculated under the patient's skin. Cupping horns were used to draw blood close to the body surface for this purpose. As this type of medication was not unfamiliar to many European observers, it was readily labelled and accepted as 'medicine' and 'therapy'. But problems arose when medicines were not recognisable as such. For instance, the elephant-hunting medicine in the form of a whistle, *opitoro* or *opitro*, reported by the administrator of Zobia post in 1918 was one such example. He complained this 'medicine' was an 'exploitation of public credulity' and that it was expensive.[35]

Liboka: *witchcraft experts*

The function of diviner-healer was fulfilled in Babua society by the *mbebe* or the *moto ma liboka*. This individual was knowledgeable in herbal remedies as well as capable of divination following a period of training or initiation. According to Calonne-Beaufaict, it was the *mbebe* alone who was capable of identifying those guilty of witchcraft (*elimba*), the *bato ba elimba*, by means of the *bondi* oracle or ritual use of *benge*. In contrast to the Azande *binza*, the *mbebe* was a highly respected member of society, often the *kumu*, or chief, of a powerful clan. In common with his Azande counterpart, the *mbebe* acquired his training in exchange for payment, although, generally, in practice, an intelligent young man was selected by an *mbebe* and invited as an apprentice for a period of several months during which he learned about the properties of an array of 'medicines' and the proper ways to manipulate them for desired effects.[36]

Thus, Babua concepts of cause and response to misfortune had significant similarities to Azande views. The Babua, like their neighbours, the Azande, perceived a dual causation of illness; and for them, like the Azande, it was imperative to discover the *ultimate* cause which was nearly always believed to be a human. Disease and death were often perceived to be indications of disrupted social relations which the society at large was compelled to resolve for the good of all. Misunderstanding the crucial necessity for such resolution by means of identification and ejection, or execution, of sorcerers and magicians in African societies, colonial administrators sought to eradicate what they perceived as superstitious and barbaric practices. At the same time they tried to replace such practices with their own notions of appropriate responses to illnesses, in the form of European practices of public health and hygiene.

The Mangbetu

The Central-Sudanic Mangbetu[37] serve as the third representative African society in this study. An important aspect of these people for the Belgians early this century was the firm conviction of many administrators that the Mangbetu had in the past been a 'demographic treasure' which was now under threat. Their first European observer, the traveller Georg Schweinfurth, rhapsodised in March 1870 that

the display of wealth, which according to central African tradition was incalculable, was truly regal, and surpassed anything of the kind I had conceived possible . . . they were comparable to the denizens of the civilised west and . . . in some respects the Franks themselves did not surpass them in the exercise of an aesthetic faculty . . . The Monbuttoo land greets us as an Eden upon earth.[38]

However, with the conquest of the region and early imposition of colonial administration, the Belgians soon fretted that the Mangbetu had since suffered serious depopulation. For instance, the Van Kerckhoven expedition had been in part rationalised by the fact that 'it was necessary to think [of protecting] well-populated and rich areas like the Momboutous (Mangbetu)'.[39]

Mangbetu ideas regarding misfortune

The Mangbetu, like the Azande and Babua, believed that most illnesses, one form of misfortune, were due to a metaphysical cause, often emanating from a fellow human within the same social group. Their equivalent of the Azande *mangu* (witchcraft substance) was *notu*.[40] It was believed that *notu* was hereditary but only passed through the same sex, i.e., from mother to daughter and father to son. Therefore, as among the other peoples discussed, it was of paramount importance to discover the source of misfortune and there were several ways in which this could be done. They included a variety of oracles, the most common being *mapingo*. *Mapingo* was consulted for a wide variety of problems ranging from personal, economic, agricultural, marital and health matters to queries from the ruler on matters involving the entire society, such as war or the appropriate treatment of criminals.[41]

The *mapingo* oracle, however, might have advised an individual to turn to another specialist, the *namamboliombe*, for help with his problem. Quite unlike the Azande or Babua, the Mangbetu believed that this individual possessed divine power which was inherited. The Azande diviner neither inherited his role nor was particularly respected, whereas the *namamboliombe* had both characteristics. In addition, the *namamboliombe* functioned as both a seer-prophet *and* a healer. Unlike the Babua and Azande concepts of diviner-healer, the concept of the *namamboliombe* incorporated the function of prediction as distinct from divination. The *namamboliombe* ministered in particular to victims of chronic illnesses. In the past, a *namamboliombe* was frequently requested to travel far beyond his local boundary to minister to many non-Mangbetu or non-Makere-speaking peoples. A *namamboliombe*, in distinct contrast to the Azande healer, could become quite rich through the payments for his services while, according to Evans-Pritchard, an Azande *avule* could never become rich.

Mangbetu faith in their own methods of dealing with illnesses is reflected in the testimony of a missionary of long residence in their region who was informed by Mangbetu in the 1920s that their medicine always worked and, without it, the sick person would be much worse or dead. Another missionary, Van den Plas, became convinced after his study of their culture that their medicines were often excellent and merited the serious attention of the administration.[42]

Mangbetu medicine, or newo

The Mangbetu concept of *newo*, medicine, included the possession by certain objects and substances of the power to cure or heal. For instance, the *nekire* whistle protected people and ensured good fortune, like the *fili* of the Azande and the *opitoro* of the Babua, One of Keim's informants explained that one might say, '*Nekire*, I am doing this because I an ill.' Again, in common with the Babua, the tree hyrax, or *nebi*, was believed to possess special powers, although among Mangbetu it seems to have been used to support the political authority of the rulers.[43]

With Mangbetu, as with the other peoples in this study, the early colonial authorities failed to understand the underlying concepts of the cause of disease and the ways to effect cures. Thus *nekire* used to ensure success, good fortune or a cure for an illness was simply one medicine among others perhaps more familiar to European minds. But whistles, as mentioned earlier, did not fit into the European idea of a pharma-copoeia. They were so misunderstood that they even became a focus of European hostility. The district commissioner of western Uele advised the administrator at Zobia, where whistles had been reported, to care-fully observe their use. He suggested that in 'certain cases we will probably be able to follow through judicially for "menacing gestures"' in the attempt to thwart the use of this medicine. Dr Thomas Parke, a member of the Emin Pasha relief expedition (1887–9) led by H. M. Stanley, described one medicine which better fitted the European con-ceptions, a Mangbetu antidote for an arrow poison. Introduced under the skin of the victim, a technique not unfamiliar to Europeans who were prepared to recognise this as an 'acceptable' medicine.[44]

Summary

African perceptions in the north-eastern Congo State of what consti-tuted, caused and cured diseases were thus radically different from most Europeans' ideas.[45] Various mechanisms existed in African societies with which to respond to misfortunes, including diseases, and among Africans, 'medicines', with their dual notion of *both* substance and inherent spirit or power, lay outside the scope of the turn-of-the-century European ideas based upon Cartesian science. Pills, potions and injections were for Africans only a small part of 'medicine'. For the Azande, there was no perceived material difference between a *real* poison which killed fish and a crocodile's tooth which was rubbed on a banana stalk to ensure growth. There was no qualitative distinction made between the two; instead, distinctions lay in the manipulation of medicines. African concepts of the cause, as well as the manifestation, of diseases were as different from European ideas as were those regarding cure.[46]

In light of all this, what happened early this century when Belgian colonial administrators of public health imposed their ideas and their medical practices upon African populations who were suffering the risk and incidence of human sleeping sickness? What attempts, if any, were made by the colonising conquerors to bridge the gulf in comprehension and communication regarding health? In what ways did Africans' responses to disease in general, and sleeping sickness in particular, conflict with the Belgian management of health?

REACTIONS TO THE DISEASE

As we have seen, the form of human trypanosomiasis which occurred in the region and time period of this study was the typically protracted, chronic, *gambiense* variety. Although the virulence and time-span of the disease varies according to a number of factors, the *gambiense* form is not as swift a killer as is the *rhodesiense* form. This means that the progression of the disease and the manifestation of a wide range of possible symptoms makes it much more difficult to clearly diagnose it as a *single* disease. Instead, it could have been diagnosed at different stages as quite different diseases. This is an important point when attempting to describe African responses.

In its advanced stage, after the central nervous system has been affected and patients decline into the classic comatose phases, few people have difficulty in recognising 'sleeping sickness'. However, the sheer variety of symptoms possible in the initial stages of the disease often make it very difficult for everyone, European medical personnel and those with an untrained eye alike, to correctly diagnose the disease. A. M. de Graer, the Dominican missionary who made a detailed study of Azande medicine, explained that they classified a disease according to its symptoms. Sometimes the same name would be used for a number of conditions possessing the same symptoms. Conversely, a disease with a great variety of symptoms would be considered as *different* diseases. Sleeping sickness was a difficult disease to identify. 'Ils n'auraient d'ailleurs que difficilement pu se résoudre à cette investigation, vu le caractère vague que présente la maladie à ses débuts et dans son développements, ils n'auraient que difficilement pu le déterminer, comme nous l'avons, vu chez eux actuellement atteints.'[47]

Did Africans believe that sleeping sickness, when it was recognised as a single disease, was a 'disease of God' or a 'disease of man'? If it were the first, then no antidotes were possible for the Azande, Babua and

Mangbetu. The only recourse was isolation of the stricken and/or flight. As we have already seen, isolation was practised in order to remove the individual beyond the range of possible harmful influences among those people around him. However, the three societies focused upon in this study tended to view slow, chronic diseases as 'diseases of man'. They were thus misfortunes which resulted from severely disrupted social relations. Such conditions required careful investigation in order to ascertain the final cause which lay behind the visible symptoms of a disease. It is vital to understand the profound importance and depth of this belief. For instance, in the 1920s a doctor explained how his microscopists perceived the cause of sleeping sickness. The African technicians were skilful at detecting trypanosomes under their microscopes, a difficult task even in good laboratory conditions. They understood perfectly well that sleeping sickness was caused by tsetses. But they *also* knew perfectly well that it was due to *likundu*, witchcraft, that the trypanosomes were present in certain individuals and not others. The ultimate cause of the disease would be located within the social group surrounding the victim. For that task, a microscope was useless.[48]

In 1903, the Liverpool researchers had questioned Europeans in the Congo Free State about sleeping sickness and about African knowledge on the subject. Several replies to their questionnaire indicated that some Africans were aware of the disease and had their own ideas about its epidemiology but this was more the case in Lower Congo where the disease had been known for a longer time. One missionary was informed by Africans in Lower Congo that the disease had arrived in their region fifty years earlier while another missionary was informed by the people that it had been present as long as they could recall. The state doctor at Leopoldville laboratory researching sleeping sickness was told by Africans that the disease was spread among people through the sharing of eating and drinking utensils.[49] In the Lado enclave the state doctor reported in 1907 that local Islamicised people knew that the bite of the tsetse fly led to a disease, which they called *amindo*, in both man and beast. Furthermore, they explained that as the disease was sent by Allah there was no cure.[50] Another group of Islamicised Africans, the so-called *Arabisés* in the region of Stanleyville, referred to sleeping sickness as *mugongio na bushinghisi*. In 1914, this term was used by the governor-general in a note to the minister explaining that 'in general, the chiefs know about sleeping sickness' and he listed some of the terms used for it: *ilo, tolo, pungi* and *busingisi*.[51]

By 1920–1, the Azande referred to sleeping sickness as *kaza rame* (*kaza*, malady) according to de Graer. Evidently, at the time he studied their ideas of disease and medicine, they did not yet have an exact idea of the disease, which made him conclude that it was of recent origin. He explained that their name for sleeping sickness derived from the descriptions provided by Africans and Europeans who came from other regions where the disease had been present longer. 'Most often, it is a white doctor who surprises them with the information that this disease is with them.' He continued, saying that the Azande knew no remedies for sleeping sickness and believed at the time that 'only the European doctor could cure them'. However, he was informed that they were convinced that if they searched among plants, as with all other maladies, they would eventually be able to find a cure for sleeping sickness.[52]

The 'cure'

Since 'civilization' was a threat with hygiene as its punishment during colonial rule, it is hardly surprising that with independence, people often did not fulfill demands that they were earlier forced to meet.[53]

It is no wonder that in the early decades of the sleeping sickness campaign many Africans perceived colonial medical practices as part of the conquest of their societies and as aimed, sometimes, at specific groups of people within those societies. After all, before 1907 there was no cure for sleeping sickness and until the introduction of tryparsamide (Bayer 205) from 1920, the highly toxic arsenicals used to kill the parasites quite often harmed the victims as well. During the first two decades of the sleeping sickness campaign, most African victims simply died.[54]

Three features of the medical practices employed by the European medical services greatly alarmed most Africans before 1930: the physical examination, the isolation or quarantine of suspected victims, and the medicines. Each of these features of European therapy could profoundly conflict with African views and practices to such an extent that little compromise was possible.

The existence of such areas of conflict should not be taken to indicate that *all* European medical practice was rejected. Africans selected and experimented with those features of colonial medicine which did not seriously conflict with their concepts; if a medicine or a technique 'worked', it could be quickly incorporated into one's culture. Thus quite early on, Belgian colonial medics as well as missionaries discovered that certain surgical procedures for men, particularly the removal of often grotesque and disabling hernias and scrotal elephantiasis, were eagerly sought.[55] Another service sometimes sought from European doctors was circumcision. One doctor reported that his skill at circumcision was very popular, and attributed this popularity to the fact that his services were free, in contrast to the high fees charged by African specialists.[56]

An important point to keep in mind is that even at the outset, or at least from 1903, two strands of European medical provision and policy were developing, and while the differences were not always clear to the Africans on the receiving end, there were those who could differentiate between the mission or state doctor who offered assistance of a general nature – bandaging wounds, ulcers, etc. – and those who were involved in the more focused sleeping sickness campaign. Even the Europeans had became increasingly confused by the two services until by the late 1920s it was often difficult for them to discern where the sleeping sickness campaign ended and general practice began. Nevertheless, the African response to specific elements of medical practice in relation to the one disease, sleeping sickness, can be demonstrated.

The physical examinations

By 1903, it was quite clear to the European investigators that diagnosis of sleeping sickness, in its earlier stages at least, depended upon a physical examination and, most probably, microscopic examination of a blood or lymph-fluid sample. Before long, and for years afterwards, the physical examination concentrated mainly upon palpation of the cervical glands located at the back of the neck. While debate continued for decades about the accuracy of diagnosis through palpation alone, it was from the beginning most often followed by examination of lymph-fluid if the glands were discovered to be enlarged. And if the latter examination were conducted, it was most likely accompanied by examination of a blood sample, usually taken from a finger prick. Later, examinations in the field also included a lumbar puncture, a painful procedure in the best of conditions.[57] The physical examinations required to diagnose sleeping sickness thus involved manipulation of the body as well as its invasion with instruments. Invasive techniques were to prove extremely troublesome for the colonial authorities because for many years most African peoples greatly resisted this aspect of European medicine.[58]

The idea of examination of the living body for symptoms to assist diagnosis of an illness was not unknown among Africans. They were often reported by Europeans to be quite skilled at identifying observable symptoms which were then treated. But individual societies possessed different ideas concerning *which* people could be examined. Some societies apparently did not approve or permit the examination of young children, the elderly of both sexes, slaves or women. Sometimes, examination was not permitted of victims with certain symptoms.[59]

Avoiding examinations

Throughout the period covered in this study, there were numerous reports throughout the north-east of people hiding or *being hidden* from physical examinations. It is not always possible to determine the reasons for the evasions, which were most likely caused by a number of factors, some of which were not 'medical'. Nevertheless, there is evidence that once Africans had some acquaintance with the methods of the colonial medical services, they were even more anxious to avoid contact with them. As early as 1907, the state doctor in the Lado enclave reported that people were hiding from his attempts to examine the area for the disease.[60] Rodhain reported of his tour of north-central Uele district in 1913 that the 1,100 people he had examined were, 'of course, the least timid ones' and in spite of their lack of timidity, 'what singular mistrust' of the colonial state they manifested. 'They only know us as conquerors and not as organisers.' He described how, during his attempts to survey the region for the disease, whole groups of people continually evaded the officials, often moving great distances overnight.[61]

African authorities themselves hid their sick people from the Belgian doctors. For instance, in 1914, Chief Bagidi was accused of hiding victims of sleeping sickness from the state officials[62] and one state doctor, writing in August of that year, explained that African chiefs were very uncooperative and concealed victims. They always found 'pretexts to excuse the absence of very large numbers of people' from the doctor's visits. One chief told him that a victim had died of sleeping sickness, but that individual was found by the Belgians 'several months later in a state of vagabondage'.[63]

As the sleeping sickness mission became a more institutionalised presence in the early 1920s, there were increasing reports of systematic evasion. In September 1923, after three years of the campaign in Uele, one doctor reported that he had a 'terrible time trying to conduct examinations' having only been able to see about one-third of the people. He explained that unfortunately 'persuasion' was the only way to get the people to attend his examinations. Such reports continued well beyond 1930.[64]

More than any other particular group in northern Congo, the Azande were most often named as evaders of the sleeping sickness missions and the colonial medical service in general.[65] There were many general statements that there was a negative response on the part of all Africans, but if a specific group in the north was singled out for comment, it was more often than not the Azande. Reasons for this might include the large Azande population, their recent political dominance in parts of the region, their typically dispersed settlement pattern which greatly irked the colonial authorities, and, perhaps we might add, their possession of a very complex set of beliefs, mechanisms and rituals for dealing with misfortune.

There is always the possibility that the Azande were specifically named by European agents as recalcitrant simply because they were the people about whom most was known. In 1924, a doctor with the sleeping sickness team commented that in addition to the Azande, other related peoples, such as the Abarambo and Pambia, made great efforts to avoid contact with European medical teams. He stressed, however, the 'distrustful' nature and scattered settlement pattern of the Azande, among whom, he added, *even* the chiefs hid. There is the implication that he was perhaps unaccustomed to African authority figures hiding from Europeans in the manner of their subjects.[66] Instructions were repeatedly issued to administrators and medical staff to elicit the assistance of the traditional authorities, the chiefs, without which the sleeping sickness mission would make little headway. In 1928, the director of the sleeping sickness mission in Uele, Dr Infante, demanded 'severe penalties' for notables representing the ruling class and chiefs who refused to cooperate as it was these figures who were 'absolutely responsible' for the flights of their subjects from the medical examinations.[67]

The colonial authorities made great efforts to impress upon ordinary Africans the necessity of cooperating with the sleeping sickness campaign by making examples of their chiefs. In March 1924, for instance, Chief Kereboro near Niangara was imprisoned for one month and fined for non-cooperation during the sleeping sickness survey. Again, in November that year, he was imprisoned for three months for infractions and soon had his chiefly authority revoked.

Perhaps a more poignant case was that of Chief Datule, a victim of sleeping sickness, in the same region. In May 1929 he was imprisoned for three months for having set a 'bad example' to his subjects by avoiding treatment for his disease. In March the following year, Datule had his authority revoked and his *chefferie* amalgamated with another. He was sent to Doruma lazaret, where he died of sleeping sickness on 1 October 1930. It is noteworthy that the amalgamation of his *chefferie* occurred at just the time an administrative policy to this effect was being carried out widely in Province Orientale; how much, one wonders, did sleeping sickness contribute to a political policy?[68]

Women and physical examinations

Maintaining control of women became a significant issue for *both* African and European men. For Africans, women played a particularly crucial role in all areas of economic life, coveted as they were for their roles in agriculture and sexual reproduction in all three societies under discussion. African men found themselves in the difficult position of trying to retain their traditional control of women as the coloniser increasingly demanded access for a variety of purposes. Medical staff involved in the early decades of the sleeping sickness campaign discovered that it was often very difficult to gain access to women. In 1908, a state physician reported that the wives of the soldiers at his post preferred to see their own African specialists and would only submit to examination by the European doctor when forced to or near death. Dr Rodhain, who conducted the first survey for sleeping sickness in the north-east, reported in April 1914 that women simply did not present themselves for the examinations. commonly, he saw twice the number of men as women. At one *chefferie* he found sixteen male victims of sleeping sickness but only one female victim. Since women would have daily visited the local water source where it was most likely that transmission of the disease occurred, this disproportion is noteworthy.[69] But when Rodhain complained about the women's reticence, the district judicial officer was unable to find an appropriate law with which to force women to submit to examinations. Missionaries involved with the sleeping sickness missions reported the same difficulty gaining access to women. While all three societies discussed here were reluctant to allow examination of their women, the Azande were particularly loathe to do so. 'It goes without saying in the Zande *chefferies* that there is always great difficulty to make the women appear.'[70] In an attempt to force women to submit to the examination, the district commissioner for Lower Uele ordered in 1918 that women be refused the obligatory travel documents. 'Be intractable with regard to their requests to travel into infected areas', he advised his agents and medical staff.[71]

As late as 1939, the situation regarding medical access to women had changed very little. Dr D. Breyne, appointed by the state to the Catholic hospital at Lolo near Ibembo, reported that young women, in particular, along with the elderly, rarely presented themselves for medical attention. They were, he said, advised by the *capitas* of their villages not to present themselves for examinations. Yet on two occasions when he informed the administrators that women and elderly people refused to cooperate, he was told, as Rodhain had been, that there was still no legal ground for punishment.[72]

The arrival of religious sisters in the mid-1920s began to made inroads to the resistance of women. Very slowly the efforts of special infant clinics, most often run by missionaries, began to attract increasing numbers of women. For instance, the Dominican hospital at Niangara reported that before 1925, when the sisters arrived, there were eighty men for every four women attending the clinics. By the end of 1925 forty women had presented themselves and, in 1929, the number had increased to 200. The important subject of maternal–infant health care lies outside the scope of this study, however. Of relevance is the fact that throughout the period under discussion here, the sleeping sickness surveys continued to have great difficulty gaining access to women.[73]

Invasive techniques: *l'aiguille*, the needle and the knife

Unpopular from the beginning, by 1920 the needle evoked horror in Africans to the extent that it had become such an obstacle to the sleeping sickness campaign that the head of the colonial medical service in Brussels wrote: 'The fear of the medical officer and his needle was such that entire villages fled and it became necessary, an unheard of thing in the Congo, to protect some medical officers.'[74] From the very beginning with the Liverpool expedition, there is abundant evidence that Africans were sceptical about European medical practices. For instance, autopsies performed by the researchers were rumoured by Africans to be a form of cannibalism.[75] It is perhaps not difficult to understand the African attitude when we learn that sometimes seven, eight or even ten cervical punctures were *not* enough to establish a diagnosis, which then necessitated a painful lumbar puncture.[76]

In 1907, the director of Stanleyville lazaret, Dr Trolli, reported that 'public rumour has it that my procedures for sleeping sickness are spreading the disease' and he continued that there were rumours of rebellion against not only him but also the state. The district commissioner went further on the rumours. He had learned that Africans in the area were not only unhappy that the doctor did not heal people, but they were convinced that he had been employed by the state to kill former African employees by means of injections and the frightening lumbar punctures. A similar rumour circulated in Barumbu lazaret in 1911 but the doctor was able to dissipate the people's fear of the needle by demonstrating cervical punctures several times on himself.[77] The fear that the invasive needle actually caused the disease was widespread and long-lived. Reports from 1914 and 1919 reveal the strength of the African fear.[78] In April 1915, the pharmacist directing Ango lazaret mounted an 'injection campaign' in an effort to 'sterilise the human reservoir' of parasites in his area. The result was mass flights of the local people across the frontier with French Congo.[79]

The continuing problem of the African fear of the needle led one doctor in 1919 to propose that diagnosis of the disease in the field be based upon palpation of the cervical glands alone, rather than by microscopic examination of gland fluid removed by means of a needle. It was his opinion that palpation was less erroneous than microscopic examination in field conditions, but in any case the African hostility towards injections was so detrimental to field surveys that he advised against them.[80]

An interesting problem arises for the historian. Documentation abundantly demonstrates the general fear that Africans had of invasive techniques in connection with the sleeping sickness campaign Yet, there is at the same time considerable evidence that with the advent of drugs like neosalvarsan, Africans *sought* injections for certain other diseases, especially yaws and syphilis.[81] By the end of the 1920s, it was noted that the rapid results of syphilis and yaws injections were 'not without favourable influence' and a decade later it was reported that injections for these diseases took up most of the doctor's time, even though, continued the same report, it was necessary 'to react against their [the Africans'] tendency to cease treatment when external symptoms disappeared'.[82]

While Africans exhibited extreme repugnance toward the use of needles in connection with sleeping sickness, we have seen that they did not fear the surgical knife for the removal of large tumours and hernias.[83] One has only to think of the widespread African practice of scarification for medicinal purposes to realise that they did not fear skin breakage; nor often did they fear the *concept* of introducing substances into the body. It may be that fear centred on the extraction of bodily fluids which occurred during the sleeping sickness examinations. Furthermore, the Azande belief that the *binza*, manipulator of *ngwa*, had the power to *both* cause and cure disease would have aroused enormous suspicion of unfamiliar techniques.[84]

Isolation and quarantine

Many African societies practised forms of isolation but to think of such isolation as 'quarantine' might be to confuse concepts regarding disease causation. More often, the African form of isolation was designed to remove the individual from possible harmful influences within his social group.[85] This was *quite* different from the European idea of protecting the group from the infected individual. Moreover, the African concept of reintegrating an afflicted individual back into the group often required the assistance of close kin. there were, however, instances of removal of afflicted individuals for fear of 'contaminating' the group. This was traditionally the case with smallpox.

With regard to sleeping sickness, there were several areas of major misunderstanding between African and European. These included the pre-1920s perception by Africans that isolation was synonymous with a death sentence because individuals were isolated from access to those very people who could possibly 'cure' them by assessing the true cause behind their apparent affliction. The importance of kin relations accompanying an afflicted individual surfaced repeatedly throughout Belgian attempts to separate sleeping sickness victims from uninfected people. The Europeans most often assumed that kin attempted to accompany afflicted individuals for reasons that they could, themselves, understand, such as affection and concern for the physical well-being of a loved one.

Yet there were frequent incidences of seriously ill victims of sleeping sickness, in the very advanced stages of the disease, being brought to the Europeans or even left in the night at the early lazarets. Thus it is wrong to make simplistic generalisations about African responses to the European practice of isolation. Why did some people thrust seriously ill victims at European medical centres while others refused to abandon a victim? This is a complex question for which a satisfactory answer may not be available. It is significant, however, that while the great majority of Africans resisted the practice of isolation of sleeping sickness victims in the early decades of the campaign, there were others who did not resist and who, in fact, used the European isolation facilities for their own reasons. For instance, in the early 1920s, the missionary, de Graer, reported that the Azande said of a sleeping sickness victim who had reached the very advanced comatose stage, *adji mpongi*, or 'he sleeps'. And it was at that stage, when the pronounced need for more and more sleep constituted for the Azande the infallible criterion of the disease, that kin presented victims to the colonial medics.[86]

African responses to isolation

A significant proportion of people deemed to be infected with trypano-somes during the surveys, in fact, felt perfectly well and among those people *correctly* diagnosed,[87] many only gradually sickened after isolation. These people in the first stages of the disease 'soon became a great obstacle in the battle against sleeping sickness provoking different rumours and a veritable mistrust among Africans'. Furthermore, as the treatment available in the early years was very ineffective, 'it happened that a man entered a lazaret feeling fine and became ill little by little only leaving the lazaret for the cemetery'.[88]

The Belgians commonly ascribed the failure of their isolation programme to 'African mentality' which they perceived as an almost deliberate rejection of European practice. One doctor differentiated between the response of those Africans already in relationship with European ways and that of the 'natives' who were still outside contact. The natives' 'habitual fatalism' meant they were quickly resigned, he explained, and even in 'the best hospital in the world' their decline was hastened by nostalgia for their families. The doctor explained that after vain attempts to escape, these Africans died early. On the other hand, the ex-soldiers and labourers made use of their 'half civilisation' and 'some-what comprehending the European attitude toward illness', these people were potentially the most uncooperative about isolation. In general, before 1930, most Africans resisted, even rejected, the practice of isolation and hospitalisation.[89]

Many patients attempted to escape from the lazarets. Since the vast majority of those isolated were employees of the state, the colonial authorities were able in many cases to recapture people. This may explain why patients did not attempt to escape either *en masse* or more often than they did. Many of those isolated in lazarets and hospitals had already lived and worked outside their own kin networks and home regions for long periods and this made it rather more difficult for them to simply 'disappear'.

The authorities made serious attempts to recapture runaways. Lazaret directors notified their district commissioners who in turn contacted the territorial administrators in the areas to which it was suspected a runaway might return. They were warned to be on the lookout for missing victims and they were instructed to inform the African authorities, chiefs and *capitas* to similarly be on the lookout for victims and all strangers.

A number of individual victims emerge in the records precisely because they did attempt to escape. We can see the mechanisms set in motion within the state in order to find these people, and we can learn a bit more about the lives of those Africans who were being increasingly drawn into the colonial world. In October 1911, a local administrator announced that two patients had run away from Ibembo lazaret and he was searching for them. When they were found, he said, they would be securely imprisoned in the lock-up *zeriba* at the lazaret. One man, Nalungwe, was recaptured, imprisoned and later died in the *zeriba*. Another, Neparata, was discovered wandering destitute around the post of Ibembo and he too was imprisoned in the *zeriba*. One can speculate about Neparata's isolation from his kin.[90]

Another interesting case was that of Djambi na Allah who was isolated at Ibembo in 1912. He escaped in 1914 and made his way over 300 kilo-metres to the post of Semio where he appeared in April. Lieutenant Defoin, the administrator at the post, explained that Djambi had come to 'collect his salary' due to him as a soldier and asked if he should pay the man or replace him. Our next glimpse of Djambi is in June when Defoin notified the district commissioner that Djambi, who had been arrested and was *en route* to Bili post, had escaped again. Other adminis-trators reported in August and September that they had not been able to relocate Djambi. So we see that considerable efforts were made to recapture one escaped patient and we begin to perceive the degree to which the coloniser affected individual lives. Yet it is significant that Djambi did not attempt to escape totally from the colonial authorities but, on the contrary, approached them with his grievance.

In some cases it is possible to follow a patient through a number of years because of his escape from a lazaret. The existence of several lazaret registers make such observation possible. The victim's name, sex, approximate age, tribal affiliation, home village, occupation, date of diagnosis and treatment were carefully recorded. Thus, when after years of isolation a patient escaped, it is sometimes possible to work out a modestly detailed history of an individual. For example, Pereke was an Azande soldier from Bima who had served in the army for five years before being sent to Ibembo lazaret in July 1907. He remained there until his escape eight years later in February 1915. Zombo and Abusa were Mangbetu soldiers from Niangara who entered the lazaret in early 1909 and escaped in March. Another Azande from Bima, Manzo, with ten years in the army was sent to the lazaret in December 1907 and escaped in February 1912. The same story was oft repeated. Banga, an Azande soldier from Bima with five years in the army, entered the lazaret in February 1909 and escaped in May 1912 while Pitanzila, a paddler from Ibembo, entered the lazaret in August 1907 and escaped in June 1909. A soldier's wife, Gandole, was a Mabinza woman from Ibemba who was sent to the lazaret in December 1907 and escaped in June 1909. It becomes apparent that isolation often meant years of imprisonment and separation from kin. Perhaps there was some truth in Dr Heiberg's observation that the reason the patients did not escape *en masse* was their hopelessness.[91]

Ibembo riots

Between March 1907 and March 1909, 33 per cent of the patients isolated at Ibembo lazaret died and 6 per cent escaped. The growing frustration and hostility of victims isolated in Ibembo lazaret was given expression in a series of riots in 1909 and 1910 much to the alarm of the authorities. Patients told the lazaret director that they viewed their incarceration in the lazaret as a life imprisonment; therefore nothing could be added to their suffering. On 22 August 1909, a group of patients attacked the lazaret guard, and the next day 'general battle reigned' with the rioters finally gaining control. Reporting on the event, Heiberg reminded his superiors that 96 per cent of the patients were former soldiers and NCOs with their families, and this background accounted for their solidarity.[92]

Five months later, on 3 January 1910, a second riot took place. It appears that, in this instance, the sleeping sickness patients from the lazaret broke out *en masse* and stormed the neighbouring administrative post to demand the release of three men who had been arrested that morning. Their numbers, some 300, and fury were such that the authorities were forced to comply. The development was viewed with great alarm by the Belgians. On 22 January, the zone chief informed the district commissioner that, in his view, the lazaret constituted a constant danger. It would be advisable to reduce the numbers of patients and to develop new village-style, open-plan lazarets in future.[93] In March the lazaret director asked for a reinforcement of 100 men to guard the patients *inside* the lazaret, yet two weeks later the local administrator had to 'restore order' in the lazaret with thirty-seven soldiers. By now it was clear to the vice governor-general that the public health policy of concentrating together large numbers of patients could be a real threat to colonisation and he advised the colonial minister that 'all groups of sleeping sickness patients, feverish and idle, are a true danger to order and security'.[94]

African cooperation

Not all Africans, however, rejected the lazarets and hospitals. In 1910, there was so much sleeping sickness in north-central Uele around Yei (today in the southern Sudan), that the Belgians reported people spontaneously presenting themselves in such numbers that the sleeping sickness service could not cope.[95] In the same year the director of Barumbu lazaret reported a 'veritable unhoped-for success' as 'masses' of people voluntarily presented themselves following the apparent cure of Malema, an important African chief, and one of his sons.[96] Keeping in mind the fact that the role of many African authorities included overseeing and ensuring the health of the people, it is not surprising that Malema's apparent cure would have had such an electrifying effect.

In 1910 and 1911 Africans were reported to be 'pouring' into Yakoma lazaret seeking help for victims of sleeping sickness. Most were coming by canoe from French territory across the Ubangi river. Dr Arthur Zerbini, in charge of the lazaret, was puzzled: 'What the reason is for this influence, I do not know: perhaps it is because they have seen the marvellous results after the treatment; perhaps it is because the houses are very decent, clean and they receive a cover and food every week.'[97] Again, in July 1911, he reported that 'the number of the patients continued to increase day by day'. With remarkable insight, Dr Zerbini made the interesting observation that chiefs and notables, that is, free men, were rarely afflicted, while most of the victims were 'those with no rights'. Far ahead of his time, Dr Zerbini perceived the political economy of health when he explained that 'sufficient food and care renders the organism more resistant to sleeping sickness'; therefore, the colonial authorities should not focus their campaign totally against the fly, 'but should also aim to ameliorate the situation of the native'.[98]

While this is an accurate observation, we must also consider the possibility that chiefs and notables, free men, might have avoided European medicine and practices with greater vigour than did the 'lower orders', who might even have been handed over to the colonials in an effort at appeasement. This would make sense in light of the fact, mentioned above, that African authorities were expected to fulfil their roles as guardians of the health of the people. There are recorded cases of chiefs, like Kereboro and Datule mentioned earlier, who attempted to evade the sleeping sickness campaign when they themselves were stricken with the disease.

In November 1912, Dr Bomstein, then directing Yakoma lazaret, reported that sleeping sickness was so serious in the region (some villages had infection rates of 60–70 per cent) that 'in some cases, victims are left in the lazaret by their relatives at night'. This doctor reported that in spite of government instructions in July that year to *reduce* the numbers isolated, he had not yet been able to succeed in persuading any patients to return to their villages. 'Some pretend to return to their villages but at night, return to the lazaret. I cannot use force or chase them away.' The administrator corroborated the doctor's story and explained that when the Africans saw that a victim was in an advanced stage of the disease, they brought him to the lazaret. 'They come to the lazaret at Yakoma in order to die', he averred. 'Since January 1912, there have been about 159 deaths.' He described the arrival of a chief, several notables and natives, all in the advanced stages, who made it clear that they wished to stay in the lazaret. Disentangling the various strands of African response to European medicine is a difficult task and, as I have stated before, generalisations can be misleading. For instance, in January 1913 Dr Bomstein bewailed the fact that 'Africans flee the examinations . . . I can only force a few individuals.' It is quite clear that the Africans' response to the physical examinations was quite unlike their response to the fact of seriously ill, dying victims.[99]

People might have responded more positively to the Belgian sleeping sickness programme for a variety of reasons, differing from place to place and over time. Evidence has been cited indicating that, following the favourable results of treating a chief, many people came forward voluntarily seeking help from the Europeans. So, it seems that when endorsed by a recognised authority figure, some aspects of European medicine were easily, or more quickly, assimilated. Another explanation might help with otherwise inexplicable positive responses of Africans. Some societies, as discussed earlier, believed that a sudden and virulent disease either was caused by a remote and inaccessible god, or was perhaps due to witchcraft practice within the social group. In either case, many people were resigned to the fact that there was no possible recourse for escape from or amelioration of the disease. When the *gambiense* form of sleeping sickness reached the advanced stages, involving the central nervous system, and when it was obviously spreading quickly among people, it is possible that some groups would have viewed it as a disease for which there was no available response beyond simply running away and/or abandoning the victims. Perhaps in such cases people would have approached the European medical services, bringing forth victims in a form of 'abandonment'.

Looking at the entire period between 1903 and 1930, however, most Africans appeared reluctant to stay in either the lazarets or hospitals. As Rodhain noted in 1924, 'The natives do not like to stay away from home several days in order to go to hospital and only do so in grave cases and when they have confidence. Usually only surgical and desperate cases arrive at the hospital.'[100]

African responses to European medications

As mentioned earlier in this chapter, the African healer derived authority in part from the fact that the client *believed* in his power to administer cures and the cures were expensive. De Graer explained that Azande *binza* had undoubtedly divulged trade secrets to him regarding their *ngwas* because he was not perceived as a potential threat. He could not compete with the *binza* because he had not passed through the long period of initiation and training during which he, like they, would have absorbed the *ngwas*. So, for the Azande, it was crucial in certain cases that medicines, *ngwas*, be administered by a recognised ritual specialist. Medicines, in these cases, were inseparable from their dispensers. There were certainly substances which anyone could administer and people were knowledgeable about which ones to use for a variety of physical complaints. But in order to deal with the true cause responsible for the physical complaint, the specialist was vital. It would be a long and difficult battle for the new, foreign doctors, and their peculiar *ngwas*.

The colonials quickly perceived certain similarities between their medicines and certain genres of African remedies. Quite naturally, it was these genres which the colonials were most prepared to take seriously as medicine. All the rest, the incantation, the ritual, the strange objects, such as the ubiquitous *filifili* whistle used throughout the Uele district, were considered by the colonial authorities and doctors to be super-stitious nonsense.

So what were some responses to the substances used by the Europeans as medications for sleeping sickness? A first immediate response was the

African lack of interest in a substance which did not produce fairly rapid, perceptible results. All through the period of this study, colonials complained repeatedly that Africans would not persevere with medications. Europeans observed many times that Africans thought they had been cured with the disappearance of their symptoms. 'One cannot count on them to continue half the regular injections!'[101] Not surprisingly, Africans always tried their own medicines first before turning to European forms. As one doctor recorded in 1905, people came for aid for their wounds and ulcers and especially for surgery, but *not* for internal medicines.[102] Dr S'Heeren had observed in 1909 that the soldiers and labourers who attended the clinic at Basoko preferred their own medicines and that 'when medicine does not please them, they take a little in my presence and throw away the rest later'.[103] Again, in 1910, the same doctor noted that the people resisted internal medicines while they appeared to 'appreciate' external treatments for conditions such as ulcers and wounds. This was a continuing pattern.[104]

One missionary recounted how, in December 1914, 'the native doctor who was so busy with his medicine yesterday, came to us this morning with skin disease asking for our medicine'. It was the missionary's opinion that 'evidently, his medicines are good enough for other folk, but not for himself'.[105] His opinion involved a misunderstanding, however, for it is clear that medications for external use could be more easily assimilated into African pharmacopoeia than could substances taken internally. The implications for the sleeping sickness campaign were serious since substances used for that disease had to be injected. Since in addition there was no immediately observable result, this medication was particularly unpopular.

But the misunderstanding between the African and European over appropriate curative procedure continued to deepen. In 1915, a missionary discussing the medical work of his mission said that 'a great difficulty is the lack of confidence of the natives in our remedies. An African who does not heal as quickly as he would like returns quickly to African medicine.'[106] A Dominican missionary who carefully studied the Azande pharmacopoeia wrote in 1924 that 'African medicines are very numerous and they always believe them to be effective . . . Without them, they say the patient would be worse, or dead.'[107]

Healing was a means to, as well as a prerogative of, power. Healing conferred authority, and medicine has throughout history been related to power. Thus healers were jealous of their power. This is an exceedingly complex subject around which revolves much polemical debate.

Some African traditional authorities were openly defiant towards the incursions of new, foreign and potentially threatening medicines. The Azande ruler Gbudwe, it will be remembered, was extremely hostile towards the introduction of new medicines into his territory. According to Evans-Pritchard, he was particularly wary of introductions emanating from the south, the region of the Belgian Congo.

What did people think about the frequent results of atoxyl injections – blindness and death? Atoxyl, in combination with a variety of substances, was the only trypanocide available until the mid-1920s. Is it any wonder that people were not only sceptical, but frightened of the European medicine and all the attendant ritual?

Atoxyl injections, blood and lymph extractions and lumbar punctures formed a most unpleasant medical experience. For masses of Africans including many people not yet drawn into the colonial network that experience of Western biomedicine was exceedingly painful. While European procedures for external conditions and medications with immediately observable results became quickly acceptable and even sought after by Africans, most of the procedures and medications used in the early sleeping sickness campaign had quite the opposite effect.

Yet, while the strictly medical features of the campaign commonly evoked negative responses from Africans, perhaps it was the administrative features of the campaign, or public health measures, which assured misunderstanding and hostility on the part of newly colonised peoples. Together, medical and administrative aspects of the sleeping sickness campaign, for the most part, were understood by the mass of Africans to be simply a part of the harsh conquest and reorganisation of their lives and societies by a foreign power.

10

Public health, social engineering and African lives

The safest place for the fly is on the flyswatter.   G. Lichtenberg

Belgian public health policy was eminently *spatial* in concept. As has been shown previously, a principal feature of the sleeping sickness campaign was the cordon sanitaire. The Belgians hoped eventually to sterilise the total human reservoir of the disease-causing pathogens, but until such time it was necessary to enforce a strict line of defence around the still uninfected portions of the colony. The health of the African population would be monitored and protected by dividing the entire colony into a pattern of zones designated as either 'infected' or 'non-infected' by sleeping sickness. A complex set of regulatory measures was produced to control the movements of people among the zones, with particular emphasis on limiting access to non-infected areas, as much of the Uele district was presumed to be. Such a global public health policy, focused on limiting movement, affected every sphere of African life – social, political and economic.

Most Congolese, however, perceived the sleeping sickness policy as simply another feature of foreign domination. Before 1930 the majority of northern Congolese would have had considerable difficulty distinguishing between medical and all other economic and political regulations imposed by the state. Most people were bewildered by the web of administrative edicts and many often found themselves caught in the dilemma of being forced by demands of one colonial department to break the rules of another department. The life of a Congolese was made no easier by public health measures intended to protect him from disease. By 1930, Uelians found their lives totally reorganised around the demands of the colonial state and, for many people, those demands resulted in the grief of disease and death.

In this chapter, I shall discuss the ways in which the Belgian public health campaign to control and contain sleeping sickness affected a number of specific areas of African life. Faced with mounting public health legislation, people found it increasingly difficult to travel in the course of their normal social and economic activities. Especially important in northern Congo was the way in which the health regulations affected African access to rivers, so central to the survival of many groups. The reader will recall the importance of the waterways which are such a prominent feature of much of northern Zaire. Denial of access to the rivers and streams and destruction of their canoes, so important to their economy for fishing, trade and travel, was disastrous for many Uelians. A widespread waterside activity, the production of salt, a scarce and essential commodity in northern Congo, became a focal point of the health regulations. Another instance of the hardship caused to Uelians by sleeping sickness regulations is revealed in the ways the regulations interfered with normal cultural practices concerning the struggle of men to retain control of their women. This is clearly illustrated by the phenomenon of husbands frustrated in their attempts to travel in search of wives who had returned to their own kin groups. The health regulations caused an impossible dilemma for Africans in connection with tax. Belgian demands for tax, in particular the collection of wild rubber, meant that people were forced to contravene sleeping sickness regulations. Perhaps the most dramatic and sweeping impact of the health regulations upon African lives was caused by the policy of totally reorganising their social and political structures by regrouping and resiting, often many miles distant, entire communities of people. Coupled with the imposition of new chiefs designated by the Belgians as the legitimate authorities, African peoples surely found their lives to be dramatically affected. By 1930, life in Uele was fundamentally changed by the Belgians, particularly in the name of their public health programme for sleeping sickness.

Sleeping sickness and travel – passports

The introduction in April 1910 of medical passports for persons not infected with sleeping sickness was another step towards the hegemony of the colonial state over African lives. The regulations surrounding the medical passports severely restricted African freedom of movement, and such restrictions naturally affected many domains of life. For instance, it became difficult for many people to maintain some kinds of kin and family relations. Mandatory medical passports particularly hindered men from the retrieval of wives who had 'run away' to their own kin for various reasons. The passport system also seriously hampered people in fulfilling the new tax obligation because regulations prevented them from entering cordoned areas where there was rubber with which to meet the tax demands. While many administrators believed the regulations to be a 'dead letter' or worse than useless because of the lack of staff with which to enforce them, there is good evidence that people's freedom of movement, in fact, was often greatly curtailed.[1]

African manipulation of the system

Examples of African response to the Belgian approach provide some idea of the widespread effects of the passport system. According to one doctor in 1912, Africans had 'many ruses' and often manipulated the passport system. For instance, they deliberately 'lost' their mandatory medical certificates on which were recorded details of recent treatment for sleeping sickness in a lazaret. Wishing to travel more than thirty kilometres from their homes, they would then visit a new doctor in order to obtain a passport. If an African had recently undergone a series of trypanocidal injections, the parasites would probably not appear in an ordinary cervical examination, with the result that the African would get a passport. Upon learning of this practice, the governor-general advised adopting the German system of permanently sealing a marked string or a metal bracelet on the wrist of all treated victims.[2]

Another form of response originated among the African clerks and *infirmiers* involved in sleeping sickness work. Some of these people took advantage of their power to issue passports in return for bribes and other favours. In August 1915, Kofi, an *infirmier* at the observation post of Bili, was found guilty of demanding gifts and payments in exchange for passports and imprisoned for three months.[3] Earlier that year, in April, the doctor in charge of the observation post at Ango had already complained that Kofi was 'lazy and careless about the regulations and appeared to take bribes'. The director of the local branch of the Société Commerciale et Minière du Congo and a Greek trader testified that Kofi had attempted to sell passports to their personnel. (In contrast to neighbouring Sudan, medical passports in the Belgian Congo were issued free of charge.) Another trader at Bili explained that when he had sent women to the observation post for their passports, they had been refused because they would not acquiesce to the *infirmier*'s 'proposals'.[4]

Another example of the manipulation of passport regulations was revealed by a local administrator in July 1916. In his experience it was common to find people with illegal passports containing post-dated visas, like that of the Kongo buyer who worked for the trader, Stagini.[5] His had been issued on 10 December 1915, and visaed only once – on 6 September 1916, two months in the *future*. The administrator strongly advised that African clerks and *infirmiers* should not be allowed to issue passports.

Nevertheless, people continued to travel widely. The continued relations among African groups in spite of restrictions on their movements are revealed in reports citing offenders against the sleeping sickness regulations. For instance, in October 1914 the district commissioner of Lower Uele addressed his counterpart in Bangala district on the problem of continued interaction among peoples on both banks of the Itimbiri river.[6] In the same year Rodhain had reported that people from the region around Doruma maintained close family relations with people as far south as the Aruwimi district, while Landeghem, the district commissioner of Lower Uele, voiced his opinion that no amount of administrative effort could succeed in totally controlling African kin relations. He pointed out that people had kin links as far afield as Ibembo, Likati and Bondo and that it would be quite impossible to prevent their interaction.[7]

People frequently crossed the international frontiers with French Congo, Sudan and Uganda; sleeping sickness was epidemic in all three colonies. It was exceedingly difficult to control such travel. Most often, it was frankly impossible and colonial frontiers remained as porous to movement as the zone borders. Dr Cuthbert Christy, employed by the Sudan Sleeping Sickness Commission to survey the Congo–Nile watershed for the disease in 1915–16, reported much movement of peoples between the two colonies in spite of the policy that 'natives were forbidden to go from the Sudan to Congo and were occasionally imprisoned'.[8] Christy reported that much of the cross-border movement was caused by trade in gunpowder, rubber, ivory and *benge* poison. 'Many have no sanction whatever for crossing or thought of obtaining any . . . those who wish to go far beyond the frontier usually took precaution to get a pass from the nearest Congo or British post or borrowed an old one from a friend or relative'.[9] In 1921 one doctor reported that 'entire families' crossed the Bomu river maintaining 'constant family and commercial relations'.[10]

In spite of the difficulty of controlling travel among kin, the sleeping sickness regulations, especially those concerning the mandatory passports, sometimes divided families. It was especially a problem for

Africans working and living within the colonial sector, and there are examples of families going to considerable lengths to remain together. In June 1914 ex-corporal Kedawo was invalided out of the army at Ibembo and repatriated home to Uele a week later. But his wife, Ingoli, who had sleeping sickness, was not permitted to enter Uele.[11] So the administrator at Ibembo, as a gesture of kindness, issued the couple a new passport and they travelled together downriver to Leopoldville. However, a senior official discovered them, fined them 55 francs for travelling aboard a state steamer and separated the man and wife. Kedawo was sent home to Niangara, while Ingoli was sent 700 kilometres away to Coquilhatville, most likely to the lazaret.

Another example of the effect of the passport regulations upon a couple occurred in May 1915 at Ibembo.[12] Like Kedawo, another soldier had been repatriated to his home in Uele, but his Kasaian wife had sleeping sickness so he had remained with her at Ibembo since 1914. Now, in May 1915, she was being transferred to Lusambo lazaret in Kasai and the soldier requested permission to accompany his wife. The local administrator requested guidance from his superior – should he allow the husband to remain with the wife, or should be simply send the husband alone to Uele?

People who had been drawn into the colonial system often found it necessary voluntarily to seek passports.[13] In 1911 the doctor at Stanleyville lazaret reported that Africans came voluntarily to his lazaret for examinations so that they could obtain the mandatory passport in order to travel on the trains. Another doctor four years later reported that most of those voluntarily seeking medical examinations were men who were in need of passports.[14]

'Runaway wives': the control of women and sleeping sickness

African men were drawn into direct confrontation with public health measures designed to prevent the spread of sleeping sickness because of their crucial need to travel freely and widely in pursuit of so-called 'runaway wives'. This is a clear example of the ways in which crises such as epidemic disease can shed light on social relations which otherwise might be more difficult to analyse. The confrontation between African men and the new colonisers revealed the important and ceaseless struggle of African males to control females. But much of the legislation involving sleeping sickness prohibited such movement. We had a hint of this in the previous chapter concerning the extreme reluctance of

Azande men to allow European doctors access to their women for physical examinations.

It was the Belgians who coined the term 'runaway women', a term mentioned repeatedly in the reports of administrators and doctors alike. These were women who had left their husbands and returned to their own kin for a variety of reasons. Belgian administrators complained of the endless discussions with aggrieved African husbands who complained of the deprivation of important capital assets – their wives. The archival record abounds with references of the complaints from those husbands who sought to retrieve either their wives or the investments they had made in the form of bridewealth as it was customary for the fathers of such 'returned' women to reimburse their husbands. In each African society mentioned in this study, a woman represented a considerable investment in potential labour and for this reason, for instance, the Babua rarely allowed women to travel alone. One contemporary observer described Buan marriage as a 'perpetual contract' by which a group of relations *hired* a woman to another group of relations, making both kin groups collectively responsible for the execution of the contract. The group was deprived of an important form of labour when it lost a woman. Disputes over males' rights to the labour of women often resulted in suffering for the women, while husbands were sometimes forced to search the whole region, often remaining absent from home for months, in order to find the women. The exchange of women in the form of wives was often an extremely drawn-out contractual relationship with 'instalments' of bridewealth spread over very long periods, and the failure of the early colonial administration to comprehend this characteristic led to serious misunderstandings indeed.[15]

Mangbetu women who left their husbands to go back to their own families were usually returned to the husband on the first occasion. She might even be beaten and forcibly returned. But if she persisted in leaving the husband, he could decide to ask her father to refund his bridewealth, thereby divorcing the wife. Any children issuing from the marriage belonged to the husband and in these cases, only a partial refund of the bridewealth was due to the husband. In difficult cases of matrimonial settlement, the *mapingo* oracle was consulted.

In cases of wives falling seriously ill, it was legally most important for African husbands to ascertain exactly *where* the illness had been contracted for several reasons, not the least of which was to establish grounds for the claim of refund of their initial investments for the wives. Married and childless Mangbetu and Azande women who returned home unauthorised and who contracted a serious illness there and died (or who died suddenly for any reason) were considered a loss to the husband who was then entitled to a refund of his bridewealth. In place of a refund of the bridewealth, he might be offered the replacement of an available sister. But, if the wife's illness had been contracted at the husband's homestead, or if she died there, the husband then lost all rights of reimbursement by the woman's father. If the woman did have children and she died or contracted an illness at her family's homestead, her father was obliged to remit only a portion of the bridewealth.[16]

Thus, the colonial public health policy exacerbated a pre-existing struggle in African societies with regard to women. Of interest here is the way in which public health regulations, specifically those for the control of sleeping sickness, were clearly manipulated by numerous men in the effort to retrieve their women.[17] For some men, not only the new administrative structure and authority, but its public health policies as well, offered novel possibilities for protection of crucial investments in women.[18]

With the implementation of the policy of a *cordon sanitaire*, the seeking of runaway wives by their husbands caused the authorities much concern in their attempts to reduce the overall movements of Africans and in spite of ever-increasing regulations against African travel, the authorities found it almost impossible to control travel for this purpose.[19] Administrators often notified their counterparts in regions to which women had fled to be on the look-out for named individuals[20] and it seems wife-seeking was an important cause of the movements of men across international frontiers. In 1914 Rodhain reported lively activity for this purpose along the French Congo border and in 1915 he went so far as to claim that it was 'the greatest cause of mobility along the frontier'.[21]

This activity might partly explain the observations made by Cuthbert Christy during his survey of the Congo–Nile watershed in 1915. He reported to the Sudanese authorities that for *each* passport issued on their side, there were at least ten or twenty Congolese passes issued.

The great majority, I think, of Congo passes are issued on the pretext of hunting a runaway woman. Forty such passes coming from the Congo have been registered . . . in one month at Yambio and many more at Tembura. These passes are issued by the Congo official either singly or in batches of half a dozen or more. In some cases the quest is genuine but in many it covers personal affairs such as trading . . . a rubber trader for instance or a gang of three or four will obtain passes on the pretext of hunting up lost women and will proceed to

Tembura district where on the strength of their passes they make the natives collect rubber for them paying nothing for it or buying it at a very cheap rate.[22]

The larger number of Belgian medical passports may have reflected not more runaway women, but more pressure upon men to collect rubber. Perhaps, the generally more stringent application of the cordon sanitaire combined with the more legalistic approach of the Belgian colonial administration could have accounted for the larger number of Congolese passports.

In any case, it is clear that Africans continued to maintain old patterns of kin and family relations in spite of the efforts by the authorities to control and even thwart such interaction. In particular, women continued to leave their husbands and return to their own kin. It is likely that this particular activity was sometimes, as Christy pointed out, the occasion of manipulation of the sleeping sickness regulations for personal advantage. Whether or not the men genuinely sought their wives or manipulated the system, the fact remains that health measures became for many Africans serious obstacles in the maintenance of important family and kin relations.

Tax demands, rubber and public health regulations

The combination of medical passports and the cordon sanitaire seriously impeded Africans in attempts to meet tax demands which came into force on a formalised basis between 1910 and 1912, although long before that time, Africans in most of northern Congo had been greatly pressured to collect wild vine rubber. As we have seen, often the only available resource with which to fulfil those demands was wild rubber. The people most involved in its collection were the 'natives' who while forming the largest proportion of the African population, most often did not come into contact with the colonial state. The state depended upon the 'native' sector to provide the most tax, while its African employees – soldiers, *capitas*, *infirmiers*, porters, mine and road labourers – could generally meet their tax requirements, when necessary, without personal recourse to rubber collection.

A number of issues arose in connection with the sleeping sickness measures and rubber collection. The 'patchwork' nature of the cordoned zones bore no correspondence to areas rich in rubber. As supplies of rubber dwindled, people were forced to search farther afield which meant disregarding sleeping sickness regulations. Unfortunately, much vine rubber grew in the gallery forests fringing small watercourses which were the favourite habitat of *Gl. palpalis*. Furthermore, the same administration which purported to restrict African travel in order to protect public health, increased its demands for rubber thereby forcing people to travel. In 1905, a *chef de poste* described how all administrators were 'continually dinned by correspondence from headquarters if rubber and ivory were not forthcoming in quantities'.[23]

In September 1907 an administrator in Rubi zone warned that sleeping sickness would be spread by people from Bangala district, east of the Itimbiri river.[24] They streamed into his district in their search for rubber. Among forty-two rubber collectors, he found seven victims. An agent in northern Uele wondered in 1908 how many unfortunate families would sicken with sleeping sickness, forced as they were to travel north towards the Bomu river to collect rubber in a region where the disease was seriously epidemic.[25]

Not long after, another administrator in the Rubi zone complained to the governor-general that rubber collectors from the southern districts of Bangala and Aruwimi were posing a grave threat in his region. He was especially concerned about the 'very numerous' caravans of people who travelled as far north as the Bomokandi river and stayed a fortnight collecting rubber. He pointed out that rubber was more often found in 'humid areas where the tsetse also lies'. He suggested that people from outside the region should be forbidden to enter his zone to collect rubber. It was the 'natives' who posed the greatest threat, according to him, since soldiers, etc. were obliged to travel with documentation and they most often travelled on state transport which meant they were carefully monitored. On the other hand, he warned, 'natives, going from village to village for private affairs are completely uncontrolled'.[26]

In 1910 the state doctor added his warning to that of the Rubi administrator. 'Natives' coming from west and south of the Itimbiri river into Rubi zone to collect rubber, he said, were a grave threat for the spread of sleeping sickness.[27] At the same time, the district commissioner complained about the numbers of Africans entering Uele from the south to collect rubber. They often travelled as far as fifty kilometres north of Buta, the district headquarters. He complained that 'advice given to chiefs and natives' regarding the danger of sleeping sickness had 'little effect'. It was necessary, he emphasised, to strictly apply the passport regulations in order to curb this movement.[28]

It was not only the state which gradually increased its demands for rubber and so forced Africans to travel farther in their searching. The concessionary companies also increased their demands for rubber and complained bitterly about the difficulties caused by the sleeping sickness regulations. In May 1913, the director of the Société Commerciale et Minière du Congo was exceedingly concerned about the closure of Uele district to free commerce because of the cordon sanitaire. While agreeing that serious measures had to be taken by the authorities because of the disease, he nevertheless insisted that his agents simply had to continue personally trading with Africans 'sur place'; otherwise, they would have to abandon business in the area because the quality of rubber would fall below their threshold.[29]

But for most of the African population in northern Congo, the collection of rubber remained an onerous burden which increasingly brought them into conflict with public health regulations. Rubber collectors were forced to be highly mobile, precisely what many sleeping sickness measures were designed to prevent. Increasingly, both medical and administrative staff commented upon the dilemma of Africans.[30]

Rubber and sleeping sickness in north-central Uele

In 1915 and 1916, when it had become apparent that sleeping sickness was epidemic and spreading in the north-central region of Uele district around the state posts of Gwane, Dakwa and Bili, concern was expressed for the fate of rubber collectors. The resource became increasingly scarce in the southern reaches of the district, yet during the war people were under pressure to supply even more. It became more necessary than ever to travel farther north to find supplies. By now, the areas of Gwane and Dakwa had been declared infected zones and subject to the cordon sanitaire, which made them out of bounds to people from zones still considered to be uninfected. When the administrator of Dakwa requested instructions concerning the incursions of people seeking rubber in his zone, the district commissioner was firm. The sleeping sickness measures must be observed.[31] Unfortunately, the north of the Gwane-Dakwa region was richer in rubber than was the south and the government continued to demand its tax and push the collection of rubber.[32]

It is obvious that, in spite of considerable administrative concern and comment that Africans would spread sleeping sickness by travelling between uninfected and infected zones, people were being *forced* to continue doing just that. Three years after the earlier warnings concerning the spread of the disease in north-central Uele by people seeking rubber, Landeghem wrote to the vice governor-general suggesting that no rubber collection should be 'tolerated' in the regions free of sleeping sickness. He pointed out that the state had never prevented the people from hunting, fishing, looking for honey, etc. in the galleries of the region, for to have done so would have been to condemn them to death or force them to emigrate. But, he added, the collection of rubber in infected zones should be absolutely forbidden. He realised that this would prevent Africans from being able to earn money, but this problem could be solved, he suggested, by the suppression of tax demands. He continued that it would be 'inhuman to add still more restrictive measures *vis-à-vis* native travel, restrictions we could not even support because of lack of personnel'.[33]

Finally, in late 1918, the central administration decided to prohibit the collection of forest rubber in infected zones by any Africans travelling from regions designated as uninfected. All rubber collection was strictly prohibited in the infected southern territories of Bumba and Mandungu and the northern regions of Gwane, Bili and Dakwa. However, rubber could still be collected in the territories of Ibembo, Bondo and Likati *but* only by people resident in those territories. While the vice governor-general hoped such a measure could be effective, he said he did not believe it would work for the simple reason that 'rubber collection was an obligation for the native' and even if he could avoid it, he still had to go into the forest to hunt and fish.[34] here is an example of the colonial administration being totally aware of the discrepancies in its own policies and both implicitly and explicitly recognising the reality. Sleeping sickness regulations might forbid the collection of a tax resource, but the tax would be paid.

During the first official sleeping sickness mission in Uele after the war, in 1921, the director of the survey reiterated the suggestion that areas in which the disease was serious should be either totally exempt from tax demands or at least subject to lower rates. The latter option was eventually put into effect in some areas.[35]

These examples show that most people disregarded sleeping sickness regulations and simply continued to collect rubber. They had little choice. That appears to have been the case judging from the number of complaints made by administrators. The complaints of local administrators that masses of people from far-distant regions were invading their zones seeking rubber generally increased as the period progressed. As rubber supplies were depleted in some areas but Africans continued to be pressured by the state to pay tax, they had no choice but to travel into zones containing rubber, and if that meant infringing public health measures, so be it.

A series of questions arises: Which agents of the colonial state did the Congolese perceive as wielding the most authority? Was it the local post administrator or the medical authority? Or was it in fact the tax collector and hence the rubber buyers, company representatives and traders who provided the cash with which to pay tax? And, in any case, how could people differentiate among colonial departments and European agents? The pervasiveness of this latter problem is well illustrated by the long list of instructions issued by Landeghem in August 1917 to the administrators in his district. He suggested that it was perfectly possible for the doctor conducting a sleeping sickness survey to be accompanied by a post administrator and a tax collector. In that manner, tax could be collected, and a census with tax registration established, complete with the distribution of identity card, at the same time as people were examined for sleeping sickness. After all, the public health programme involved every single human being – what better time to conclude other necessary administrative business?[36]

Rivers: bridges, canoes, fishing and salt

Northern Congo, stretching southwards from the Congo–Nile watershed, bounded by the Bomu, Aruwimi and Itimbiri rivers, and with the Uele river traversing it, is richly veined with waterways. It is a haven for the riverine *Gl. palpalis*. From the beginning, scientists stressed the importance of guarding against invasion of trypanosomes along the waterways and the colonial authorities often acted upon that advice in connection with the Africans' travel. But, before 1912, the regulations mainly concerned Africans within the state sector, people who were *allowed* to travel aboard state watercraft. From 1912, there was a shift of emphasis as concern increased that sleeping sickness was being spread by natives operating outside the state economy.

Much of the sleeping sickness legislation dealt with controlling African access to waterways in any form, from crossing rivers and travelling and trading in canoes to fishing and bathing. The regulations also affected residence patterns near water, and riverine pursuits such as the collection of salt-bearing aquatic grasses. They caused great hardship to groups of people whose livelihood was based upon river activities – people like the so-called Bakango of Uele. As the sleeping sickness campaign progressed, increasing numbers of small streams and rivers were declared off limits as the cordon sanitaire was extended to include them. Waterways where sleeping sickness had reached epidemic proportions were 'closed' or strictly regulated, while those where *Gl. palpalis* was particularly prevalent were placed under close surveillance. Obviously, in a region like Uele with its profusion of waterways, it would be impossible to totally control African access to water. Yet this aspect of the public health policy affected quite large numbers of people in a variety of ways.

Before 1910–12, most pressure upon African access to rivers centred on people who would have reason to travel aboard European craft – people like soldiers and clerks. The earliest public health regulations had stressed the importance of carefully controlling access to state steamers, and special river sanitation police were appointed at strategic ports of call. Water travel and ports were traditionally central in public health programmes aimed at the control and prevention of infectious and epidemic diseases in Europe, so it is not surprising that the initial health policies in the colonial setting focused upon the spread of disease along waterways.

Increasingly, the colonial authorities became concerned that sleeping sickness would be, and was, spread by those groups – fishermen, canoe paddlers, etc. – whose lives were spent on or near tsetse-infested waterways. A note on the sleeping sickness campaign prepared in 1911 by the colonial hygiene department contained a paragraph on the difficulties encountered by the authorities when trying to regulate African fishing activities.

Theoretically, native fishing methods should be forbidden on all *Gl. palpalis* infested rivers and this has been implemented along certain watercourses in Katanga [province]. But to extend this prohibition to the entire colony, beginning with the destruction of canoes, would be practically impossible, and it would present grave economic inconvenience.[37]

The government's apparent hesitancy to impose such drastic measures in the north-east was soon overcome.[38] The Itimbiri and Uele rivers had been subject to restrictions because of sleeping sickness since 1907 but from 1912 there was a marked increase in emphasis on controlling the waterways. In July 1912, Governor-General Fuchs issued a new set of sleeping sickness measures in an attempt to coordinate the burgeoning campaign throughout the colony.[39] The new regulations included strict controls on access by Africans to waterways. Watercraft personnel were obliged to have medical examinations *fortnightly* and to possess a valid medical passport. Africans could only board rivercraft upon presentation of a valid passport. If there was no doctor present at a post to issue this document, then the administrator was obliged to undertake this duty among all his others. All rivercraft had to stop at the sanitary posts *en route* so that all personnel and passengers could be examined for the disease. Sleeping sickness victims were not normally permitted to travel aboard rivercraft, with certain exceptions such as travelling to lazarets. Victims who were 'apparently cured' could travel, as could other non-infected natives, but never into non-infected zones behind the cordon sanitaire. All doctors had the right to examine Africans on all rivercraft, whether state-operated or not. There were fines and punishments for any individual, black or white, who was party to any infraction of the regulations.

Measures referred to by the governor-general as 'radical' were imposed in regions which were either heavily infected or not yet infected. These more radical measures included the right of the authorities to forbid or strictly supervise traffic and fishing. For instance, fishing might be allowed only at certain times and places.[40] In August 1912, the administrator of Buta announced that natives could no longer fish during daylight hours on the Itimbiri river, its tributaries and nearby ponds. Administrators now had the right to confiscate and destroy canoes used by Africans for fishing and transport, and there are numerous accounts of such destruction in the records. Bridges were also destroyed on occasion.[41]

The administrator at Bondo was incensed to discover in November 1912 that despite his strict orders to the contrary, Africans with medical certificates were still crossing the Bili river. 'I warn the *chefs de poste* that if any Africans – natives, boys, courriers, etc., still cross the Bili to reach the left bank, I will severely punish the guilty *chef de poste* according to the regulations' – by docking him ten days' salary. He demanded that the administrator at Lebo inform all of the private company agents who were working in his region that judicial steps would be taken against all transgressors.[42]

But Africans did not acquiesce feebly in these actions of the state. They quite naturally continued to use the rivers so vital to their existence and made great efforts to retrieve confiscated canoes which had required much labour to construct. For instance, in 1914, all but two of forty-five confiscated canoes were retrieved from the observation post of Ango where they had been impounded.[43]

A particularly well-documented case is that of an Azande notable, Onga, whose story is related in the proceedings of his tribunal hearing on 19 October 1914. Onga was charged with having broken the sleeping sickness regulations during August and September of that year by travelling in and out of an infected zone. He did so by means of a vine bridge which he had thrown across the Angu river. Onga explained that he and other people were forced to cross the river in order to procure certain products unavailable in their region. Amazingly the charges against Onga were dismissed by the judge, Charles Smets. He ruled that the district commissioner's decree of 5 December 1913, which Onga was charged with disobeying, conflicted with the governor-general's ordinance of 8 September 1910. Therefore, the district commissioner's decree was ruled to be illegal and invalid for he could not simply declare local rules in conflict with central government.

This was an amazing decision but it revealed the typically thorough nature of Belgian legal concerns in remote northern Congo. After all, Onga travelled to and fro between territories designated by the local administration to be cordoned off from each other in the bigger concern of preserving public health. The local administrator at Gwane post, Fredrickssen, related in his report of 30 September 1914, how he had removed all canoes from the Uere river between Ango and Dakwa and how he had destroyed the vine bridge built by Onga. Sleeping sickness was very serious in the area, and it had already 'ravaged' the *bakomba*, or fieldhands, employed by the Azande. He named two groups of people who traditionally acted as *bakomba* which had been almost totally destroyed by the disease in 1912–13. 'I am talking about what I have seen. Extended groups – entire families have died, disappeared.'[44]

But the judge pointed out that as the central government and the governor-general had not yet *officially* declared the region to be an infected zone on the grid of the cordon, the district commissioner did not have the legal right to override, as it were, his superiors' decisions. Thus, Onga's vine bridge, while in an infected region, was not an infraction because the local ruling was voided by the ruling of the central government.[45]

The Uere river was finally 'closed' officially in September 1914.[46] One month later, the administrator at Dakwa (on the Uere river) reported that although he had not yet been able to stop all of the traffic on the river, his 'patroller with escorts' had arrested six natives and confiscated six canoes.[47] These offenders, like five arrested previously, had been issued a *procès verbal* and sent to the Buta tribunal. In December 1917,

Landeghem reported that all but two commercial firms had obeyed his decision to prohibit canoe transport on the Upper Likati river.[48]

Belgian efforts to control African access to waterways, with consequent frustration of vital economic activities, continued for decades. Gradually, legislation proliferated extending wider powers of control over African lives to members of the medical community. For example, an ordinance of 6 March 1929 extending the judiciary sanctions available to doctors to cover all waterways meant they no longer had to seek the assistance of the local administrator in implementing the regulations.

Salt and sleeping sickness

The harvesting of salt-bearing aquatic grasses provides an excellent example of the way in which the sleeping sickness regulations intruded deeply into African life. Through much of Uele district, there were no deposits of salt, which made it a much sought-after item. Some people processed salt from plants which grew along rivers, and access to, as well as control of, those grasses was an economic factor of importance.[49] As one official observed in 1910, 'the riverine peoples reside near fields of aquatic grass in the ways others seek oilpalms'.[50] The salt industry was hindered in two ways by state action.[51] First, like the activity of fishing, salt manufacture came to be forbidden during daylight hours as part of the campaign against sleeping sickness. Secondly, the salt-bearing grasses were often destroyed during compulsory brush clearance undertaken as part of the same effort.

We have seen that what some colonial administrators referred to as a 'paper war' against sleeping sickness was, in practice, for many northern Congolese a serious upheaval on the levels of economic activities and kin relations. But the upheavals did not stop there. Sleeping sickness control programmes extended to the level of entire communities, which were often restructured and forced to move from time-honoured sites.

Regrouping and resiting population

From quite early on, the regrouping and resiting of Africans as a public health measure was recognised as a radical action by the colonial authorities which would most likely be strongly resisted by the people. The sheer size of the colony and the geographical obstacles it presented, as well as the widespread presence of *Gl. palpalis*, generally militated against this policy. More importantly, the policy of regrouping and resiting

African populations proved to be even more unpopular than the government had expected, a difficult situation for an understaffed administration with sometimes no more than a tenuous control of Africans. A note from the colonial hygiene department in September 1912, when such policies were contemplated, pointed out that in most of the colony such an action would be useless because the flies were everywhere; and, besides, 'Africans would only return to the rivers to fish and tend their agriculture.'[52] Some administrators, like one general commissioner in Uele in 1913, were deeply concerned that the government should make quite clear its policy regarding moving Africans since such a policy was bound to cause 'economic difficulties' to some peoples, such as the fishing populations along the Uele. He suggested that such a policy would, in fact, lead to a 'grave economic crisis' which the government would be forced to resolve.[53]

The pattern of Azande settlements became a particularly contentious and oft-discussed issue with both the Belgian and British administrations, especially in relation to public hygiene and the sleeping sickness campaigns. Typically, each adult man lived in isolation with his wife or wives, young children, close relations and domestic slaves in *kpolo*, or 'scattered homesteads' as the Europeans labelled them. This settlement pattern was very unlike that of the majority of Bantu-speaking peoples such as the Babua, who tended to congregate with groups of families in villages. Azande *kpolo* were most often separated from each other by at least several hundred metres. Colonial administrators often described the peculiarity of the narrow winding pathways which connected the *kpolo*, *not* to each other, but to the central authority. Occasional stretches of forest bordering a chief's region were unoccupied; these were known as *ngbokungbo*.[54] The major exceptions to this settlement pattern were the residences of chiefs who possessed many wives. For instance, Gbudwe's own *kpolo* in Sudan was said to have extended five miles.[55]

The Azande insisted on living near a minor river or a stream which frequently meant close contact with tsetse flies. E. E. Evans-Pritchard, the British anthropologist who studied the Azande of the southern Sudan between 1926 and 1930, observed that each family had its private water supply. This preference meant that *kpolo* were most often established along a gallery forest, a location which had serious implications in the epidemiology of *T. gambiense*, the pathogen which caused the common form of sleeping sickness in the area. While Azande sought minor watercourses for settlement, they usually avoided major waterways; this was for political reasons. A traveller noticed in 1906, a period of great strife, that seldom was an Azande village located close to a major river such as the Kibali or Uele as the people preferred to keep away from lines of communication.[56]

Azande commitment to this residential pattern caused tremendous problems in both Congo and Sudan when the colonial authorities insisted that they live in more centralised groups, preferably along the recently established road networks. As late as 1931 the director of the sleeping sickness survey in Uele discussed at length the unsolved issue of Azande resettlement. Previous attempts to implement this policy had failed, with people fleeing the confines and authority of both the district and the Congo State – they simply moved into the French or British territories. The Belgian doctor reported Azande authorities as being anxious to retain their influence since subjects who fled to Sudan and French Equatorial Africa considered themselves 'unconquered'. Revealing the interplay between political and social (medical) policies, the doctor insisted that the Azande should not continue to suffer the consequences of sleeping sickness through high morbidity and mortality 'simply in order to protect their customs'.[57]

Nevertheless, many people in northern Congo were reorganised and moved to new locations. Such policies began to be applied actively in 1913. The declared position of the central government of the colony was that *only* district commissioners were authorised to order these measures although they were to take into consideration the advice of medical authorities.[58] While many people negated these attempts by later simply returning to their original locations, others were harassed by the colonial authorities into remaining in the new spots by a variety of means including destruction of the old villages and relocations so far from the original sites that return was difficult. In other cases Africans were made to regroup in larger settlements.

From 1913 onward, the records of local administrators revealed numerous moves, successful and not, of African populations in northern Congo. We can quickly see that the motives for moving people did not always concern the promotion of public health. Sometimes the emphasis was upon forcing the 'stubborn' Azande to forgo their penchant for 'scattered', isolated homesteads and instead conform to the Belgian idea of a more conveniently administered large village situated near or beside a major communication route. At other times, the emphasis was less transparently political and apparently more concerned with public health and the control of sleeping sickness. In these cases, Africans were forced to move at least one kilometre away from a river to a spot chosen for its freedom from tsetse flies, or at least from infected flies.

Often the decision to move people appears to have been made by lesser administrators, in disregard of the May 1913 directive from central government that *only* district commissioners had the authority to decide such moves.[59] In October 1913 a sector chief announced that he had moved a *chefferie* away from the Bomu river and seized all of its canoes.[60] In November, he explained that although he had decided to move *all* of the villages under the authority of one Azande chief in north-western Uele, the chief refused to cooperate.

It was not always simply a matter of forcing people to move to new locations. Sometimes people moved in a manner not acceptable to the Belgians. Great emphasis was placed upon the *controlled* movement of all people. So when some Bakango fishermen on the Uere river moved before a doctor could examine them and issue the required *feuille de route*, the local administrator complained to the general commissioner.[61]

Moves of populations were complex affairs the effects and local politics of which the Belgians had only the slightest understanding. For instance, the administrators of Buta reported that a chief, requested by the doctor to relocate some of his people, agreed that one of his head-men would move. But when assigned a new location by the chief, the headman refused to budge.[62] Neither coloniser nor colonised very often comprehended each other's motives. One of the major problems encountered during any public health programme, at any time, is the fact that policies purporting to protect the community must avoid overtones of political expediency or coercion. In the northern Congo where political authority had been 'reshuffled' in such a cavalier manner, any further upheavals, such as those related to sleeping sickness measures, were bound to encounter opposition.

Sometimes African agreement to relocate their villages was evidently motivated by the wish to avoid the even more arduous labour of brush clearance.[63] There are many examples of orders given to evacuate and destroy villages or settlements which were too near tsetse-infested brush and water. On some occasions, the colonial authorities were only concerned to move a few dwellings within a village and this was some-times acceptable to the people.[64] At other times, the orders to move villages involves significant numbers of people as was the case when the district commissioner gave instructions that all the villages of five *chefferies* around the post of Monga be evacuated and destroyed.[65]

There are fewer examples of administrators carrying out the

instruction to regroup scattered hamlets into larger villages. Possibly, this can be explained by the fact that Africans most strongly resisted such attempts to radically restructure their societies. Moving people to new locales was disruptive but restructuring societies was more likely to be traumatic. An administrator in 1923 reported that he was having great difficulty implementing such reorganisation which had been advised by the sleeping sickness team. He reiterated the oft-expressed view that the scattered settlement pattern of the Azande was *the main* reason for the catastrophic effects of sleeping sickness upon them and that it was imperative that they eventually be grouped together in carefully situated, large villages. But at the same time he feared that forcing the issue would have such an adverse effect on neighbouring communities that there would be serious economic and political repercussions.[66]

In the late 1920s doctors were advocating another form of mass move, the creation of no man's lands along colonial frontiers. In 1927 the general inspector informed the colonial minister that Dr Rodhain and the president of the Kilo-Moto gold mines had advised measures to halt the spread of sleeping sickness which included the evacuation of all the African populations from the frontier zones of the colony, leaving a cleared strip fifteen kilometres wide. Furthermore, it was necessary, they advised, to collect the hamlets of Africans along chosen routes and arrange them in larger settlements in the shape of *boucles* (bows).[67]

By 1930, most territorial administrators in northern Congo had encountered such resistance from Africans to the public health policy of regroupment and relocation that they were extremely reluctant to attempt to continue implementing these measures. Dr L. Fontana, the provincial doctor for Province Orientale, devoted a considerable portion of his annual report on the medical service in 1931 to a discussion of this policy. Dr Marone, one of the directors of the 1931 sleeping sickness mission in Uele, devoted sixteen pages to a detailed discussion of the problems encountered by medical staff when trying to gain the cooperation of territorial administrators in implementing it. Bertrand, an official with many years of experience in the north, said that he had no faith in the policy of regroupment and resettlement because Africans who were already hesitant or evaded European medical services in general, would certainly resist such restructuring of their societies. Another administrator astutely pointed out that a family chief with a dozen people under his authority would not want to merge them with other groups, thereby losing his little authority. The administrator of Doruma near the frontier with the Sudan said that forcing such measures would cause people to flee into the bush and cross the borders with the Sudan and French Congo. Moreover, Africans who rebelled against regroupment might well consider themselves to be 'unconquered', an impudent attitude no colonial power dared tolerate.

Finally, in May 1931, Bertrand, then the district commissioner of Uele-Nepoko, declared that the public health policy of regroupment had proved impractical and would be henceforth abandoned.[68] The policy of regroupment and resettlement of African populations to protect them from sleeping sickness had been attempted by many medical and territorial officials in northern Congo for well over two decades. It was supported by the medical men, but it was almost consistently resisted by the people for a variety of reasons. By 1931, a senior administrator felt forced by the constant African opposition to abandon the policy for fear of paying the greater price of political and economic disruption brought on by an unpopular public health measure.

African authorities and the sleeping sickness campaign

The effects of the sleeping sickness regulations upon African societies were often revealing of social and political relations and tensions in those societies. As R. J. Morris asserted in his study of the 1832 epidemic of cholera in England, sometimes the deeper springs of social processes are only revealed during periods of severe stress. This proposition is certainly demonstrable in the case of the northern Congo early this century.

One subject which surfaces extensively in the records is that of the difficulties caused for African authorities through the imposition of public health measures. Repeatedly, local administrators and medical staff engaged in the sleeping sickness campaign complained that without the cooperation of the African authorities – chiefs and *capitas* (headmen) – the implementation of many public health measures was almost impossible.[69] And when African authority figures assisted people, either directly or indirectly, in their evasion of the public health measures, then the colonial administration was at an extreme disadvantage. From the central government in Brussels and Boma to the provincial and district levels, there were repeated instructions to all colonial agents to gain the confidence and cooperation of African authorities in connection with the campaign.

African authorities faced several sorts of difficulty because of the pressure imposed on them by the colonial administration to help enforce the public health regulations. For instance, in the realm of kin and family relations, African authorities were expected by the Europeans to intrude into, limit, control and even prevent, forms of social interaction not so 'traditionally' within their powers. An administrator of Uere-Bili zone complained in late 1913 that chiefs did nothing to prevent relations between people in the Belgian Congo and French Congo. Some chiefs were extremely uncooperative when asked to assist the doctors in gathering people for examination.[70]

Not all African authorities remained uncooperative. Some assisted the Europeans with the public health programme. Dr Wille, who toured three *chefferies* in north-central Uele during the 1914 sleeping sickness mission, examined 9,235 people and made 411 lumbar punctures, reported that in all of the *chefferies* he 'had no difficulty examining the natives . . . I was very well assisted by the chiefs and sub-chiefs who for the most part had a lot of authority over their subjects.'[71] This success in Wille's case may have been due to his working in an area where the authority of the precolonial chiefs had been retained under the Belgians.

An example of one way in which the sleeping sickness programme revealed tensions within African societies is provided by the political report of the administrator of Angu post in 1913. Among Bakango villages, especially in the villages of the 'new chiefs', there was great lack of compliance with the regulations. The administrator explained that some of the *former* chiefs, who had been demoted to sub-chiefs during political reorganisation, were particularly unwilling to aid the newly appointed chiefs in their task of carrying out public health measures. This administrator said that he threatened the recalcitrant sub-chiefs with deportation if they continued to resist.[72] It must be remembered that the Belgians pursued a political policy of restructuring African societies along what they conceived to be 'traditional' lines and that in that process many authorities legitimate in the eyes of their people were either demoted or removed and replaced by individuals whom the people did not recognise as authorities. This was obviously the case at Angu and it was revealed through the attempt to enforce extremely unpopular public health regulations.

In December 1913, Bertrand, who had accompanied Dr Rodhain during part of his sleeping sickness survey in Uele, described the great difficulties encountered when trying to examine people. In parts of the territory, he explained, it was only thanks to the power of the chiefs that examinations could be accomplished – for instance, in most of the Azande territory. 'Elsewhere, among the Ababua, Bakango, Alarambo [*sic*], Mokeret, Magogo, etc., traditional authority, stripped of

Table 5. *Exiled African authorities, 1911–1918*

1911	1	
1912	2	(17 during the pre-war period)
1913	7	
1914	7	
1915	28	
1916	14	(62 during the war)
1917	15	
1918	5	

all coercive sanction, was only exercised in the most precarious fashion . . . '[73] It had only been through the force of insistence, menaces and numerous judicial summonses that in certain *chefferies* they had been able to gather together even 10 to 15 per cent of the population. As late as 1924 the state doctor at Doruma reported that the 'Barambo, Pambia and true Bantu' populations all still hid at the approach of the doctor: 'even their chiefs hide'.[74]

The Belgian system of appointing and dismissing chiefs also played an important role in the sleeping sickness campaign. The colonial administration was well aware of the impact such actions could have on the general population, and they sometimes employed such measures intentionally to persuade people to take seriously the sleeping sickness regulations. Chiefs were used by the Belgians to set memorable examples. That was the case in 1924 with Chief Kereboro and in 1929 with Chief Datule, both of whom were punished and eventually stripped of their positions for failing to comply with sleeping sickness regulations.[75] The statistics in Table 5 for the period 1911–18 in Uele district demonstrate the frequency of such dismissals by the colonial administration. The Belgians themselves mentioned that most often the *relégués*, as they called dismissed chiefs, were those newly appointed. In all fairness it must be added that Vice Governor-General de Meulemeester reprimanded the district commissioner of Lower Uele for the 'irregular, even illegal' use made of this sanction. It was Meulemeester''s opinion that about sixty of the dismissals had been effected simply in order to simplify the reorganisation of Africans into *chefferies*. I suggest that the quadrupling of dismissals during the war reveals the response of Africans to greatly increased pressures from the state. The newly created chiefs, *chefs médaillés*, most often possessed no legitimate claim to authority in the eyes of the people and their weak status was soon shattered when they found themselves forced to pressure the people to collect more of the hated rubber.[76]

At the same time, the prestige and authority of some chiefs, those recognised as legitimate by their people, was revealed by their involvement in the sleeping sickness programme. In 1910, one state doctor was amazed at the positive reaction of the local people to the campaign following the apparent cure of an important chief and his son. Vice Governor-General Malfeyt toured the lazarets that year and was most concerned about the use of force and coercion in connection with public health. He believed that such force would in the end make the entire campaign useless. Thus, he was delighted to learn of the effect of an apparently successful cure by the doctor at Barumbu lazaret. The treatment of a chief and his son gained not only the confidence of the patients, but also the confidence of all of the chief's subjects. When the chief, Mokondji Kati, had returned to his village after a series of injections over several months, the people proclaimed him cured. The doctor found himself unable to cope with the 'floods' of sleeping sickness victims who them came to the lazaret. Another result of the doctor's success with the chief was that 'all the native chiefs wanted the doctor to visit their villages and they offered to construct lazarets and to feed and care for the victims'. The vice governor-general exclaimed, 'it was a veritable, unhoped-for success . . .'[77]

But it was not a widely repeated success, and the sleeping sickness campaigns usually continued to face varying degrees of resistance from Africans throughout the period covered in this study. The combination of the medical campaign to contain the disease *and* the public health measures implemented to prevent its spread, meant that the impact of colonial rule upon African populations in northern Congo in the early part of this century was indeed harsh and debilitating. As it increased in scope and scale, the public health programme for sleeping sickness affected nearly every aspect of life from marital relations to the supply of sorely needed salt. Sleeping sickness regulations formed an effective tool for social engineering, which helped to ensure that Africans served the needs of the coloniser.

11

Conclusion and legacy

Belgian pride in medical services – best in Africa

When their colonial venture came to an abrupt end in June 1960, the Belgians were convinced of the success of at least one aspect of their half-century administering the Congo – they were confident that their medical service was outstanding in all of colonial Africa. Many agreed. In 1958 a European Common Market survey described the medical infrastructure in the Belgian Congo as the best in tropical Africa and a 1959 US government report agreed that the Belgian programme was one of the best on the continent with more hospital beds in the Congo than in all the rest of tropical Africa.[1] Most Belgian administrators would have explained that their paternalistic administration had been a resounding success in the area of public health; this success, they would argue was exemplified in part by the near-conquest by medical means of at least one disease, human sleeping sickness.

Sleeping sickness and 'vertical' health programme

They believed that their policy of concentrating efforts and resources in a campaign aimed at one disease, sleeping sickness, was responsible in large part for this success. In public health parlance, such concentration of resources is described as a 'vertical' model of health-care delivery. As we have seen, their approach to control of the disease, unlike that of the British for instance, had been the attempted medication of the entire population of the colony in order to systematically 'sterilise' the human reservoir of the disease-causing parasites, the trypanosomes. The campaigns of mass chemotherapy were aimed at the parasite while the basic ecology of the disease remained unaltered. In contrast, a 'horizontal' health care programme aims to cope with a broad spectrum of public health issues which might range from infant and maternal care to sanitation engineering while responses to endemic and epidemic diseases would form only one part of the overall programme. Indeed, this latter approach was from the 1930s encouraged in parts of the Belgian Congo, especially Province Orientale, where much emphasis was placed upon developing a network of rural primary health clinics. Nevertheless, by 1930, there existed throughout the colony a considerable medical and administrative infrastructure, much of which was concerned specifically with the control and eradication of human sleeping sickness. With these points in mind, can we agree with those administrators who believed that Belgian colonisation of the Congo had been a blessing for African health?

Public health and imperialism – domination?

Or, as more radical critics claim for other regions of Africa, must we see colonial health provision as a powerful tool for the domination and control of African peoples which outweighed, even negated, the medical advantages? Was the cost to Africans too high?[2] 'Apologists for colonialism often look myopically at the medical services, proclaim their humanity and even argue that their philosophy ran counter to that of imperialism.'[3] Perhaps medical practitioners are subject to unrealistic expectations? The critique is indeed hard. Yet, many who study the history of health in former European colonies would agree readily with the following comment concerning Morocco: 'While medical authorities did not produce the worst atrocities committed in the imperialist cause, they did participate in them and support them.'[4] But is it fair to accuse colonial doctors in the Belgian Congo or having been 'medical operatives', or 'agents of imperialism' because their work was unavoidably interwoven with the conquest and domination of Africans? And blessing or otherwise, was colonial medicine used in the Belgian Congo to dominate people? The question is not purely academic for it seems that some of the problems encountered today in the areas of public health and medical provision in parts of Africa can be understood only in light of their historical roots.

The history of the Belgian Congo before World War II concerns not only real epidemics of sleeping sickness but also the ways in which this disease stirred the imagination of those involved in colonisation. It is a history which demonstrates vividly the complex interplay of disease and the state.

The state and epidemics

First, it is the state which defines an epidemic through its organised responses to such crises. While medical specialists may be responsible for identifying an epidemic situation, it is the state which provides the necessary sanctions for organised responses to that situation. Thus, the declaration of an epidemic becomes a political as well as a medical matter. Consequently, disease, especially when epidemic, can affect directly the very form of an emerging state. The crisis presented by an epidemic disease becomes not only a political issue but itself becomes a factor affecting political developments in the state. Sleeping sickness was an important factor which helped to shape the colonial state of the Belgian Congo.

This was clearly demonstrated in 1943 when the director of the colonial medical service, Dr A. Duren, rationalised that the dreadful health conditions of the Africans in the Congo basin had not formed part of King Leopold's initial motivation to create his African empire.[5] Nevertheless, continued Duren, the poor health of Africans, exacerbated by the process of conquest itself, became in time a clear rationalisation, *after the fact*, for having colonised the region. Belgians invaded the Congo basin, conquered its residents and in the process caused the increase and spread of diseases, some of which like sleeping sickness became epidemic. The same conquerors then made medical provisions which in retrospect could be regarded by the administration as adequate compensation for the terrible upheavals caused the Congolese. This is a clear example of the way in which health, disease and medicine are highly political matters. For the director of the colonial health service in 1943, the medical response to disease adequately compensated millions of Africans for their total subjection and exploitation.

Thus, in answer to the question whether medicine was a form of imperialism – an effective mechanism used by Belgians to impose their authority over subject peoples, the answer must be yes. The web of relations among sleeping sickness, the state and epidemics and the development of the colonial state early this century in the Belgian Congo cannot be ignored.

It would be incorrect, however, to assert that Belgian medical provision was solely a tool used to dominate subject peoples as has been claimed for the former Portuguese colonies in Africa.[6] This study has shown that such sweeping generalisations are inappropriate for the Belgian colonial medical services or their public health policy. The tensions within the medical sector and between it and the political and economic administrative sectors reveal a lack of any coordinated public health policy. As in other areas of administration, public health policy and the medical services evolved in a more piecemeal, *ad hoc*, manner and involved a range of motivations which varied from time to time and place to place. Nevertheless, it is the nature of historians to press for underlying trends, directions and movements in their efforts to make sense of otherwise overwhelming particularities. In this sense, with the advantage of the 'long view', I can make several summarising statements about the Belgian colonial medical services and the role of sleeping sickness in the formation of a public health policy.

By the 1930s a vertical health-care system was beginning to emerge out of the highly bureaucratised, cumbersome sleeping sickness campaign. In large parts of the Belgian Congo, that campaign with its specific infrastructure had been the basis for the colonial medical service. By 1930, however, the medical service was autonomous enough to occasionally come into direct conflict with its 'parent' organisation. In fact, the boundary between the two organisations was unclear, sometimes non-existent. Furthermore, by 1930 the more general medical service began developing in ways now referred to as 'horizontal', expressing concern in a broad range of health-related issues such as infant and child care, nutrition, public health and sanitation, major endemic and epidemic diseases and vaccination campaigns – in effect, the spectrum of health issues which are today the concern of primary health clinics throughout the developing world.

Epidemics and social relations

This study has also demonstrated the ways in which disease, especially when epidemic, illuminates or mirrors social relations. The historian, tempted by the plethora of data generated by crises such as epidemics, can easily produce a rather warped view of the past. This is particularly problematic for historians attempting to reconstruct the past of societies for which there is limited and uneven documentation and sources. Nevertheless, I believe that examination of the epidemic of sleeping sickness in north-central Uele district early this century helps to reveal the otherwise obscure social relations among African societies and between them and their new colonial masters. Furthermore, that epidemic can be legitimately considered a 'social product', stemming as it did from the radically changed social relations in the region. Africans experienced a series of tumultuous upheavals resulting in the imposition of Belgian colonial rule. Coinciding with the establishment of the new and very unequal relations of power was the increased incidence and spread of human trypanosomiasis, sleeping sickness. But not all Africans suffered the disease in equal measure. We have seen that a few colonial administrators noticed differences in the degree of affliction suffered by social groups, or classes. For instance, it was observed that those Africans who were better nourished and less stressed by state demands seemed to fare better than others. Africans in different regions of the colony had sometimes quite different responses to both the disease and the European management of the disease, which is another proof that epidemic disease can reveal social relations. The authority structures within African societies were seriously strained because of sleeping sickness and the myriad public health measures imposed upon those authorities and their subjects.

The epidemic of sleeping sickness which occurred during the first decades of this century in north-central Uele district is an excellent example of the ways in which social relations affect health. The colonial conquest of that region was protracted and brutal. Large numbers of people became refugees, many of whom were threatened by famine. At the same time, ecological conditions were excellent for two events. First of all, endemic foci of the chronic *gambiense* variety of sleeping sickness flared into epidemic proportions. Secondly, the same strain of the disease was introduced into new environments suitable for its existence and spread.

In May 1912, the doctor travelling with a military expedition north of the Uere river noticed victims of sleeping sickness in an area recently the scene of fierce combat and much turmoil. For the Belgians, it was an alarming observation since for nearly a decade the district of Uele had been considered by the authorities to be uninfected by the dreaded disease. Much attention had been devoted to elaborate measures designed to protect the district from infection and, from December 1905, an ever-increasing amount of public health legislation had been aimed at creating a cordon sanitaire.[7]

Over the next fifteen years until 1927, the disease became increasingly entrenched and epidemic in the region.[8] Nevertheless, although much effort was aimed at control of the movements of people in the region through elaboration of the cordon sanitaire, nothing was done to alleviate the social conditions. There was particular hardship during World War I when the people were forced to collect more and more wild rubber, a much-needed resource for the war effort. It was exceedingly difficult work. While not rich in rubber, north-central Uele contained many gallery forests – fringing forests along well-watered ravines – which contained wild rubber vines and which were also superb biotopes for *Glossina palpalis*, the main vector of human sleeping sickness in the Congo.

It was not until the mid-1920s that the first medical services *began* to appear in the region and, a short five years later, the authorities claimed that as a result of their medical campaign, the epidemic was under control. I suggest, however, that research into the changing nature of social relations in north-central Uele reveals the true causes of the decrease in sleeping sickness.

Improvements in nutrition and hygiene were the first and most important reasons for the decline of many diseases in the developed world.[9] Thomas McKeown led the way in declaring the relative lack of impact of biomedicine on the incidence of diseases like tuberculosis, poliomyelitis and even smallpox in the Western world. He argued convincingly that it was improved socio-economic conditions, rather than medical therapies, which accounted for the overall improvements in the health of Western populations. Many people now believe that the same solutions remain to be provided for widespread diseases in the Third World. Improved social conditions, more than medications and medical services, will lead to improved health, according to this view. Protein-energy malnutrition is perhaps the most important 'pathogenic' factor in sub-Saharan Africa. The synergism of protein-energy malnutrition and infectious and parasitic diseases is certainly among the greatest causes of early childhood mortality.

The legacy of the public health programme and medical services

What then are we to make of the apparent irony that the Belgian colonists helped to cause a disease to become epidemic, made provisions in the form of medical services to combat it, and finally rationalised their colonial venture in part by claiming credit for that medical provision? It can be demonstrated that sleeping sickness did increase and spread in northern Congo as a direct consequence of the changed relations brought about among African societies during the protracted military conquest and harsh economic exploitation of the region by the Belgian colonists. It can also be demonstrated that after two decades of increase and spread, epidemic sleeping sickness in the region was clearly on the wane by 1930. But it is far more difficult to confirm the Belgian view that the decrease of sleeping sickness was due solely, or even primarily, to the medical efforts of their elaborate campaign to effect control over this disease.

It is only through examination of the total set of social relations in the region and the changes wrought among them during the early decades of this century that we can begin to understand why sleeping sickness became epidemic and why it then subsided. In other words, it is necessary to study the total context in which health and disease occur.

Historians of medicine in Africa often argue that biomedicine and improved public health comprised the most valuable legacy left by the colonial powers. Indeed, beginning in the 1920s with the introduction of effective drugs, there were some notable success stories. For example, yaws or pian, a disease widely endemic in sub-Saharan Africa until the 1940s,[10] responded well to sulphadones, especially neosalvarsan (Bayer 914, or neoarsphenamine) and from 1944, penicillin. Immediate results were spectacular, with Africans eagerly seeking injections, which resulted in the near eradication of yaws in some regions. The medical success of yaws was a critical factor which enhanced the power of biomedicine and helped to establish it as a viable choice for Africans. However, there is evidence that yaws was declining in incidence by the 1950s because of improved socio-economic conditions, and quite independently of the availability of effective drugs.[11]

Yet even where biomedical solutions proved effective and successful there remained the serious problem of finance for public health in colonial Africa. 'Vertical' campaigns like those aimed at sleeping sickness, yaws, malaria and, more recently, smallpox are expensive in terms of infrastructure, staffing and supplies. More general, or 'horizontal', health programmes aim to address a broad spectrum of public health issues such as control of major endemic and epidemic diseases, infant and mother care, vaccinations and primary health clinics, and are usually far more cost-effective in their use of personnel, infrastructure and supplies. Throughout much of the colonial period in sub-Saharan Africa, medical services tended to be more vertical than horizontal in their operation. The big campaigns launched against single diseases like sleeping sickness were extremely costly, absorbing scarce resources and drawing finance away from other crucial needs of health provision. Another significant aspect of health economics is the fact that many pharmaceutical companies were in the past, and remain today, reluctant to invest heavily in the research and development of medicines for diseases which afflict mainly impoverished, often rural, populations in underdeveloped regions of the world. During most of the past century, the combination of these two factors, vertical medical campaigns and reluctance of pharmaceuticals to invest in research with so little prospect of profit from their drugs, has had profoundly adverse effects on the health of millions of sub-Saharan Africans.

By the 1960s, vaccination campaigns in many countries were routine. In some regions, more often urban centres, public health programmes had imposed a degree of control over malaria. Maternal and child health programmes were well established in Belgian Congo and in many other colonies. Employers of mass labour such as mines and plantations had expressed some concern for the well-being of their workers and in some regions conditions were improved marginally. In the interwar period, Africans were increasingly perceived as an important source of wealth, 'human capital', to be protected like other forms of investment. By the time of their independence in the 1960s many African populations experienced considerably better health than had their predecessors during the early stages of colonial contact. Mortality and morbidity rates were lower than ever and major epidemics occurred less frequently than before. Departing colonial administrations tended to account for these improvements by citing the ameliorating effects of the medical services which, as noted above, many believed to be the most valuable portion of the colonial legacy. In other words, most colonial rulers, like the Belgians, believed that disease incidence had been decreased through the beneficial effects of Western biomedical staff, infrastructure and techniques. Very few colonials would have credited improvements in the standard of living of many millions of Africans for the decreased disease incidences. After all, it was not until the 1970s that McKeown made his provocative observations.

By the 1930s, many Congolese populations no longer suffered the intense social and economic disruption of the earlier contact period. The patterns of Belgian rule had stabilised, and Africans had learned better how to cope with and, if need be, get around Belgian controls on their lives and livelihoods. At the same time the Belgians had begun to back away from the use of the more disruptive of their social engineering practices, most notably the abrupt resiting of whole communities. These factors are likely to have had as much, if not more, to do with the decline of sleeping sickness as the medical campaigns.

Postscript: AIDS

I cannot conclude this study of the social history of sleeping sickness without making at least a few comments on the appearance of another alarming epidemic disease in the early 1980s, human immuno-deficiency virus, or HIV. It is not certain just what percentage of persons carrying HIV will go on to develop the disease syndrome referred to as AIDS (Acquired Immuno-deficiency Syndrome). However, with no cure available and none expected in the near future, AIDS is a fatal disease. Every premature death is sad in personal terms and a loss for the wider society. Death from AIDS, however, is particularly tragic, affecting as it does large numbers of young adults in their productive and reproductive prime. This is a factor which could have an enormous impact on the development potential of sub-Saharan African nations, many of which already experience severe shortages of trained and professional citizens. Many agree with World Health Organisation projections that AIDS might constitute over the next several decades the major disaster of the African continent.

Unfortunately, the advent of HIV/AIDS has helped to exacerbate an already increasingly negative view of sub-Saharan Africa held by a large portion of the public. For many, crises like the droughts and famines of the 1970s and 1980s have reawakened images of Africa, the 'dark continent', home of diseased and dying people. This has led to some hysteria in the media reporting of the potential demographic impact of HIV/AIDS. It cannot be denied that there is ample cause for concern, but a more judicious view is required.

We should not discount the real possibility that African AIDS is and will continue to be overestimated in its current magnitude. Rumours abound, many local areas are inaccessible to systematic data collection, diagnostic facilities are rare, and a host of deaths from other causes can be mistakenly attributed to AIDS.

On the other hand, it would be just as imprudent totally to discount the possibility of African AIDS triggering epidemics and destabilizations to rival those initiated by the Black Death, which in the fourteenth century helped depopulate Europe and its food-producing regions by one-third.[12]

Have we come full circle then in the history of medicine and disease in Africa? Almost a century has passed since the discovery of epidemic sleeping sickness in Uganda and the Congo Free State and a number of analogies with the present AIDS epidemic are worth noting. They might even provide us with important lessons from the past.

AIDS is a fatal disease because there is as yet no cure, and sleeping sickness too, if left untreated, leads ultimately to death. The *gambiense* form of sleeping sickness is especially analogous with AIDS in that both diseases are chronic with a variety of increasingly destructive clinical manifestations. In the secondary, or advanced, stages of sleeping sickness, when there is central nervous system involvement with frequent dementia and other forms of neurological deterioration, sleeping sickness shares similarities with the latter stages of many HIV infections. A major difference between the two diseases, which reflects the significant advances which have been made in biomedical research, has been the impressively rapid understanding of the aetiology and the epidemiology of AIDS. This knowledge made it possible for some public health authorities to implement measures aimed at controlling the spread of HIV far more quickly than would have been possible for fledgling colonial authorities in Africa at the beginning of the century in the case of sleeping sickness. Nevertheless, the awful fact remains that at present AIDS is an incurable disease and the only defence involves attempts to affect the behaviour of people in order to contain the spread of the virus. The major public health message of the late 1980s has been 'safe sex', with sporadic campaigns around the world propounding the use of condoms.

A second important analogy between the two epidemics concerns the fear of many that an epidemic disease will decimate African populations. Of course, the epidemiology of the two diseases is significantly different. Thus far, the AIDS epidemic has appeared[13] to be more prominently an urban problem while sleeping sickness is clearly a disease of the rural sector, even a disease of the 'frontier' between sylvan and man-controlled biotope. I agree with those who believe that, upon closer scrutiny and with more careful research by social scientists and medical experts, it will most likely become clear that AIDS is closely related to a wide range of socio-economic factors. Socio-economic factors are especially important to the epidemiology of diseases in Africa, as stressed throughout this study. It cannot be a surprise that an immuno-deficiency disease like AIDS could wreak havoc among highly susceptible populations already suffering high levels of background infections in combination with disruptions and upheavals associated with the political tensions experienced since the 1960s in many parts of sub-Saharan Africa.

A third important analogy between the two diseases can be identified in the degree of response of the international scientific community and its effect on African leadership and statecraft. As with sleeping sickness earlier this century, regions of sub-Saharan Africa are experiencing the influx of Western-trained biomedical and scientific experts who either directly or indirectly will affect the course of public health for some time. Today virologists rather than parasitologists are centre stage, but with both sleeping sickness and HIV/AIDS, the role of the epidemiologist is crucial indeed. Fears expressed earlier this century, sometimes real, sometimes exaggerated, that sleeping sickness would decimate African populations are once again reflected in much reporting of HIV and AIDS in Africa, with the difference that contemporary media possess enormous power through the instantaneous message. It is not my intention to argue the validity or otherwise of projections concerning the potential impact of HIV/AIDS on African demography but it is most relevant to the social history of health in Africa to recognise the potential impact on African societies of the contemporary concerns and policies regarding HIV and AIDS. And here the role of the international scientific community will be crucial in much the same way that many decades ago the influence of the Western biomedical community was such that it affected the shaping of colonial states like the Belgian Congo.

Defined by the state and medical authorities, disease epidemics generate a momentum of their own which stretches far beyond the immediate illness and death of those afflicted. As we have seen in this study, public health authorities respond to epidemics in ways which affect societies at many levels, from the personal to the more broadly economic and political. The high profile involvement of state authorities sometimes required in the management of epidemic disease can pose enormous problems in countries suffering other forms of social, economic and political weakness or disorder. Disease management can become inextricably linked in the minds of stressed peoples with other forms of intrusion on the part of the state.

The social history of HIV/AIDS in Zaire and Uganda will be further proof of the necessity to examine carefully the total socio-economic and political context of an epidemic disease in order to appreciate fully the complexity of the never-ending struggle between man and his pathogens. Such understanding is a fundamental prerequisite for the improvement of the overall quality of life for millions of sub-Saharan Africans.

Appendix A

Health legislation and instructions, 1888–1934

Following are some of the more relevant items of legislation and instructions which pertained to human trypanosomiasis in northern Congo. It can be observed that the medical service itself was a direct outgrowth of the campaign against sleeping sickness.

5 Aug. 1888 *Decree*. A sanitary service organised.

22 Aug. 1888 *Ordinance*. Obligatory notification of contagious/epidemic diseases.

20 Oct. 1888 *Decree*. Upgraded 22 August ordinance; until 1926, this was the basis of the health legislation of the colony.

22 Feb. 1892 *Decree*. Created three-man Hygiene Commissions (Boma, Matadi, Banana).

13 Nov. 1895 *Arrêté*. Created Commissions d'Hygiène in all zone/district headquarters. Three-man including a doctor. Three reports a year.

1899 Research laboratory established at Leopoldville.

24 Apr. 1899 *Ordinance*. Altered Commissions d'Hygiène in district headquarters.

Jan. 1903 *Circular*. Travel restrictions.

5 May 1903 *Circular*. Isolation of sleeping sickness suspects on advice of Liverpool [MAEAA 846.20].

26 May 1903 *Arrêté*. Upgraded 5 May circular.

16 Jun. 1903 [WIHM Ms. 2268]. Re: isolation/no Africans on steamers.

26 Aug. 1903 *Arrêté*. Notification of sleeping sickness mandatory according to ordinance of 22 August 1888.

7 Dec. 1903 *Circular*. Lantonnois, 'Sleeping Sickness Instructions' [MAEAA 847.112; 858; MRAC Fuchs 114].

7 Dec. 1905 First comprehensive Sleeping Sickness Instructions based upon advice from Liverpool researchers. (No drug available, thus isolation only.)

1906 School of Tropical Medicine Formed in Brussels (31 March 1931: replaced by l'Institut de Médecine Tropicale Prince Léopold).

24 Mar. 1906 *Circular*. First on village sanitation.

17 Apr. 1906 *Circular*. Africans with sleeping sickness, in state service or not, forbidden to travel in uninfected territories (GG Wahis to all agents).

3 Jun. 1906 King Leopold II offered a prize of 200,00 francs for a cure for sleeping sickness and he established a *crédit* of 300,000 francs for research. (The

funds were never used and fell into desuetude. In July 1953 the funds were reactivated and were worth 1,000,000 francs.)

24 Aug. 1906 *Circular.* Three lazarets created (N. Anvers, Stanleyville, Lusambo; already one at Leopoldville); use atoxyl and trypanroth.

5 Dec. 1906 New sleeping sickness measures systematising all previous legislation: created Ibembo (as defence for the north-east) and Yakoma lazarets/observation posts. Now six lazarets in state. Atoxyl and strychnine sulphate were available drugs.

8 Feb. 1907 *Circular.* Requesting reports on drug therapy [MAEAA 847.273].

18 Feb. 1907 *Report.* Dr Heiberg's thirty-four page 'Report on Sleeping Sickness' for the Secretary-General with proposed programme. Need sanctions against recruitment of labour from infected areas. Establish a series of examination points through which Africans would be obliged to pass in the manner of a 'sieve'. Establish *mobile* teams to deal with flies, brush, parasite reservoirs (victims in first stage). Doctor should begin tours farthest from centres of state 'and in that way brush ahead of him like the hunter *all* suspects and expel them through the post which is the "key" to the district'. The doctor should educate Europeans and Africans to be on lookout for victims. He proposed three regions be especially examined for the disease: Lado-Uele, Haut-Ituri and Lake Kivu districts [MAEAA 847.259].

4 Dec. 1907 Secretary of State, Brussels, recommended as measures: invalid out and repatriate all second-stage victims except those from uncontaminated regions. They should go to lazarets nearest their home regions. All first-stage victims should have two periods of treatment – lazaret and long follow-up treatment by special units; careful surveillance of labour recruitment and of all rivercraft. He explained that while atoxyl caused 'some' blindness, it should nevertheless be continued and dosages should be researched.

27 May 1908 *Circular.* All religious missions to assist with search, isolation and injections.

14 Jul. 1908 *Circular. Re:* recalcitrant victims. Doctors now aided by army [MRAC 58.20.46].

15 Jul. 1908 *Circular.* Africans not to disembark from steamers in areas not yet examined by doctors for sleeping sickness. Africans not employed by state not to travel without medical papers. Can travel to lazaret if injected with 50 cc atoxyl at embarkation.

18 Sep. 1908 *Measures. Re:* cordon sanitaire. Special precautions to protect the north-east from infection by Uganda, Sudan and French Congo. All natives require route passes to travel. All natives wishing to enter Congo State from either Uganda or Sudan to pass through Lado while those from French Congo must use Yakoma, and all those coming from infected regions require permits obtained after exams. The same applies to Europeans. All trade caravans are forbidden to pass through infected regions. And, provisionally, *no* porterage through the Ubangi-Uele region [MRAC 58.20.46].

15 Nov. 1908 Congo Free State became a Belgian colony.

2 Feb. 1909 *Circular.* Clothing for victims.

19 Apr. 1909 *Ordinance.* Closed Uganda border.

29 Apr. 1909 *Ordinance.* Observation posts at borders [MAEAA 848.82].

30 Apr. 1909 *Circular.* Provisionally, no porterage in Uele [MAEAA 843.46].

1 Dec. 1909 *Royal Arrêté.* Established Hygiene Department in Brussels while doctors remained directly under authority of territorial administrators.

20 Dec. 1909 *Ordinance.* Fuchs relaxed 19 April ruling.

8 Jan. 1910 *Circular.* Missionaries to follow tropical medicine course at Brussels and practical lab. course at Leopoldville.

15 Apr. 1910 *Circular.* Reorganised sleeping sickness regulations; Africans loathed isolation – created open-style village-lazarets with room for families – only for incurables, very ill and insane; out-patients continue labour; created line of observation posts to screen [MRAC Fuchs 830: MAEAA 849.273; 859.15].

30 Apr. 1910 *Circular.* Obligatory medical passports valid 18 months and visaed every three months by doctor. Medical certificates were to indicate diagnosis of sleeping sickness [MAEAA 850.260].

22 Jul. 1910 *Circular.* Instructions to trap tsetse flies by using African or animal walking about slowly with a cloth on the back, the cloth impregnated with a glue-like substance to attract flies; this technique to be used between 11 a.m. and 4 p.m.

8 Sep. 1910 *Ordinance.* New sleeping sickness measures to replace those of 5 December 1906 and upgrade circular of 15 April; all state employees responsible to detect victims; none to evade regulations, isolation, treatment; none to refuse exams; none to enter contaminated area without permit; not to employ in uninfected area anyone who had resided in infected area during previous twelve months; persons from infected area prohibited to travel through uninfected areas; no steamer or rail transport for Africans without permit; force sanctioned for exams – use army; doctors sanctioned to enforce isolation; solicit aid of African authorities – educate Africans; tsetse fly eradication, moves of villages, brush clearance policy, ten observation posts, sanitary brigades, clearance.

9 Sep. 1910 *Ordinance.* Established cordon sanitaire around north-eastern uninfected triangle: Aba for Sudan and Uganda, Yakoma for French Congo were only points of entry.

24 Sep. 1910 *Circular.* All state agents instructed to issue passports to Africans as too many were found to be travelling about freely.

30 Sep. 1910 *Ordinance.* Instructions to monitor and control the travel of Ugandan porters across Congo borders [MAEAA 843.546].

10 Oct. 1910 *Arrêté.* Missionaries to attend tropical medicine school for short course [Tongerloo Abbey Archives, Uele file 4].

23 Jan. 1911 *Ordinance.* Updated to ordinance, arrêté of 1 December 1909 establishing Hygiene Department. Observation posts placed under authority of doctors.

15 Mar. 1911 *Circular.* Warning all territorial administrators that those who neglected application of the 8 September 1910 ordinance would be held accountable [MRAC 50.30.385].

20 Apr. 1911 *Circular.* Warning all administrators to follow sleeping sickness regulations, cooperate with doctors, see to village hygiene and agglomerate

small groups of people as well as move villages away from rivers [MRAC 50.30.215].

26 Apr. 1911 *Ordinance. Re:* African travel across frontier with French Congo.

28 Jun. 1911 *Ordinance. Re:* uninfected triangle (modified 9 and 30 September 1910).

28 Jul. 1911 *Ordinance.* Moved back the eastern frontier of infected area of Uele [MAEAA 843.25].

29 Jul. 1911 *Ordinance.* Kivu infected.

20 Sep. 1911 *Ordinance.* Uganda border.

20 Sep. 1911 *Circular.* Minister Renkin ordered maximum number lazaret patients in colony to be 850 or 30 per lazaret. Lazarets should evolve into hospitals thus freeing doctors who could then tour [MAEAA 842.119].

20 Oct. 1911 *Ordinance.* Closed Uele district to all Ugandans.

21 Oct 1911 *Decision.* Forbidden for employers to take locally recruited porters out of the colony, i.e., do not cross foreign boundaries [MRAC 50.30.83].

9 Dec. 1911 No pack-animals to cross eastern frontier into Uele.

12 Jan. 1912 Closed Uele to Africans from *all* neighbouring territories.

1 Feb. 1912 *Ordinance.* Sleeping sickness measures for Ituri.

6 Jun. 1912 *Ordinance.* Sanitary Police for all navigation on rivers in State.

23 Jun. 1912 *Circular.* Africans from neighbouring colonies in north-east absolutely forbidden entry into Uele [MRAC 50.30.221].

25 Jun. 1912 *Circular.* Measures concerning relocation of villages.

30 Jun. 1912 Sudan closed its border with Belgian Congo [MRAC 50.30.222].

4 Jul. 1912 *Circular.* 'Absolutely' forbidden by ordinance to allow porters from neighbouring colonies to enter Uele [MRAC 50.30.221].

22 Jul. 1912 *Ordinance.* New sleeping sickness regulations replaced those of 8–9 September 1910. This thirty-nine-page document covered the following: all aspects of cordon sanitaire (passports, infected regions, observation posts); all state agents obliged to participate in *la lutte*; detailed section on regroupment of Africans and relocation of villages at discretion of doctor with obligatory cooperation of local administrator and army. Sanctions for uncooperative African authorities; abandoned habitations to be burned and surveillance of old sites to prevent re-entry. Travel and canoeing forbidden or regulated and canoes eventually seized and/or destroyed. Discretion to be used; thus, when fishing forbidden, certain individuals should be issued permits to fish during *certain* hours, but permission withdrawn if abused. Doctors now possess rights to examine anyone, anytime and anywhere.

4 Aug. 1912 *Decision.* Region between Uere river and Bili post decreed infected. Non-resident Africans and porters from uninfected regions strictly forbidden to enter, while those from infected areas must possess medical passport [MRAC 50.30.222].

6 Aug. 1912 *Circular.* Daytime fishing and salt-grass collection on Itimbiri river and all affluents forbidden [MRAC 50.30.117; 50.30.387].

30 Aug. 1912 *Circular.* Dr Grenade named Director of Medical Service, Uele, especially for sleeping sickness [MRAC 50.30.221].

4 Sep. 1912 *Circular.* Train African medical auxiliaries.

5 Sep. 1912 *Circular.* All state agents to follow measures and cooperate with doctors.

21 Sep. 1912 *Circular.* Obligatory monthly palpation of soldiers at state posts by agents [MRAC 50.30.222].

26 Sep. 1912 *Ordinance.* Declared part of northern Uele infected. Bili created observation post.

3 Oct 1912 *Circular.* Apply sleeping sickness measures continually; involve African chiefs in *lutte*; uncooperative agents will be fined [MRAC 50.30.222].

16 Oct. 1912 *Circular.* All territorial administrators to make effort to involve African authorities in sleeping sickness measures [MRAC 50.30.221].

31 Oct. 1912 *Circular.* Territorial staff must observe hygiene rules.

11 Nov. 1912 *Circular.* Palpate all soldiers; instruct Africans in this; educate Africans about tsetse flies, etc. [MRAC 50.30.222].

14 Nov. 1912 *Circular.* Africans forbidden to enter infected region north of Bili river and any who do so, to be severely punished [MRAC 50.30.133].

13 Dec. 1912 *Circular.* Sanitary brigades.

15 Dec. 1912 *Ordinance.* Closed Uele to *all* Africans from neighbouring colonies [MRAC 50.30.154].

26 Dec. 1912 Uele closed to free trade.

20 Jan. 1913 *Circular.* Relocation of villages.

21 Jan. 1913 *Circular.* Sleeping sickness measures.

4 Mar. 1913 *Circular.* Sanitary brigade allocations for eighteen districts. Uele to have 7 teams with 340 people in total.

6 Mar. 1913 *Circular.* Brush clearance.

18 Mar. 1913 *Circular.* Sleeping sickness map.

28 May 1913 *Ordinance.* Modified village relocation.

3 Jul. 1913 *Decree.* No river traffic on Rubi–Itimbiri and affluents [MAEAA 855.46].

17 Jul. 1913 Landeghem forbade *all* (including European) canoe traffic during day on Likati river [MRAC 50.30.84].

1913 King Albert allocated 1,250,000 francs for a sleeping sickness campaign. The funds consisted of interest which had accrued on 50 million francs designated by an Act of 28 November 1907. A sum of 115,000 francs was given by the Queen in addition to an annual sum of 804,000 francs allocated to the colony to organise a special service to fight sleeping sickness. Before the service could be established, however, World War I began.

20 Jan. 1914 Using ordinance of 28 May 1913, Landeghem forbade canoe traffic on Upper Rubi river [MRAC 50.30.379].

16 Feb. 1914 *Circular.* Vital that *even* natives, organised by *chefferies* participate in the campaign. Territorial administrators must contact chiefs. Plantation, commercial and religious missions likewise. Each native must be able to recognise a *glossina* and understand its role. All Europeans should help educate Africans. Stir their apathy. Convince chiefs to regroup populations and move them [MAEAA 4403.435].

29 Sep. 1914 Doctors given powers of territorial administrators in regard to sleeping sickness [MRAC 58.20.55].

18 Jan. 1915 *Ordinance.* North-central region of Uele declared infected zone [MRAC 50.30.156].

21 Jun. 1915 *Ordinance.* Established observation post at Bondo with all powers of the Judicial Police in hygiene matters.

26 Sep. 1915 *Circular.* The district commissioner refused to allow a religious mission to send Africans north of the Bomu river to 'perfect their French' as importation of sleeping sickness must be guarded against.

12 Jan. 1916 *Ordinance.* Commissions d'Hygiène organised (modified ordinance of 24 April 1899).

27 Jun. 1916 *Decision.* Travel forbidden on Uere river and *all* travellers except those from the observation post at Ango to be stopped. All riverine villages on Uere up to Api to be moved at least one kilometre from river.

5 Sep. 1916 Uere river closed [MRAC 50.30.379]. Villages near river must be moved at least one kilometre away.

27 Dec. 1917 *Decision.* Forbade canoe paddlers above Likati.

3 May 1918 Closed Uele between Voro and Bondo to canoe traffic [MRAC 50.30.379].

3 May 1918 *Circular.* All travel forbidden on Uele river above Bondo. Move all villages which threaten spread of the disease. Proscribe all travel of women and children.

1919 Dr Trolli explained that in this year, the postponed campaign against sleeping sickness was able to begin. The basic elements of the campaign were to be: a census of victims of sleeping sickness; a programme to treat ambulatory patients; African auxiliaries would be trained; European *agents sanitaires* would assist; dispensaries would be established.

8 Jul. 1920 *Ordinance.* Established sleeping sickness (public health) policy for some time to come (Trolli, *Exposé*). A medical service at last established. Passports required for travel more than thirty kilometres outside home region; villages, posts to be located at least one kilometre from river banks; strict regulation of fishing and river travel in infected regions.

End 1920 *Ordinance.* Established two special sleeping sickness missions, or surveys: Uele and Kwango (later another at Yakoma).

25 Aug. 1921 Landeghem decree prescribed brush clearance and village moves two kilometres from rivers [MAEAA R/CB 149.4; report of 1923 sleeping sickness survey].

Oct. 1921 Landeghem suspended 25 August 1921 decree as he foresaw political problems.

End 1922 Two more sleeping sickness missions at Bangala and Mayumbe with another later in Katanga.

4 Dec. 1922 *Royal Arrêté.* Medical Service became autonomous with a chief medical officer directly under the governor-general and principal medical officers for each province.

9 Jul. 1923 *Decree.* Doctors could have temporary powers of police magistrates.

16 Sep. 1923 Sleeping sickness regulations.

26 Sep. 1923 Sleeping sickness regulations.

3 Jun. 1924 *Ordinance.* Judiciary status available to certain members of Hygiene Service.

27 May 1925 *Ordinance*. African *infirmiers* and medical assistants.

10 Jun. 1925 *Ordinance*. African auxiliaries in Medical Service.

22 Jun. 1926 *Ordinance*. GG Rutten replaced 8 July 1920 ordinance. Treatment must be available within twenty kilometres; six-month provisional passport upon cure; identity cards will make note of the passport; forbidden to employ state labourer without identity card. All second-stage victims isolated in lazaret or hospital [MAEAA 2934].

26 Jul. 1926 *Decree*. *Re:* hygiene and public health.

23 Apr. 1927 *Royal Arrêté*. Conseil Supérieur de l'Hygiène Colonial established.

17 Aug. 1927 *Decree*. Modifications to 26 July 1926 hygiene and public health legislation.

26 Aug. 1928 GG Tilkens' proposed ordinance to establish sanitary brigades: each province capital to have 'Technical Department of Hygiene Works' under governor composed of hygienist-doctor and provincial engineer of public works; to deal with hygiene of population centres; to study epidemic control.

15 Dec. 1928 *Ordinance*. Hygiene and public health.

25 Feb. 1929 *Circular*. Dr Van den Branden of Leopoldville laboratory established rules for administration of atoxyl, tryparsamide and tryponarsyl because of number of 'accidents' recently reported by doctors enthusiastically experimenting.

6 Mar. 1929 *Ordinance*. Doctors' judicial sanctions now extended to cover waterways. New regulations for Sanitary Police at the frontiers and ports.

10 Feb. 1930 *Ordinance*. Established cadre of 'sanitary guards' – African auxiliaries to assist hygiene measures in urban centres.

24 Sep. 1934 *Arrêté*. Basic organising principles of Medical Service under authority of governor-general.

Appendix B

Sample documentation

50. 30. 200

CONGO BELGE

District d *Abele.-*

N° .... (1)

MODÈLE N° 1.

CHEFFERIES INDIGÈNES

PROCES-VERBAL D'INVESTITURE

L'an mil ....

le .... jour du mois de .... ,

Nous, Commissaire de district d .... , avons

confirmé (²) .... *Bôle* .... , chef de (³) *village Bôle*

.... et de la région de(⁴) *village Etuau, Oesi, Dengi,*
Douli, Oili, Zauebago, Balaueba, Cazu, Lungba, Dingih et Zuuu
relevant du chef de (⁵) .... , dans l'autorité qui lui est
attribuée par la coutume indigène, pourvu qu'ele ne soit pas contraire aux règles d'ordre public
universel, ni aux lois de la Colonie qui ont pour but de substituer d'autres règles aux principes de la
coutume indigène, et lui avons fait remise de l'insigne décrit à l'article 8 de l'arrêté du 16 août 1906.

Le chef prédésigné a déclaré fixer son principal établissement à .... *Bôle* .... ;
il s'est engagé à se conformer à toutes les dispositions du décret du 3 juin 1906, sur les chefferies
indigènes.

De tout quoi nous avons dressé le présent procès-verbal en double original aux jour, mois et an
que dessus.

Le Chef,   Le Commissaire de district,

N. B. — Ce chef est le successeur du chef .... *Effulu* .... confirmé suivant le
procès-verbal n° ....

(1) Numéro d'ordre du procès-verbal.
(2) Nom du chef.
(3) Nom du village ou des villages sous la dépendance du chef.
(4) Région sur laquelle il exerce son autorité avec désignation des villages en faisant partie ainsi que des chefs de ceux-ci. — Mentionner
si l'investiture lui a été donnée pour toute cette région.
(5) Nom du chef auquel il peut être soumis.   2586

(a) Chefferies indigènes: procès verbal d'investiture.

GOUVERNEMENT LOCAL

1ʳᵉ Direction
SECRÉTARIAT GÉNÉRAL

Nᵒ 855

Deux annexes

OBJET :

Maladie du sommeil. — Certificats et
passeports à délivrer aux indigènes
pour le contrôle du mouvement des
populations.

Messieurs,

En vue de combattre, plus efficacement, les progrès de la maladie du sommeil, on a signalé, à diverses reprises, tant au Congo que dans les autres Colonies, l'impérieuse nécessité de pouvoir contrôler d'une manière certaine les mouvements des populations indigènes.

J'ai l'honneur de vous faire savoir que, pour renforcer le contrôle qui se fait actuellement dans la Colonie, le Gouvernement a décidé l'emploi, sur tout le territoire, de passeports et de certificats médicaux dont vous trouverez ci-joint un exemplaire. Il vous en sera expédié en quantité suffisante.

Pour surveiller les déplacements des porteurs, courriers, soldats, etc., le passeport sera délivré, sur simple demande et sans frais, tant pour les employés de la Colonie que pour les indigènes au service des particuliers ou ceux voyageant librement. Pour ces derniers, il faudra s'assurer l'aide des chefs indigènes ; la mesure a une importance capitale dans les régions frontières de l'extension de la maladie du sommeil.

Le passeport sera valable pour une année et demie ; il devra être visé par un médecin de la Colonie, tous les trois mois au moins. L'identité du porteur du passeport sera suffisamment garantie par les renseignements fournis et par l'impression digitale du pouce gauche.

Tout agent de la Colonie, médecin ou non médecin, aura pour devoir de vérifier, à toute occasion, si les porteurs ont leur passeport et si la pièce produite est régulière (date, contre-visite, etc.).

Le certificat médical à délivrer aux malades qui ont été traités pour trypanose, soit au lazaret, soit en dehors de celui-ci, permettra de suivre utilement les convalescents dans la suite. Cette pièce pourra aussi servir de billet de sortie pour un malade qui serait transféré dans un autre lazaret ou dans un autre poste.

Si le médecin qui a procédé à la deuxième contre-visite jugeait que le malade devrait se représenter ultérieurement, il pourra l'indiquer sur le certificat et le médecin, qui l'examinera par la suite, établira, au besoin, un nouveau certificat.

Je vous serais obligé, Messieurs, de bien vouloir au reçu de la présente, délivrer les passeports et certificats médicaux dans le sens indiqué ci-dessus.

LE VICE-GOUVERNEUR GÉNÉRAL,

F. FUCHS.

(b) Circular from Vice Governor-General Fuchs, 30 April 1910: 'Maladie du sommeil. – certificats et passeports à délivrer aux indigènes pour le contrôle du mouvement des populations'.

1470
Bute

CONGO BELGE

PASSEPORT MÉDICAL [1]

Le présent certificat a été délivré le _27 7 11_ , au nommé _Ragudu_
tribu _Bargbe_ , race _Aberbure_, village _kwele_

Signes caractéristiques : _____

Qualité : _Cook_
Au service de : _Mr l'ingenieur Monti_
ou position actuelle : _____
Destination (route à suivre) : _Gamba_

Age et sexe : _27 ♂_
Taille : _155_
Périmètre thoracique : _98_

Impression
digitale
du pouce gauche

CONSTATATIONS MÉDICALES

DATES	le _27 7 11_	le _____	le _____	le _____	le _____	le _____
	1	2	3	4	5	6
Impressions digitales du pouce gauche						
Etat des ganglions lymphatiques	normaux					
Ponctions de ganglions et résultats	0					
Examen du sang : 1° entre lame et lamelle.........	0					
2° en couche épaisse						
3° sang centrifugé..						
4° autoagglutination						
Symptômes divers : Fièvre..........						
Hyperesthésie.....						
Céphalalgie......	0					
Amaigrissement...						
Décisions du médecin et signatures						

(1) Le présent passeport est valable pour la durée d'une année et demie et devra être visé par un médecin de la Colonie, tous les trois mois au minimum.   4266

(c) Passeport médical.

MINISTÈRE

DES

COLONIES

—

5ᵉ DIRECTION GÉNÉRALE

—

2ᵉ DIRECTION

—

2ᵉ Division

CERTIFICAT MÉDICAL

Je soussigné, Médecin du Ministère des Colonies, déclare avoir visité

le nommé Omakayn amrkyn .

et estime que sa constitution physique

est bonne

; sa constitution mentale est bonne

Il peut donc être admis au service du Ministère des Colonies,

en Afrique.

Bruxelles, le 5 novembre *19 40*

Signature du Candidat :

(d) Certificat médical.

ETAT INDEPENDANT DU CONGO

Feuille de route pour l'agent dénommé ci-après qui se rend de _____ Buta _____ à _____ Gomba et retour .

NOM ET PRÉNOMS GRADE OU FONCTION	NOMBRE de porteurs mis à sa disposition	OBJETS DE CAMPEMENT UTILISÉS	DATE et heure de départ au poste d'origine	DATE ET HEURE d'arrivée et de départ aux routes intermédiaires	VISA des commissaires de district ou chefs de poste	OBSERVATIONS (indiquer dans cette colonne le motif de la réserve)
Ponti Ingenieur en chef de section			Buta 27/7 à 1h			Est accompagné de son boy Jacqui .

Reçu les objets ci-dessus :

Vu à _____ , le _____

pour arrivée le _____

Le _____

N. B. — Les agents voyageant avec des objets de campement appartenant à l'État, les remettront le lendemain de leur arrivée au chef du poste indiqué dans la colonne « Observations » de la feuille de route. L'agent qui ne se sera pas conformé à cet ordre pourra être puni disciplinairement. — Les objets non reproduits seront portés au compte de l'agent responsable. — Les agents rentrant à Boma remettront ces objets dans les magasins du Service Administratif à Boma-rive.

(e) Feuille de route.

CONGO BELGE
BELGISCH-CONGO

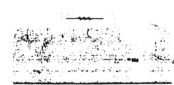

LIVRET D'IDENTITÉ
EENZELVIGHEIDSBOEKJE

429

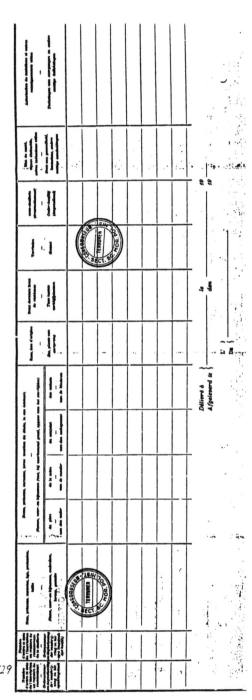

(f) Livret d'identité.

Notes

1 Disease and medicine in the history of Africa

1 A. Beck, *A History of the British Medical Administration of East Africa, 1900–1950* (Cambridge, Mass., Harvard University Press, 1970); A. Bayoumi, *The History of the Sudan Health Services* (Nairobi, Kenya Literature Bureau, 1979); D. F. Clyde, *History of Medical Services in Tanganyika* (Dar-es-Salaam, Government Printer, 1962); E. E. Sabben-Clare, D. J. Bradley and K. Kirkwood, eds., *Health in Tropical Africa During the Colonial Period* (Oxford, Clarendon Press, 1980); M. Gelfand, *Tropical Victory: An Account of the Influence of Medicine on the History of Southern Rhodesia, 1900–1923* (Cape Town, Juta, 1953); O. Ransford, *Bid the Sickness Cease: Disease in the History of Black Africa* (London, John Murray, 1983).
2 P. Curtin, 'Epidemiology and the slave trade', *Political Science Quarterly*, 83 (1968), 190–216; H. Kjekshus, *Ecology Control and Economic Development in East African History: the Case of Tanganyika, 1850–1950* (London, Heinemann, 1977); G. W. Hartwig and K. D. Patterson, *Disease in African History: An Introductory Survey and Case Studies* (Durham, N.C., Duke University Press, 1978); World Health Organisation, Resolution WHA.30.49 of 1977, *World Health Chronicle*, 31 (1977), 428–32.
3 The collected papers of two conferences (sponsored by the Joint Africa Committee of the Social Science Research Council and the American Council of Learned Societies), 1978: J. M. Janzen and S. Feierman, eds., 'The social history of disease and medicine in Africa', *Social Science and Medicine*, 13b (December 1979); J. M. Janzen and G. Prins, eds., 'Causality and classification in African medicine and health', *Social Science and Medicine*, 15b (July 1981); P. S. Yoder, ed., *African Health and Healing Systems: Proceedings of a Symposium* (Los Angeles, Crossroads Press, 1982).
4 Founded in 1885 as the Congo Free State, the territory became the Belgian Congo in 1908 when it was transferred to the administration of the Belgian government. With independence in June 1960, the name was changed to the Republic of the Congo which it remained until 1974 when it was renamed Zaire as part of President Mobutu's policy of *authenticité*. I shall use Belgian Congo and Congolese.
5 London, Public Record Office [PRO], FO 367.215.42829, Campbell

to Grey; J. du Plessis, *Thrice Through the Dark Continent: A Record of Journeyings Across Africa During the Years 1913–16* (London, Longman, Green and Co., 1917), p. 143.

6 An endemic disease is present in a community and the social circumstances do not offer any effective barrier to its spread. Thus the common cold but not malaria, for instance, is likely to be endemic in a northern European city. An epidemic disease is one which appears among a population which has no immunity having not recently encountered the infection. The infection quickly spreads throughout the population until it 'peaks' and gradually subsides. Those people who survive will possess some degree of immunity but those people born in the intervals between outbreaks of that disease will most likely possess no immunity beyond that briefly inherited from their mothers. These new generations provide the physiolgical environments for new epidemics. In the mid-nineteenth century, however, 'epidemic' meant not that a disease was transmitted from the sick to the healthy but that it was simultaneously 'affecting large numbers of people under the influence of certain atmospheric or climatic and soil conditions to which "filth" was often added and the whole known as an "epidemic condition"'. N. H. Jones, *The Scientific Background of the International Sanitary Conferences, 1851–1938* (Geneva, World Health Organisation, 1975).

7 P. Curtin, S. Feierman, L. Thompson and J. Vansina, *African History* (London, Longman, 1978), p. 554.

8 J. Ford, *The Role of the Trypanosomiases in African Ecology: A Study of the Tsetse Fly Problem* (Oxford, Clarendon Press, 1971), p. 9.

9 D. H. Molyneux and R. W. Ashford, *The Biology of Trypanosoma and Leishmania, Parasites of Man and Domestic Animals* (London, Taylor and Francis, 1983), pp. 97–8; C. Lucasse, 'Present control of human sleeping sickness', *Annales de la Société Belge de Médecine Tropicale*, 44 (1964), 285–94, 287; P. G. Janssens, interviews 10 April 1982, 20 July 1982 and 11 April 1984.

10 N. E. Gallagher, *Medicine and Power in Tunisia, 1780–1900* (Cambridge University Press, 1983); W. McNeill, *Plagues and People* (Oxford, Basil Blackwell, 1977); F. F. Cartwright, *Disease and History* (London, Hart-Davis, 1972).

11 R. J. Morris, *Cholera 1832: The Social Response to an Epidemic* (London, Croom Helm, 1976); A. Briggs, 'Cholera and society in the nineteenth century', *Past and Present*, 19 (April 1961), 76–96; C. M. Cipolla, *Christofano and the Plague: A Study in the History of Public Health in the Age of Galileo* (London, Collins, 1973); M. W. Dols, *The Black Death in the Middle East* (Princeton University Press, 1977); P. Richards, 'Ecological change and the politics of African land use', *African Studies Review*, 26 (1983), 1–72.

12 D. Arnold, ed., *Imperial Medicine and Indigenous Societies* (Manchester University Press, 1988); R. MacLeod and M. Lewis, eds., *Disease, Medicine and Empire: Perspectives on Western Medicine and the Experience of European Expansion* (London, Routledge, 1988); R. Headrick, 'The impact of

colonialism on health in French Equatorial Africa, 1880–1934' (Ph.D. thesis, University of Chicago, 1987).

13 M. Shapiro, 'Medicine in the service of colonialism: medical care in Portuguese Africa, 1885–1974' (Ph.D. dissertation, University of California, Los Angeles, 1983); F. Fanon, 'Medicine and colonialism', in J. Ehrenreich, ed., *The Cultural Crisis of Modern Medicine* (New York, Monthly Review Press, 1978); Gallagher, *Medicine and Power.*

14 T. O. Ranger, 'Godly medicine: the ambiguities of mission medicine in southeast Tanzania, 1900–45', *Social Science and Medicine*, 15B (1981), 261–78; M. Worboys, 'Science and British colonial imperialism, 1895–1940' (Ph.D. dissertation, University of Sussex, 1979), p. 83.

15 T. McKeown, *The Role of Medicine: Dream, Mirage or Nemesis?* (Oxford, Blackwell, 1979).

16 A. Learmonth, *Patterns of Disease and Hunger* (Newton Abbot, David and Charles, 1978), p. 54.

17 L. Doyal and I. Pennel, *The Political Economy of Health* (London, Pluto Press, 1979); McKeown, *The Role of Medicine*; A. S. Wohl, *Endangered Lives: Public Health in Victorian Britain* (London, Methuen, 1984).

18 Learmonth, *Patterns of Disease*, p. 15; J. M. May, *The Ecology of Human Disease* (New York, MD Publications, Inc., 1958), p. xxiii; M. Howe, 'Environmental factors in disease'. in J. Leniham and W. W. Fletcher, eds., *Health and Environment* (London, Blackie, 1976), p. 21; L. D. Stamp, *Some Aspects of Medical Geography* (Oxford University Press, 1964); see articles by C. M. Good, M. J. Azavedo, M. De Lancey in Hartwig and Patterson, *Disease in African History.*

19 McKeown, *The Role of Medicine*, p. xvi.

20 F. Marti-Ibanez, 'Medical geography and history', in May, *The Ecology of Human Disease*, p. xi.

2 From private empire to public colony

1 J. Stengers, 'The Congo Free State and the Belgian Congo before 1914', in L. H. Gann and P. Duignan, eds., *Colonialism in Africa, 1870–1960*, vol. I (Cambridge University Press, 1969), p. 274.

2 Ford, *The Role*, p. 463; Curtin *et al.*, *African History*, p. 554.

3 In 1930 the Belgian Congo consisted of 2,350,000 square kilometres.

4 Archives of the Musée Royal de l'Afrique Centrale, Tervuren, Belgium. Section Historique [MRAC] 50.30.372, 1 December 1913. Dr Jerome Rodhain report of Uere-Bili sleeping sickness survey; Ministère des Affaires Etrangères, Archives Africaines, Brussels. Service de l'Hygiène [MAEAA] 4408.2, 12 June 1912, District Commissioner [DC] Meulemaere, Bambili to Governor-General [GG][MAEAA 4408.2, 2 August 1912, GG to Minister [Min.]. This epidemic is discussed in chapters 7 and 8.

5 On Afro-Arab traders, see P. Ceulemans, *La Question Arabe et le Congo (1883–1892)* (Brussels, Académie Royale des Sciences Coloniales, 1959). Traders from the north, or the Sudan, were known variously as

'Khartoumers' (where many had been based since the early 1820s), Soudanese, Danaqla or Jallaba. *Danaqla* were people of Dongolawi ancestry who often formed the military escort for the traders. *Jallaba* were traders from the northern provinces of Kordofan and Darfur, themselves often of Dongolawi ancestry. P. M. Holt, 'Egypt and the Nile Valley', in *The Cambridge History of Africa*, vol. V, 1790–1870, ed. J. E. Flint (Cambridge, Cambridge University Press, 1976), 36–8. Those coming into Congo from the south-east were called variously Zanzibaris, Waungwana, Panga-panga and Matamba-tamba. For the Waungwana, see D. K. Bimanyu, 'The Waungwana of Eastern Zaire: 1880–1900' (Ph.D. dissertation, University of London, 1977). See also P. Salmon, 'L'Etat Indépendant du Congo et la Question Arabe (1885–1892)', *Le Centenaire de l'Etat Indépendant du Congo* (Brussels, Académie Royale des Sciences d'Outre-Mer, 1988), 437–60.

6 For traders' *zeribas*, or fortified encampments, see J. R. Gray, *A History of the Southern Sudan, 1829–1889* (Oxford University Press, 1961), 58–69. *Zeribas* usually contained thirty to eighty 'settler-agents' together with their slaves. Some controlled extensive areas. For instance, the traveller, Georg Schweinfurth in 1869 estimated that the Coptic trader, Ghattas, controlled some 3,000 square miles with about 13,000 people. W. Junker, *Travels in Africa, 1879–1889* (London, Chapman and Hall, 1890–2), vol. II, pp. 372, 432; L. Lotar, 'Souvenirs de l'Uele', *Congo*, 1 (1933), 658.

7 Based in Cairo, this southerly extension of the Ottoman Empire had by the mid-nineteenth century reached present-day northern Zaire.

8 For a discussion of the effects of traders on pre-colonial African society, see C. A. Keim, 'Long-distance trade and the Mangbetu', *Journal of African History*, 24 (1983), 1–22. Other sources include: R. O. Collins, 'Sudanese factors in the history of the Congo and Central West Africa in the nineteenth century', in Ysuf Fadl Hasan, ed., *Sudan in Africa* (University of Khartoum, 1971), and for the southern Sudan, Gray, *A History of the Southern Sudan*; Junker, *Travels in Africa*, vol. II, p. 255.

9 Later known as Stanleyville; in 1974 renamed Kisangani.

10 Between 24 and 27 October 1891, Captain Ponthier was said to have commented on victims at the conclusion of a massive battle at the Bomokandi river. H. L. Duke and L. Van Hoof, 'Epidemiology of sleeping-sickness in the Upper Uele (Belgian Congo)', *Final Report of the League of Nations International Commission on Human Trypanosomiasis* (Geneva, 1928), p. 346. Their source was Dr Emile Van Campenhout of the Belgian colonial medical service who, himself, reported that he had seen a victim of sleeping sickness at Djabbir in Uele district in 1892. E. Van Campenhout, 'Prophylaxie de la maladie du sommeil', in *XIII Congrès Internationale d'Hygiène et de Démographie* (Brussels, 1903), vol. VIII, p. 2.

11 The colonial literature on the so-called 'Arab wars' stressed the benevolent role of the Congo Free State in ridding eastern and northern Congo of 'evil slave traders'. Examples of the titles which convey the 'crusading' flavour include E. Muller, *Ouelle: Terre d'Héroisme* (Brussels, Editions l'Essor, 1941); Dr Meyers, *Le Prix d'un Empire* (Brussels, Charles Dessart, 1943);

Ch. Liebrechts, *Léopold II: Fondateur d'un Empire* (Brussels, Office Publicité, 1932); S. Hinde, *The Fall of the Congo Arabs* (London, Methuen, 1897); Commandant Renier, *Héroisme et Patriotisme des Belges: l'Oeuvre Civilisatrice au Congo* (Ghent, Heckenrath, 1913); and Ligue du Souvenir Congolais, *A Nos Heros Morts Pour la Civilisation (1876–1908)* (Brussels, Ligue, 1931).

12 J. Stengers and J. Vansina, 'King Léopold's Congo 1886–1908', in *The Cambridge History of Africa*, vol. VI, eds. R. O. Oliver and G. N. Sanderson (Cambridge University Press, 1985), p. 334.

13 B. T. Fialkowski, *John L. Todd 1876–1949. Letters* (Senneville, Quebec, privately printed, 1977) (henceforth Todd, *Letters*), letter of 2 October 1903 to his family in Canada.

14 Leopold to reporter on 30 August 1892. J. Stengers, 'The Congo Free State and the Belgian Congo before 1914', *Colonialism in Africa 1870–1960*, vol. II, eds. L. H. Gann and P. Duignan (Cambridge University Press, 1969), p. 286.

15 Stengers, 'The Congo Free State', p. 274.

16 Ministère des Affaires Etrangères et du Commerce Extérieur. Archives Africaines. [Madame Van Grieken], *Décrets de l'Etat Indépendant du Congo Non-Publiés au Bulletin Officiale (1886–1908)* (2 vols., Brussels, 1967).

17 Great Britain. Intelligence Report, Egypt (Confid.), no. 8, November 1892 stated that there were 'some 4,000 well-armed natives, with several guns, under command of Capt. Vander Kerkhove [sic] and some 50 Belgian officers'. The Egypt and Sudan Intelligence Reports are useful in this regard as the British kept a particularly close watch between 1892 and 1910 on all Congo Free State movements in the disputed territory known as the Lado enclave. To give an idea of the numbers involved, in 1900, 1,500 Free State troops were reported to be posted among the three stations of Kiro, Lado and Redjaf on the Nile. In April 1902 there were 200–300 men with guns at Dufile; in January 1903, estimates of total troops in the enclave were between 1,500 and 2,000, while February 1904 estimates gave 2,300 infantry, including two battalions with Krupp guns and between six and twelve maxim guns. In April 1904, 2,600 members of the Congolese army, the Force Publique, including 200 artillery men were reported present in the enclave. On 9 May 1906, the Congo Free State, under pressure from the British to withdraw from their occupation of the enclave, agreed to limit the number of troops to 450. See Sudan Intelligence Reports: 107, 108, 115, 117, 132, 135 and 149; PRO, FO 403.304.93, 5 March 1900, Captain Moreton F. Gage, Fort Berkeley, Equatoria, memorandum on Belgium administration on the Upper Nile.

18 Rhodes House, Oxford. Lt. Alexander Boyd Mss., 20 April to 18 November 1906; PRO, FO 367.259.2447, 21 January 1911, J. P. Armstrong to Sir E. Grey, 'Report on conditions of natives in the Uele District'; FO 367.323.31211, 3 July 1913, H. C. Johnson to Gen. Wilson; De Keyser article of 29 July 1906 in *La Belgique Coloniale*; MRAC 54.95.70, 22 November 1892 and MRAC 54.95.75, 12 December 1895, Emile Christiaens' letters to brother Felix.

19 Founded in 1886 the Force Publique became the largest colonial army in sub-Saharan Africa. By January 1891 there were 3,127 troops and 49 per cent of the Congo Free State budget was devoted to the army. In the early days the State recruited large numbers of men from West Africa and these men were often referred to by the generic term, 'Houssas', or Hausas. Between 1883 and 1901, 12,452 recruits came from the Gold Coast, Liberia, Abyssinia, Somalia, Egypt, Dahomey, Zanzibar, Hausaland and Sierra Leone. By 1914, there were about 18,000 men in the army. F. Flament, ed., *La Force Publique de sa Naissance à 1914* (Brussels, Académie Royale des Sciences d'Outre-Mer, 1952); see also: S. J. S. Cookey, 'West African immigrants in the Congo in the nineteenth century', *Journal of the Historical Society of Nigeria*, 3 (1965), 261–70.
20 J. S. Galbraith, 'Gordon, MacKinnon and Leopold: the scramble for Africa, 1876–84', *Victorian Studies*, 14 (1971), 369–88. G. Casati, *Ten Years in Equatoria and the Return of Emin Pasha* (London, Frederick Warne & Co., 1891; reprinted ed., New York, Negro Universities Press, 1969), vol. I, p. 288. Casati reported that the Danaqla had armed their slaves who moved 'north . . . robbing and spreading terror'.
21 Flament, *La Force Publique*, p. 125; Brussels, Belgium. *Archives Palais Royal* [APR] 102/79. 30 December 188. Leopold II to H. M. Stanley. After congratulating Stanley on having reached Emin Pasha, Leopold expressed the hope that he had 'improved' the frontier of the Congo State either by means of treaties with chiefs 'or any other way dictated by your great experience and unparalleled ability'. Leopold continued that he wanted harbours on the different lakes in the east and a 'few good positions in the Bahr el-Ghazal to prevent the Mahdi invading the Congo'. D. Bates, *The Fashoda Incident of 1898: Encounter on the Nile* (Oxford University Press, 1984), p. 57. 'It was said in the competition for control of upper Nile whoever had the Azande on their side would come out on top.'
22 See C. Denuit-Somerhausen, 'Les traités de Stanley et de ses collaborateurs avec les chefs africains, 1880–1885', in *Le Centenaire de l'Etat Indépendant du Congo: Receuil d'Etudes* (Brussels, Académie Royale des Sciences d'Outre-Mer, 1988), 77–146.
23 Flament, *La Force Publique*, annexe 14, 'l'Expédition Van Kerckhoven dans l'Uele', p. 519; *Le Mouvement Géographique*, 9 (27 November 1892). In 1891, there were eight doctors in the Congo Free State. Dr J. Emile Van Campenhout, assigned to the Van Kerckhoven expedition, had few medical supplies, consisting only of a little quinine, no chloroform, many purgatives and no microscope; and instead of his surgical instruments, he had been provided with veterinarian tools by mistake.
24 MAEAA, Affaires Etrangères, [AE] 288, Mission Lemaire 1903–7. 16 January 1906, C. Lemaire to GG; MRAC 54.95.73, 18 June 1894, DC Francqui, Makrakas, arrived at Surango post with 225 coastal reinforcements; Intelligence Report, Egypt, no. 8, November 1892, reported Van Kerckhoven in south-west Bahr el-Ghazal with fifty Belgian officers and 4,000 well-armed Africans.

254   *Notes to pp. 18–23*

25 Ceulemans, *La Question Arabe*, pp. 326–30; *Le Mouvement Géographique*, 9 (18 September 1892).
26 MRAC 54.95.74, 10 October 1893, E. Christiaens to brother. D. Vangroenweghe and J.-L. Vellut, eds., 'Le rapport Casement', *Enquêtes et Documents d'Histoire Africaine*, 6 (1985), i.
27 C. Janssen in A. de Calonne-Beaufaict, *La Pénétration de la Civilisation au Congo Belge et les Bases d'une Politique Coloniale* (Brussels, Institut de Sociologie Solvay, 1912), p. 76; Ceulemans, *La Question Arabe*, pp. 329–30.
28 MRAC 50.30.25, 13 January 1917, TA Hurlet, Zobia, Rapport Annuel 1916; MRAC, Section Ethnographique, Etudes 69 and 73, 17 July 1914. A. Landeghem, 'Etude sur Babua'; *Le Mouvement Géographique*, 16 (22 April 1906); R. du Bourg de Bozas, *Mission Scientifique du Bourg de Bozas de la Mer Rouge à l'Atlantique à Travers l'Afrique Tropicale (Octobre 1900–Mai 1903)* (Paris, F. R. de Rudeval, 1906), pp. 423–4. He reported that there was 'severe war' and he saw terrible devastation between Libokwa and Buta.
29 12 September 1898, Post Chief [PC] Bima, Sous-Lt. E. Boone; 24 December 1899, Letter to *Le Mouvement Antiesclavage*, 6 (December 1899, pp. 239–41).
30 FO 403.304.93, memorandum of 5 March 1900, Capt. Gage, 'On Belgian administration on the Upper Nile'; Sudan Intelligence Report, 87, Jan.–Mar. 1900. Evidence of Mr Grogan, Capt. Gage and Dr Milne; Bozas, *Mission Scientifique*, p. 372.
31 Rhodes House, Oxford. Hobbis Harris Papers, J. C. McLaren, 'Congo Atrocities'; *Western Daily Mercury*, Plymouth, 7 March 1907; Lt. A. Boyd Mss., entries for 2, 4 and 22 August 1906.
32 P. Salmon, *Les Zandes Sous l'Administration Belge 1908–1980* (Paris, Comptes Rendus Séances de l'Académie des Sciences d'Outre-mer, 1971), pp. 99–100; P. Salmon, *La Reconnaissance Graziani Chez les Sultans du Nord de l'Uele, 1908* (Brussels, Centre Scientifique et Médical de l'Université Libre de Bruxelles en Afrique Centrale (Cemubac), 1963); see chapter 7, 'The Uele survey and Gwane epidemic'.
33 FO 367.69.24474, 4 June 1907, G. B. Michell to C. F. Cromie.
34 MAEAA, Affaires Indigènes, [AI] 1372, 15 January 1911, Zone Chief [ZC] Acerbi, 'Rapport annuel 1910, Zone Bomokandi'; Armstrong, 'Report on conditions of natives'.
35 MAEAA, AI 1372, 15 January 1911, ZC Acerbi, 'Rapport annuel 1910, Zone Bomokandi'; AI 1372, DC de Meulenaer, 'Rapport annuel 1912, Zone Bomokandi'; AI 1422, 31 January 1910, DC Bertrand, 'Rapport mensuel, Zone Bomokandi', Bomokandi zone was some 1,000 kilometres by 3–4,000 kilometres with a total of twenty-five State agents, one *chef de zone*, one *chef de secteur* and 470 soldiers spread among twelve posts. There was no doctor in 1911.
36 MRAC 50.30.156, 12 July 1915, DC Acerbi, Niangara to DC Landeghem, Buta; MRAC 50.30.156, 1 March 1915, Acerbi to Landeghem; MRAC 50.30.156, 27 February 1915, Acerbi to Landeghem;

MRAC 50.30.91, 5 February 1915, Territorial Administrator [TA] Thuysbaert, Bondo to Landeghem; MRAC 50.30.90, 16 March 1915, Landeghem to TA, Ibembo; MRAC 50.30.91, 16 March 1915, Landeghem to TA Bondo; MRAC 50.30.91, 5 April 1915, TA Brussels, Belgium to TA Thuysbaert, Bondo; MRAC 50.30.93, 6 June 1918, Vice Governor-General [VGG] de Meulemeester, circular to all administrators, re: 'Lugwaret Rebellion'.

37 MRAC 50.30.27, December 1918, TA Bambili, annual report; MAEAA R/CB 150.1, 5 February 1932, Dr Marone's report of the 1931 sleeping sickness survey; R/CB 151.1, 21 May 1932, Dr Fontana's report of the 1931 survey.

38 K. R. S. Morris, Letter to the Editor, *East African Medical Journal*, 38 (September 1961), 432–4; K. R. S. Morris, 'The epidemiology of sleeping sickness in East Africa. Part 5: Epidemics on the Albert Nile', *Transactions of the Royal Society of Tropical Medicine and Hygiene*, 56 (1962); J. J. McKelvey Jr, *Man Against Tsetse: Struggle for Africa* (Ithaca, Cornell University Press, 1973), pp. 34–5.

3 *Mise en valeur*: economic exploitation

1 J. Wauters, *Le Congo au Travail* (Brussels, l'Eglantine, 1924); A. Bertrand, *Le Problème de la Main de l'Oeuvre au Congo Belge: Province Orientale* (Brussels, Ministère des Colonies, 1931); C. F. A. Lemaire, *Au Congo: Comment les Noirs Travaillent* (Brussels, Bulens, 1895); S. J. S. Cookey, 'West African immigrants in the Congo, 1885–1896', *Journal of the Historical Society of Nigeria*, 3 (1965), 261–70; Dr Daco, 'Le problème de la main d'oeuvre indigene au Congo belge', *Bruxelles-Médical*, 21; 22; 23 (March–April 1929); Dr Daco, 'The problem of native labour in the Belgian Congo', *International Review of Missions*, 14 (1925), 536–44.

2 Wellcome Institute for the History of Medicine, London [WIHM]. Manuscript collection. Diaries and notebooks of J. L. Todd and J. E. Dutton, 1904–5 Congo Free State; J. E. Dutton and J. L. Todd, 'The distribution and spread of "sleeping sickness" in the Congo Free State with suggestions on prophylaxis: being the fourth progress report of the expedition of the Liverpool School of Tropical Medicine to the Congo, 1903–05', in *Memoir XVIII* (Liverpool School of Tropical Medicine, March 1906), pp. 25–38.

3 MAEAA 4461.230, December 1926, Report by Drs Duke and Van Hoof, enclosed in 15 February 1927, Van Campenhout to Minister [Min].

4 Lemaire, *Au Congo*, p. 64; Capt. A. M. G. Daenen, *Le Mouvement Géographique*, 12 (1895), 92–3.

5 MRAC 5495.75, 24 October 1893, Emile Christiaens, Commandant, Niangara to Lt. Verstraeten, re: Ch. Lemaire.

6 MAEAA, AI 1370, 31 October 1898, Sector Chief [SC] Tengele, Yakoma Post, 'Renseignements sur la main d'oeuvre au Congo' (21 pages).

7 MRAC 50.30.1, 28 July 1910, Rodhain's 1916 report on this question;

MRAC 50.30.218, 1 June 1915, DC Landeghem, Bondo, circular. Tax defaulters were forced to act as porters for the state; MRAC 50.30.91, 5 May 1915, TA Heinzmann, Buta. Thirty *corvéed* people rescued by kin; MRAC 50.30.25, 13 January 1917, TA Hurlet, Zobia, annual report for 1916; MRAC 50.30.378, 22 September 1917, Dr Fauconnier, Buta, first semester report.

8 MRAC 50.30.146, 14 December 1914, DC Acerbi, Niangara to DC, Buta. Acerbi reported that the Kilo-Moto mines offered chiefs a ten franc bonus per labourer or twelve francs if the wife accompanied him during a three-year contract; MRAC 50.30.166, 24 March 1916, Sous-Directeur, Moto mines to DC Landeghem. Chiefs' bonuses were now ten francs for each three-year contract undertaken; FO 367.259.2447, Armstrong, 'Report on conditions of natives'; MAEAA, AI 1422.1, 'First semester 1928, District de l'Uele-Nepoko, Rapport sur l'administration générale'. For instance, in 1928 Kilo-Moto recruiters operated around Dungu, Niangara, Doruma and Poko and the district commissioner asked his administrators to act as intermediaries for them. Recruiters met Africans in the headquarters of the district and saw to it that they received a medical examination. They arranged an allowance for food and arranged transport by lorry (although most often the Africans had to walk) to a 'camp de concentration' from where the Africans were later assigned to specific mining sites.

9 MRAC 50.30.539, 1 October 1918, list of *corvées*.

10 A. Bakonzi, 'The gold mines of Kilo-Moto in northeastern Zaire: 1905–1960', (2 vols., Ph.D. dissertation, University of Wisconsin, 1982); FO 367.363.56226, 1 December 1918, Kitchener to Grey re: Kilo-Moto gold mines' 'difficulties of labour' in 1912. Approximately 1,000 Africans were working there then and women often engaged in heavy labour; G. Moulaert, *Vingt Années à Kilo Moto, 1920–40* (Brussels, Charles Dessart, 1950).

11 MAEAA 839.23, 31 January 1913, Kilo-Moto second semester medical report, 1912; Bakonzi, 'Gold mines', vol. II, pp. 148–9 and 158, reports that between 1905 and 1919 Africans did *not* volunteer but were sent by their chiefs and administrators to the mines; MAEAA, Main d'Oeuvre Indigène [MOI] 3603.167, 12 November 1919, Ch. Scheyraerts' report of his inspection of the Kilo-Moto mines; J.-L. Vellut, 'Mining in the Belgian Congo',in D. Birmingham and P. M. Martin, eds., *History of Central Africa* (Harlow, Essex, Longman, 1983), p. 141; MRAC 50.30.146, 14 December 1914, DC Acerbi, Niangara to DC, Buta; L. J. Vanden Bergh, *On the Trail of the Pigmies* (London, Fisher Unwin, 1922), p. 229. This eyewitness described the scarcity of African labour at the mines, which retarded their exploitation; MAEAA, Rapports Congo Belge [R/CB] 151.1, Dr Marone's 1931 report of sleeping sickness survey of Uele; MRAC 50.30.90, 29 June 1915, DC Landeghem to VGG; MRAC 50.30.156, 2 December 1915, VGG Malfeyt to DC; MRAC 50.30.16, May 1916, Landeghem's annual report for Bas-Uele, 1915; MRAC 50.30.166, 24 March 1916, Sous-Directeur, Moto Mines to DC

Landeghem. The wages were six francs per month plus an indemnity of six francs for a cover, salt and food.

12 Bakonzi, 'Gold mines', vol. II, pp. 148–9 and 410; MAEAA R/CB 151.1, Dr L. Fontana, Annual report of Medical Service for Province Orientale, 1931. He reported that forty-six firms in the province employed 61,190 labourers. In 1928 a subsidiary company, Minière de Tele, operated eight mining camps in the Nepoko region and employed 2,081 labourers; MAEAA AI 1422.1, 'First semester 1928, District de l'Uele-Nepoko. Rapport sur l'administration générale'.

13 MAEAA 838.23, 1906, Dr Grossule, Basoko, Sanitary report; MAEAA R/CB 149.4, Dr Mouchet, Annual report of Medical Servcice, 1923; MAEAA 839.4, 5 May 1909, Dr Abetti, Kilo, Medical report.

14 MRAC 50.30.166, 24 March 1916, Sous-Directeur, Moto mines to DC Landeghem; MRAC 50.30.156, 23 December 1915, General Commissioner [GC] Mertens, Stanleyville, to DC, Buta; MRAC 50.30.91, 4 May 1915, DC Landeghem to TA, Buta.

15 M. Mulambu, 'Cultures obligatoires et colonisation dans l'ex-Congo Belge', *Cahiers du Cedaf*, 6–7 (1974), pp. 7; 15–16 and 28; A. Moeller de Laddersous, 'Les origins et l'introduction de la culture de coton au Congo Belge', in A. de Bauw, ed., *Trente Années* (Brussels, Compagnie Cotonnière, c. 1945), 14–18.

16 J.-L. Vellut, 'The "classical" age of Belgian Colonialism: outline for a social history (1910–40)', paper presented at African History seminar, School of Oriental and African Studies, London, 1978, p. 6; Laddersous, 'Les origins'; MAEAA 156.1, Annual report for Uele-Nepoko, 1930.

17 17 August 1982, Brussels. Interview with M. Houssiau, former director of Compagnie Cotonnière Congolaise (Cotonco), Province Orientale. He implemented the cotton scheme in Lower Uele in 1927 and remained in the region until 1970, eventually becoming a company director; 2 August 1982, Brussels. Interview with Francis Busschots, Administrateur-Délégué, Cotoni, Brussels. Busschots was in Province Orientale from 1945 until 1972. Cotoni sold its Uelian interests in 1972. In the area from which Cotoni had extracted 50,000 tons of cotton before independence in 1960, the new company extracted only 5,000 in 1981.

18 American University, *Area Handbook for the Democratic Republic of the Congo* (Washington, US Government Printer, 1971), p. 379; L. Franck, *Le Congo Belge* (2 vols., Brussels, La Renaissance du livre, 1930), vol. I, p. 223; Mulambu, 'Cultures', pp. 6–7; American University, *Area Handbook*, p. 492; Bertrand, *Le Problème*, p. 27; MAEAA R/CB 156.1, 'Rapport sur l'administration général de la District de l'Uele-Nepoko, 1930'.

19 H. Waltz, *Das Konzessionwesen im Belgischen Congo* (Iena, 1917), vol. I, p. 20.

20 A. Boyd, diary entry for 29 July 1906.

21 FO 367.259.2447, 21 January 1911, Armstrong to Grey; FO 367.215.42829, 25 November 1911, Acting Consul Campbell to Grey, Confidential report on changes under new Belgian government. Until Uele was 'opened' to free trade on 1 July 1912, annual tax was ½–1

kilogram of rubber in the Uere-Bili zone; ⅕–2⅖ kilograms in the Bomokandi zone and 1–2 kilograms in the Rubi zone. All adult males' tax was five to twelve francs per annum plus two francs for each wife up to a maximum of sixty francs.

22 MRAC 50.30.156, 23 July 1915, VGG Malfeyt, circular.

23 MAEAA 850.9, 1917 fourth quarter, DC Landeghem, Report on general administration of Bas-Uele, containing note to Bertrand.

24 MRAC 50.30.167, 20 December 1915, TA Hurlet, Zobia to DC, Buta.

25 MRAC 50.30.26, First semester 1918, DC, Bas-Uele, Report on general administration. The forced labour used for hygiene works could not have endeared public health policy to Africans.

26 MRAC 50.30.218, 1 June 1916, DC Landeghem, Bondo, public notice.

27 MRAC 50.30.91, 5 May 1915, TA Heinzmann, Buta.

28 Ford, *The Role*, p. 463; MAEAA 855.13, 20 April 1910, A. Bertrand, Note appended to Drs Neri, Nagels and Marchal, Hygiene Commission, Bomokandi zone report. 'Our workers . . . are only children'.

4 Epidemiology and ecology of human sleeping sickness

1 Epidemiologists have proposed a number of models to explain disease patterns. Evocative terminologies such as 'epidemiological triangle' (J. P. Fox, C. E. Hall and L. Elveback, *Epidemiology, Man and Disease* (London, Collier-Macmillan, 1970)), the 'web of causation' (Brian MacMahon and Thomas F. Pugh, *Epidemiology: Principles and Methods* (Boston, Little, Browne & Co., 1970)) and 'the wheel of causation' (Judith S. Mausner and Anita K. Bahn, *Epidemiology: an Introductory Text* (Philadelphia, W. B. Saunders, 1974)), describe vividly the idea of interaction among factors. Interview with Professor R. Mansell-Prothero, Liverpool, England, 14 February 1985.

2 N. H. Jones, *The Scientific Background to the International Sanitary Conferences, 1851–1938* (Geneva, World Health Organisation, 1975), p. 12. Between 1852 and 1903 there were thirteen international hygiene conferences – three in Belgium. The mid-nineteenth century was a period of 'reform' in Europe. R. Sand, *La Belgique Sociale* (Brussels, 1933), p. 72.

3 Maria Lancisi published a book on the subject in 1717, *De Noxiis Paludum Effluviis*. The French term for malaria, *paludisme*, from the Latin *palus* (swamp) is another example of the underlying idea of disease causation. Wohl, *Endangered Lives*, p. 87; G. Harrison, *Mosquitoes, Malaria and Man: A History of the Hostilities since 1880* (London, John Murray, 1978), pp. 24–5; A. Briggs, 'Cholera and society in the nineteenth century', *Past and Present*, 19 (1961), 76–96; F. F. Cartwright, *A Social History of Medicine* (London, Longman, 1977), pp. 20, 123, 138–41; R. J. Morris, *Cholera 1832: the Social Response to an Epidemic* (London, Croom Helm, 1976).

4 A. Palmberg, *A Treatise on Public Health and its Applications in Different European Countries* (London, 1893), pp. 229, 255; Sand, *La Belgique Sociale*, p. 72. Cholera epidemics in Belgium occurred between 1832 and 1892/3; Wohl, *Endangered Lives*.

5 Lazarets derived from the Italian practice in the Middle Ages when, during time of plague, a building was designated as a 'pest-house', or *lazaretto*; earlier still, lepers (Lazarus) had been isolated in these places. See C. M. Cipolla, *Christofano and the Plague: a Study in the History of Public Health in the Age of Galileo* (London, Collins, 1973), p. 24. The Belgians and the French concentrated at home more on a dispensary system than a sanatorium system like Germany's to deal with tuberculosis victims. There were Belgians, however, who strongly propounded more direct state intervention with the provision of sanatoria or hospitals for the poor. *XIII Congrès International de l'Hygiène et Démographie* (Brussels, 1903), vol. VI, pp. 82, 85.

  The 1885 Epidemiology Conference at Antwerp concluded that the main measures the state should utilise were those of isolation and disinfection. However, because Belgium was so densely populated (1885: 5,853,272; 1900: 6,693,100 (*XIII Congrès*, annexe B, vol. VI, 6th Section) it was recognised that the practice and control of isolation would be imperfect, at best. So the theory evolved of the cordon sanitaire with observation posts to check all travellers, and lazarets in which to isolate the infected persons. By 1893, Brussels still did not possess *one* isolation lazaret and victims of contagious diseases were kept either at home or in special sections of hospitals. By 1903, European epidemiologists were still debating the value of sanatoria. The Germans pursued this policy and one establishment was under way at Liège in Belgium near the German border.

6 M. Worboys, 'Tropical medicine and colonial imperialism, 1895–1914', in 'Science and British colonial imperialism, 1895–1940' (Ph.D. dissertation, University of Sussex, 1979). The author suggests that by describing problems in the colonial context as 'technical' rather than 'structural', the administration could rationalise making adjustments to its policies rather than admit the deeper socio-economic problems. In this way, it could justify simply transferring to Africa European-derived ideology and technology.

7 MAEAA 839.4, 1 November 1907, Dr Hosselet, 'Rapport sanitaire', Meridi Territory; MAEAA 834.15, 9 July 1908, Dr Grossule, 'Rapport Sanitaire', Basoko-Aruwimi Territory; MAEAA 841.6, 10 October 1908, Dr Haavik, 'Rapport Sanitaire', Rubi Territory. See also John Ford, the British entomologist, on 'invasion' theory which was long accepted by most medical thinking: 'Ideas which have influenced attempts to solve the problem of African trypanosomiasis', *Social Science and Medicine*, 13b (1979), p. 272; Ford said that it was a principal object of his seminal study, *The Role of the Trypanosomiases in African Ecology*, 'to show that notions of the circumstantial epidemiology of trypanosomiasis put forward in the first quarter of the century, even in its first decade, are long out of date' (p. 467).

8 On population movements see: R. Mansell-Prothero, 'Population mobility and trypanosomiasis in Africa', *Bulletin of the World Health Organisation*, 28 (1963), 615–28; R. Mansell-Prothero, *People and Land in Africa South of the Sahara: Readings in Social Geography* (Oxford University Press,

1972); R. Mansell-Prothero, 'Disease and human mobility: a neglected factor in epidemiology', *International Journal of Epidemiology*, 6 (1977), 259–67; K. R. S. Morris, 'The epidemiology of sleeping sickness in East Africa', *Transactions of the Royal Society of Tropical Medicine and Hygiene* 54 (1960); K. R. S. Morris, 'The movement of sleeping sickness across Central Africa', *Journal of Tropical Medicine and Hygiene*, 66 (1963), 159–76. A typical example of the misinformed view that pre-colonial Africans dared not venture far from their locales before the arrival of the 'civilising white man' is presented by O. Ransford, *Bid the Sickness Cease: Disease in the History of Black Africa* (London, John Murray, 1983); Ford, *The Role*, p. 390; J. N. P. Davies, Letter to Editor, *East African Medical Journal* (January 1961), 55. Davies suggests an alternative to the theory that it was Stanley who introduced sleeping sickness to eastern Africa.

9 J. Ford, 'Early ideas about sleeping sickness and their influence on research and control', in E. E. Sabben-Clare, D. J. Bradley and K. Kirkwood, eds., *Health in Tropical Africa During the Colonial Period* (Oxford University Press, 1980), p. 272; Morris, 'The movement'.

10 Morris, 'The movement'; H. H. Johnston, *George Grenfell and the Congo* (London, Hutchinson & Co., 1908), vol. II, p. 547; Great Britain, Colonial Office, Cd 7350 (London, 1914), Sleeping Sickness Committee. 'Minutes of evidence taken by the Departmental Committee on sleeping sickness', testimony of Sir H. H. Johnston, 25 November 1913. For the Sudanese left behind by the Emin Pasha relief expedition on 10 April 1889, see: F. R. Wingate, *Mahdism and the Egyptian Sudan* (London, 1891), p. 464; K. R. S. Morris, Letter to Editor, *East Africa Medical Journal*, 38 (1961), 432–4. The geographer, Brian W. Langlands, reported that some 8,000 people were introduced from the Congo–Nile watershed into Uganda. 'The sleeping sickness epidemic of Uganda 1900–1920: a study in historical geography', Paper presented to WHO course in parasitology, Makerere University College, May 1967.

11 W. B. Johnson, *Notes on a Journey Through Certain Belgian, French and British African Dependencies to Observe General Medical Organisation and Methods of Trypanosomiasis Control* (Lagos, Government Printer, 1929).

12 MAEAA 855.50, 12 December 1913, CG Zobia to GG Bertrand; MAEAA 849.336, 28 September 1912. Dr Van Campenhout recommended the destruction of the wild game reservoir based upon a report of the work of the British researchers, Kinghorn and Yorke. On 4 October 1912, the GG gave instructions to 'freely issue' hunting permits, especially for antelope, buffalo and boar; MAEAA 4403.408, 14 November 1913. Dr Van Campenhout suggested a predatory spider.

13 H. L. Duke and L. Van Hoof, 'Epidemiology of sleeping-sickness in the Upper Uele (Belgian Congo)', in *Final Report of the League of Nations International Commission on Human Trypanosomiasis* (Geneva, 1928).

14 F. M. J. C. Nevens, "Projet de plan général de l'organisation de la lutte contre les trypanosomiases en Afrique', *Bulletin de l'Académie Royale des Sciences d'Outre-Mer*, 17 (1965), 7.

15 Two forms of human sleeping sickness occur in Africa, the *gambiense* and

the more acute *rhodesiense* caused by *T.b. rhodesiense*. The latter is more common in the savannah woodlands of eastern and southern Africa, and is commonly transmitted by tsetse flies of the genus, *G. morsitans* (*G. morsitans, G. pallidipes* and *G. swynnertoni*). The *rhodesiense* form of the disease can cause death within weeks and, if left untreated, most victims die within a few months.

16 'Protective immune responses can be mediated by antibodies or by T cells. Antibodies protect by neutralizing the toxins of infecting agents, blocking penetration of microbes into cells, promoting inflammation and phagocytosis, inhibiting biochemical pathways of parasites or directly destroying parasites . . . and . . . A vaccine has to circumvent or overcome the strategies developed by parasites to evade the host's immune response.' UNDP/WorldBank/WHO, Special Programme for Research and Training in Tropical Diseases [TDR], 'Tropical disease research: a global partnership' (Geneva, WHO, 1987), p. 4. Humans are resistant to *T. brucei, T. congolense* and *T. vivax*, strains of trypanosomes which cause disease in animals, but they are susceptible to infection by *T. rhodesiense* and *T. gambiense* in Africa and to *T. cruzi*, which causes Chagas disease, in South America.

17 This characteristic has helped to make the trypanosome one of the most researched pathogenic parasites and a particular favourite with molecular biologists today. K. S. Warren, personal communication, 24 February 1988.

18 J. Ford, *The Role*, pp. 86–90; J. C. Boothroyd, 'Antigenic variation in African trypanosomiasis', *Annual Review of Microbiology*, 39 (1985), 475–502. Beyond the biological difficulty lies an economic obstacle, the reluctance of pharmaceutical firms to commit large sums to research and development on a disease which afflicts mainly rural, impoverished populations in Africa. L. G. Goodwin, 'Chemotherapy and tropical disease: the problem and the challenge', in M. Hooper, ed., *Chemotherapy of Tropical Diseases* (Chichester, Wiley, 1987), 1–18.

19 McNeill, *Plagues and People*. It should be noted that an important variant of this disease is its animal form, *nagana*. While the wild ungulate herds become trypotolerant, with few exceptions domestic cattle succumb to the disease. It should also be mentioned that the vast proportion of research and funding has been aimed at solving the problem of animal, not human, sleeping sickness.

20 F. L. Lambrecht, 'Aspects of evolution and ecology of tsetse flies and trypanosomiasis in prehistoric African environment', *Journal of African History*, 5 (1964), 1–24.

21 Ford, *The Role*, p. 90.

22 Ford, *The Role*, pp. 87, 243.

23 As recently as 1987, the World Health Organisation's Special Programme for Research and Training in Tropical Diseases urged the submission of proposals from scientists on the role of immunodepression as a possible cause of disease manifestation following infection by trypanosomes. *TDR News*, 24 (1987), WHO, Geneva, p. 6.

24 A. M. Jordan, *Trypanosomiasis Control and African Rural Development* (London, Longman, 1986).
25 Professor P. G. Janssens, personal interviews at Antwerp and Brussels, 10 April 1982, 20 July 1982 and 11 April 1984; Lambrecht, 'Aspects of evolution'; B. W. Langlands, 'The sleeping sickness epidemic of Uganda 1900–1920: a study in historical geography', presented to the World Health Organisation course in parasitology at Makerere University College, May 1967; C. Lucasse, 'Control of human sleeping sickness at present times', *Annales de la Société Belge de Médecine Tropicale*, 44 (1964), 285–94; M. T. Ashcroft, 'A critical review of the epidemiology of human trypanosomiasis in Africa', *Tropical Diseases Bulletin*, 56 (1959), 1073–93. The Russian epidemiologist, Pavlovski, regarded a natural focus of infection as biocoenosis: 'a linking together at a single locus, defined in terms of the inanimate environment ("landscape ecology") and the vegetation (basic food and shelter) of the parasite, its natural hosts, the vectors, and the adventitious hosts, in circumstances favouring maximum circulation of the parasite', in Ford, *The Role*, p. 311. It was from Pavlovski's work in Russia that the concept of 'natural foci' of infection, the 'nidality of disease', emerged. Epidemic conditions arise where the various organisms involved interact so that there is continual circulation of the pathogenic agent, via the vector, between the natural and the adventitious hosts. Such a biocoenosis can only occur where the environment is such that all its components can meet in favourable conditions of time and space. Ford, *The Role*, p. 10.
26 P. G. Janssens, personal interview, 20 July 1982; A. J. Duggan, 'An historical perspective', in H. W. Mulligan, ed., *The African Trypanosomiases* (London, Allen & Unwin, 1970).
27 C. Lucasse, 'Control of human sleeping sickness at present times', *Annales de la Société Belge de Médecine Tropicale*, 44 (1964), 285–94; J. F. Ruppol and L. Kazyumba, 'Situation actuelle de la lutte contre la maladie du sommeil au Zaire', *Annales de la Société Belge de Médecine Tropicale*, 57 (1977), 299–314.
28 Lucasse, 'Control', p. 287; interviews with P. G. Janssens.
29 Ford, *The Role*, p. 458.
30 Alphonse Jerome Rodhain (1876–1956) began his colonial career in Ubangi in 1903. He was Chief of the colonial Medical Service in 1920–4 and then returned to Belgium to become Director of the Prince Léopold Institute of Tropical Medicine in Belgium (1925–47). He suggested the possibility that a small focus of TB in Uele district, called *dingo* by the Azande, might have been introduced from the Sudan. J. Rodhain, 'Rapport sur la tuberculose humaine au Congo Belge', *Revista Médica de Angola*, 4 (August 1923), 203–125.
31 A. J. Rodhain, 'Quelques aspects de la pathologie indigène dans l'Ouelle', *Bulletin de la Société de Pathologie Exotique*, 8 (1915), 734–45, 739.
32 Believed to have been introduced into Uele district in 1918 from Uganda by African porters accompanying troops returning from the East African campaign. From there it spread through the districts of Ituri and Maniema

in 1919–20 until by 1925 it was present in endemic foyers in each province of the colony. Belgium, Colonie du Congo Belge, *Rapport sur l'Hygiène Publique pendant l'Année 1925; Rapport, 1928.*

33 C. C. Reining, *The Zande Scheme* (Evanston, Ill., Northwestern University Press, 1966), pp. 6–7.

34 D. Livingstone, *Missionary Travels and Researches in South Africa* (London, John Murray, 1857), pp. 80–3; J. E. Dutton and J. L. Todd, 'The distribution and spread of "sleeping sickness" in the Congo Free State with suggestions on prophylaxis: being the Fourth Progress Report from the expedition of the Liverpool School of Tropical Medicine to the Congo', 17 October 1905; MAEAA 831.383, 20 February 1912, ZC Ermingen, Uere, 'Rapport annuel Uere-Bili – Service Médical et Hygiène', re: Azande practices; WIHM, Western Manuscripts Collection, Ms. 2268, J. E. Dutton and J. L. Todd, Congo Expedition Diary, vol. 2, 2 July 1904 to 12 May 1905: entry of 12 July 1904 at Lukolela.

35 F. Lambrecht, Review of *Disease in African History* by G. W. Hartwig and K. D. Patterson, in *African Economic History*, 9 (1980), 163–4; P. G. Janssens, interview, Brussels, 11 April 1984; George S. Nelson, interview, Liverpool School of Tropical Medicine, 14 February 1985, discussed the dramatic ecological change in northern Kenya. Due to epidemic sleeping sickness in the 1920s, Acholi people were evacuated *en masse* from a large area east of the Nile and the region became an elephant sanctuary (Murchison Falls National Park). By the time Professor Nelson visited the area in 1962, an astonishing transformation had taken place: 'entire forests with chimps, colubus, lianas, forest guinea fowl . . . all the birds . . . had totally disappeared' and it was now all grassland. P. Gourou, *L'Afrique* (Paris, Hachette, 1970), p. 60.

36 A. J. Duggan, interview, London, 2 December 1983; Dr Adetokunbo O. Lucas, 'New strategies for controlling tropical diseases', 38th Ciba Foundation annual Lecture, 1 December 1988. Dr Lucas made the important point that it makes more sense to refer to so-called tropical disease as 'environmentally determined' diseases.

37 David Bruce made the important discovery in 1896 of the connection between a trypanosome and the animal form of sleeping sickness, *nagana*. A. D. P. Hodges, P.M.O., 'Report of East Africa and Uganda Protectorates', 22 December 1908. Only man and the fly should be considered agents for the spread of sleeping sickness – no animal reservoirs had been pinpointed; see also: Balfour, *Third Report of the Wellcome Research Laboratories* (supplement), 'Review of the recent advances in tropical medicine', p. 174; also: Great Britain, Colonial Office, Sleeping Sickness Committee, *Minutes of Evidence Taken by the Departmental Committee on Sleeping Sickness* (Cd 7350, June 1914), which concerned itself almost entirely with this issue.

38 WIHM, Ms. 2262, J. E. Dutton and J. L. Todd, Congo Expedition Diary, vol. 1, 1903–4: entry of 30 January 1904 based on information from Dr A. Broden, Director of the Leopoldville laboratory.

39 J. Van Riel and P. G. Janssens, 'Lutte contre les endémo-epidémies', in

Livre Blanc, vol. II (Brussels, Académie Royale des Sciences d'Outre-Mer, 1962), p. 917; McNeill, *Plagues and People*, pp. 20–1; P. E. C. Manson-Bahr, *Manson's Tropical Diseases*, 18th edn (London, Balliere Tindall, 1982), pp. 73, 795–6.

40 Ford, *The Role*, pp. 456, 458, 467, 473.

41 See G. D. H. Carpenter, *A Naturalist on Lake Victoria with an Account of Sleeping Sickness and the Tsetse Fly* (London, T. Fisher Unwin, 1920); W. F. Fiske, 'A history of sleeping sickness and reclamation in Uganda' (Entebbe, Government Printer, 6 May 1926); D. H. Molyneux and R. W. Ashford, *The Biology of Trypanosoma and Leishmania, Parasites of Man and Domestic Animals* (London, Taylor and Francis, 1983), ch. 3.

42 J. D. Tothill, 'A note on the origin of the soils of the Sudan from the point of view of the man in the field', in J. D. Tothill, ed., *Agriculture in the Sudan* (Oxford University Press, 1952 [1948]), pp. 102, 125.

43 E. L. Ladurie, *The Mind and Method of the Historian* (Brighton, Sussex, The Harvester Press, 1981), ch. 9, 'The crisis and the historian', pp. 270–89.

44 E. Stark, 'The epidemic as a social event', *International Journal of Health Services*, 7 (1977), 681–705.

45 Ford, *The Role*; Kjekshus, *Ecology Control*; Hartwig and Patterson, *Disease in African History*.

46 Ford, *The Role*, p. 494; Ford, 'Ideas', p. 272.

47 Kjekshus, *Ecology Control*, p. 160.

48 K. Hodnebo, 'Cattle and flies: a study of cattle-keeping in Equatoria province, the southern Sudan, 1850–1950' (Thesis, University of Bergen, November 1981).

49 Kjekshus, *Ecology Control*, p. 15; R. Mack, 'The great African cattle plague epidemic of the 1890s', *Tropical Animal Health and Production*, 2 (1970), 210–19; T. P. Ofcansky, 'The 1889–97 rinderpest epidemic and the rise of British and German colonialism in eastern and southern Africa', *Journal of African Studies*, 8 (1981), 31–8.

50 A. J. Duggan, interview, London, 2 December 1983.

51 Bakonzi, 'Gold mines', p. 39; E. Verleyen, *Congo: Patrimoine de la Belgique* (Brussels, Editions de Visscher, 1950), p. 155.

52 G. Schweinfurth, *The Heart of Africa*, 2 vols., translated by Ellen E. Frewer (New York, Harper & Brothers, 1873), vol. I, p. 493.

53 Junker, *Travels in Africa*, vol. I, pp. 114, 117; G. Schweinfurth, R. Ratzel, R. W. Felkin and G. Hartlaub, eds., *Emin Pasha in Central Africa: Being a Collection of His Letters and Journals* (London, George Philip & Son, 1888), p. 200.

54 Gourou, *L'Afrique*, p. 288; FO 367.259.2447, Armstrong to Grey, 'Report', 21 January 1911.

55 Lucasse, 'Control', p. 287.

56 Great Britain, Foreign Office, Africa no. 4, 'Correspondence respecting Mr Stanley's expedition for relief of Emin Pasha', February 1890.

57 Van Riel and Janssens, 'Lutte', p. 917. *Bilé* signifies forests in which water is found, particularly a river gallery. Azande referred to those among them

who lived in such forested regions near the Uele river as *abile*. V.-H. Vanden Plas and C.-R. Lagae, *La Langue des Azande*, 2 vols. (Ghent, Editions Dominicaines, 1921), vol. I, p. 37.

58 Junker, *Travels in Africa*, vol. II, pp. 115, 117.
59 Tothill, *Agriculture*, p. 50; P. M. Larken, 'Zande background', compiled and edited by T. A. T. Leitch (typescript, 1954), School of Oriental and African Studies Library.
60 Schweinfurth, *Heart of Africa*, vol. II, pp. 504–8; Junker, *Travels in Africa*, vol. II, p. 117.
61 Chorley, 'Effect of cloud on the behaviour of tsetse-fly', *Uganda Journal*, 5 (1938), 245–51; Wellcome Tropical Institute (WTI) Archives, 22 June 1962, A. J. Duggan to Secretary, Royal Observatory, Herstmonceux Castle, Herstmonceux, Sussex. Dr Duggan had noticed cyclical epidemics of sleeping sickness across western Sudan around 12 degrees north between 1850 and 1953 and as the temperature pattern is important for the development of the insect, he queried the possibility that there might be a correlation between sunspot activity and the appearance of epidemics. A response from P. S. Laurie, Royal Greenwich Observatory of 29 June 1966 revealed no such correlation between solar activity and epidemics. This query demonstrates the interesting type of questions raised in an examination of epidemiology.
62 A. W. Ireland, 'The climate of the Sudan', in Tothill, *Agriculture*, pp. 875–918; M. Robert, *Le Congo Physique* (Liège, Vaillant-Carmanne, 1946), p. 287.
63 Robert, *Le Congo Physique*, pp. 284, 286,. 291; Gourou, *L'Afrique*, p. 38. Temperatures can reach 38 degrees Centigrade. Ireland, 'Climate', pp. 62–83; Dominican House, Louvain, Belgium, *Le Propagateur du Rosaire*, 25 December 1913. R. P. Van Caloen, Amadis, to sister. Temperatures ranged from 32 degrees to 35 degrees Centigrade in the day to between 14 and 15 degrees Centigrade at night and the Africans complained of the cold.
64 McKelvey, *Man Against Tsetse*, p. 88; Molyneux and Ashford, *The Biology*, p. 65, say three to five months.
65 P. C. C. Garnham, 'Arthropods and disease', in J. Leniham and W. W. Fletcher, eds., *Health and Environment* (London, Blackie, 1976), p. 62.
66 The first food is often reptilian but man is always acceptable.
67 Ford, *The Role*, pp. 77–9.
68 Molyneux and Ashford, *The Biology*, p. 71.
69 Casati, *Ten Years*, p. 234.
70 Robert du Bourg de Bozas, *Mission Scientifique du Bourg de Bozas de la Mer Rouge à l'Atlantique à Travers l'Afrique Tropicale* (Paris, F. R. de Rudeval, 1906), p. 404. Emile Brumpt, later a noted parasitologist, travelling with this expedition was, in 1903, the first to comment upon the ubiquitous *Gl. palpalis* along the Uele valley.
71 Ford, *The Role*, pp. 53, 114.
72 Garnham, 'Arthropods'.

5 'The Lure of the Exotic': sleeping sickness, tropical medicine and imperialism

1 *La Belgique Coloniale* (26 June 1898), 305–7; *La Mouvement Géographique* (25 August 1901), 442; MAEAA 846.34, Mbanza Banteke, District des Cataractes, Dr C. Mabie, response to Royal Society questionnaire on sleeping sickness of August 1903; MAEAA 846.34, 11 August 1903, Matadi, Dr A. Sims, response to questionnaire; MAEAA 846.34, September 1903, Stanley Pool (Kitwa), Madimba District, Rev. P. Frederickson, American Baptist Missionary Union, response.

2 London School of Hygiene and Tropical Medicine, Archives [LSHTM], Correspondence of G. C. Low with Patrick Manson, Director of the School, June–October 1902; Wellcome Institute for the History of Medicine, Contemporary Medical Archives Centre [WIHM: CAC] Lt. Col. A. E. Hamerton, Ms. notebook and photo album while serving on Sleeping Sickness Commission, 1908–10; Royal Commonwealth Society, Archives [RCS], Cuthbert Christy Papers, Mss. notebooks of Royal Society Expedition to Uganda, 10 June 1902–12 April 1903; Wellcome Tropical Institute, Archives [WTI], A. J. Duggan papers, Correspondence re: Ugandan epidemic and C. Christy, 8 October 1902–27 May 1903; WTI, G. Hale Carpenter Mss. 'History of sleeping sickness in Uganda', 13 August 1924.

3 D. J. Bradley, 'The situation and the response', in E. E. Sabben-Clare, D. J. Bradley and K. Kirkwood, eds., *Health in Tropical Africa during the Colonial Period* (Oxford, Clarendon Press, 1980), p. 9.

4 MAEAA 846.34, August 1903, Dr Catherine Mabie.

5 J. Burke, 'Historique de la lutte contre la maladie du sommeil au Congo', *Annales de la Société Belge de Médecine Tropicale*, 51 (1971), p. 466; WIHM Ms. 2268, 27 August 1904. Baptist Missionary Station, Upoto. Note of K. Smith, 31 May 1905 – quite certain that there had been cases of the disease in Stanley's time. It had never quite disappeared at Upoto where the Africans called it *litukutuku*. Smith's careful research showed that since 1898, 80 to 100 people of a total population of some 600–700 had died in Upoto village.

6 MAEAA 4408.1, 7 March 1912, A. Bertrand to GG.

7 J. Ford, 'Ideas which have influenced attempts to solve the problem of African trypanosomiasis', *Social Science and Medicine*, 13B (1979), p. 272.

8 MAEAA 846.1, 4 November 1902, VGG Felix Fuchs to Secretary of State [SS] Liebrechts.

9 C. Neujean and F. Evens, *Diagnostique et Traitement de la Maladie du Sommeil à T. gambiense* (Brussels, Académie Royale des Sciences d'Outre Mer, 1958), p. 5; H. H. Johnston, *George Grenfell and the Congo* (2 vols., London, Hutchinson & Co., 1908), vol. II, p. 547, gives the twelfth century.

10 John Atkins in 1734 described sleeping sickness along the Guinea Coast. *Voyage to Guinea, Brasil, and the West-Indies: In His Majesty's Ships, the Swallow and Weymouth* (London, 1735), p. 180 and *The Navy-Surgeon: or,*

A Practical System of Surgery (London, 1734); T. Winterbottom, *An Account of the Native Africans in the Neighbourhood of Sierra Leone to Which is Added an Account of the Present State of Medicine Among Them* (London, 1803) and *The Medical Directions for the Use of Navigators and Settlers in Hot Climates* (London, 1803). H. W. Mulligan, *The African Trypanosomiases* (London, Allen & Unwin, 1970), p. 588. There are variations in the pathological types of sleeping sickness. For instance, the swelling of the glands in the posterior triangle of the neck occurs frequently in some, but not all, areas in West Africa; McKelvey, *Man Against Tsetse*, pp. 7–8.

11 Todd, *Letters*, letter to brother, 8 July 1903.

12 P. E. C. Manson-Bahr, *History of the School of Tropical Medicine in London (1899–1949)* (London, K. K. Lewis, 1956), p. 9.

13 'Lines by an insomniac', *Punch* (16 September 1903), p. 185.

14 H. H. Scott, *A History of Tropical Medicine* (2 vols., London, Edward Arnold, 1939); M. Worboys, 'Tropical medicine and imperialism, 1895–1914', in 'Science and British colonial imperialism, 1895–1940' (Ph.D. dissertation, University of Sussex, 1979), p. 127.

15 L. Doyal and I. Rennell, *The Political Economy of Health* (London, Pluto Press, 1979); M. Turshen, *The Political Ecology of Disease in Tanzania* (New Brunswick, N.J., Rutgers University Press, 1984). M. Worboys, 'The "discovery" of colonial malnutrition: the colonial problem as a technical problem', in Worboys, 'Science', note 9.

16 D. Bruce, 'Sleeping sickness in Africa', *Journal of the African Society*, 7 (1908), p. 249. The parasite which Bruce observed was named in his honour *T. brucei.*

17 A. J. Duggan, Director of the Wellcome Museum of Medical Science (retired), interview, 9 August 1983; E. Stark, 'The epidemic as a social event', *International Journal of Health Services*, 7 (1977), 681–705; J. Boothroyd, quoted by G. Kolata, 'Scrutinizing sleeping sickness', *Science*, 226 (1985), p. 226.

18 Todd, *Letters*, Todd to brother Bert, 8 July 1903.

19 *Ibid.*, Todd to mother, 13 July 1903.

20 Dr L. Sambon, quoted in 'Tropical medicine and the Congo State', *West Africa* (22 August 1905), p. 195.

21 LSHTM, J. L. Todd, 'Tropical medicine, 1898–1924', n.d., 25th Year Commemorative Talk for the United Fruit Company.

22 G. Philips, 'Historical record, 1920–47' (unpublished typescript, n.d., in the Liverpool School of Tropical Medicine Library), 'Tropical medicine'; B. G. Maegraith, 'History of the Liverpool School of Tropical Medicine', *Medical History*, 16 (1972), 354–68; M. F. Lechat, 'L'expédition Dutton–Todd au Congo 1903–05. De Boma à Coquilhatville, Septembre 1903–Juillet 1904', *Annales des Sociétés Belges de Médecine Tropicale, de Parasitologie et de Mycologie*, 44 (1964), 493–512.

23 W. R. Louis and J. Stengers (eds.), *E. D. Morel's History of The Congo Reform Movement* (Oxford, Clarendon Press, 1968); MAEAA 847.356, A. L. Jones to Secretary of State Liebrechts, 13 January 1908; E. D. Morel, *Red Rubber* (London, T. Fisher Unwin, 1906); E. D. Morel, *Great Britain*

and the Congo (London, Smith, Elder & Co., 1909); R. Harms, 'The end of Red Rubber: a reassessment', *Journal of African History*, 16 (1975), 73–88.

24 S. J. S. Cookey, *Britain and the Congo Question, 1885–1913* (New York, Humanities Press, 1968), pp. 94–8.

25 Louis and Stengers, E. D. *Morel's History*, note 18, p. 50.

26 C. Christy, 'Sleeping sickness', *Journal of the African Society*, 3 (1903), p. 4. He gave 20,000 dead; H. G. Soff, 'A history of sleeping sickness in Uganda' (Ph.D. dissertation, Syracuse University, 1971), pp. 21, 30–1. Soff explains that the statistics provided by the African chiefs showed the number of deaths in Busoga as 13,565 but the commissioner, Colonel James Hayes Sadler agreed with the sub-commissioner that this figure represented only the confirmed deaths and that, in fact, 20,000 was most likely a 'low estimate' of the actual deaths.

27 Soff, 'History', note 20, p. 27; Christy, 'Sleeping sickness', note 20, pp. 1–11; J. E. Eyers, 'A. D. P. Hodges and early scientific medicine in Uganda, 1898–1918: with a select bibliography on the early history of sleeping sickness in Uganda, 1900–1920' (M.A. thesis, Loughborough University of Technology, 1982), p. 27.

28 WTI, Duggan Papers. G. C. Low to Royal Society, 15 October 1902. Castellani had found the 'germ' causing the disease; LSHTM, Entebbe, G. C. Low to P. Manson, 15 October 1902; A. Castellani, 'Etiology of sleeping sickness', *British Medical Journal*, 1 (14 March 1903), 617–18.

29 Soff, 'History', note 20, p. 24; on the fears for India, see WTI, A. J. Duggan Papers: 15 March 1903, A. C. H. Gray, Sleeping Sickness Laboratory, Entebbe to Col. Bruce; 30 June 1903, Lt.-Col. Bruce, Sleeping Sickness Commission, Uganda to H.M. Commissioner-General, British East Africa.

30 The Sleeping Sickness Bureau was initiated by Lord Elgin, Secretary of State for the Colonies, and was housed temporarily at the Royal Society in 1908. From then until 1912, it issued a large number of important bulletins on sleeping sickness, but in 1912, having broadened its scope to tropical diseases, it moved to the new Imperial Institute and changed its name to the Tropical Diseases Bureau. Since that time, it has published the extremely important abstracting journal, *Tropical Diseases Bulletin*. In 1926, the organisation became the Bureau of Hygiene and Tropical Disease.

31 WTI, Duggan Papers, 12 May 1903, minutes of meeting of Royal Society Malaria and Tsetse Fly Committee.

32 WTI, Duggan Papers, 5 December 1902, minutes of meeting of the Royal Society Malaria Committee.

33 Carpenter, *A Naturalist*, p. 7.

34 Bruce, 'Sleeping sickness in Africa', p. 251; Dr Nabarro quoted in J. L. Todd, 'The distribution, spread and prophylaxis of "sleeping sickness" in the Congo Free State', *Transactions of the Epidemiological Society of London*, 25 (1905–6), p. 23.

35 B. W. Langlands, 'The sleeping sickness epidemic of Uganda, 1900–1920', paper presented to World Health Organisation course in parasitology,

Makerere University College, May 1967; WIHM, Western Manuscripts Collection, Ms. 2268, Congo Expedition Diary, vol. 2. Todd was informed on 23 April 1905 by Major E. Wangermee of the Congo Free State that within four years about 250,000 Africans had died around Entebbe. Dutton and Todd believed that most of the recent figures of deaths in both the Congo Free State and Uganda only approximated the truth because about 30 to 50 per cent of the population in many villages had trypanosomes and only a small number could be expected to recover. Therefore, one-third of the population would probably die (Dutton and Todd, 'Distribution and spread'). For the early demography of Uganda, see D. W. Cohen, *The Historical Tradition of Busoga* (Oxford, Clarendon Press, 1972). Cohen asserts that the most important causes of the tremendous demographic upheavals in Busoga during the colonial period were famines and epidemics. The sleeping sickness epidemic continued in full force until 1910 and 'as a result, the most densely populated region of Busoga, the homeland of perhaps 200,000 persons in the late nineteenth century, was totally cleared of population in ten years' (pp. 24–5).

36 Bruce, 'Sleeping sickness in Africa'.

37 F. D. Lugard, *The Rise of our East African Empire* (2 vols., London, 1893), vol. II, pp. 205–25, 559; Soff, 'History', pp. 8, 450; WIHM, A. Balfour Papers. Typescript note to A. Balfour from a member of Lord Desart's Commission, re: sleeping sickness; K. R. S. Morris, letter to *East African Medical Journal*, 38 (September 1961), 433. Morris took seriously Emin Pasha's testimony that there was nothing like sleeping sickness around Wadelai and Dufile between 1885 and 1889. As Dr Grieg of the Sudan Sleeping Sickness Commission found the disease at both spots in 1904, Morris concluded that the disease *must have arrived* on the upper Bomu, Uele and Nile rivers *c.* 1890–1900.

38 J. S. Galbraith, 'Gordon, MacKinnon and Leopold: the scramble for Africa, 1876–84', *Victorian Studies*, 14 (1971), p. 373.

39 Todd, *Letters*, 2 October 1903, Todd to family.

40 Dutton and Todd, 'Distribution and spread', pp. 25–38; MAEAA 847.143, 23 April 1906, Todd to Dr Van Campenhout, Department of Colonial Hygiene, Brussels.

41 Louis and Stengers, *E. D. Morel's History*, pp. 158–68.

42 Vangroenweghe and Vellut, *Le Rapport Casement*.

43 Todd, *Letters*, 23 August 1906 and 27 August 1906, Todd to family.

6 Discovery: Liverpool scientists in the Congo

1 Todd, *Letters*, p. 121; LSTM Archives. TM/8/SX.1.1, 'Liverpool School of Tropical Medicine. Register of Students 1899–1923'; WIHM, Autograph Letters Collection, Ms. 314522, 5 November 1903. J. E. Dutton to sister, Ethel Davies; F. Cornet, *Bwana Muganga: Hommes en Blanc en Afrique Noire* (Brussels, Académie Royal des Sciences d'Outre-Mer, 1971), p. 126; A. Dubois, 'Le développement de la médecine expérimentale au Congo Belge', IRSAC, 1949, p. 95.

2 Liverpool School of Tropical Medicine, *Fourth Annual Report* (1906), p. 7.
3 Duke and Van Hoof, *Final Report*, p. 346.
4 MAEAA 861.54, 14 November 1903, VGG Fuchs to SS Liebrechts.
5 Todd, *Letters*, 10 August 1903, Todd to family.
6 Todd, *Letters*, 8 July 1903, Todd to brother Bert.
7 Todd, *Letters*, 13 July 1903, Todd to mother.
8 LSTM Archives, TM/14/DUJ 10, 1 February 1904, Dutton to Professor Ross; J. E. Dutton and J. L. Todd, 'Prophylaxie de la malaria dans les principaux postes de l'Etat Indépendant du Congo' (Liverpool School of Tropical Medicine, 1906).
9 WIHM, Western Manuscripts Collection, Ms. 2262, 1 October 1903; Todd, *Letters*, 2 October 1903, Todd to family note: Ms. 2262, 21 November 1903. Leopoldville had 150 Europeans (various) and about 2,000 labourers; RCS, Cuthbert Christy Papers, Notebook 15, 21 November 1903. Christy reported 150 and 1,500 from Upper Congo according to Dr Grenade, Principal Medical Officer.
10 Todd, *Letters*, 29 January 1905, Kasongo, Todd to family.
11 Dutton and Todd, 'Distribution and spread', pp. 1–2; Lechat, 'L'Expédition'.
12 LSTM Archives, TM/14/DUJ 10, 1 February 1904, Dutton to Professor Ross.
13 Todd, *Letters*, 24 December 1903, Todd to family.
14 WIHM, Autograph Letters Collection, Ms. 314522, 5 November 1903, on the road to Lutete, Wathen Mission, Dutton to his sister, Ethel Davies; RCS, Cuthbert Christy Papers, Notebook 15, 14 November 1903.
15 RCS, Cuthbert Christy Papers, Notebook 15, 13 November 1903.
16 MAEAA 846.27, 1903 example of questionnaire; 846 . . . , 13 February 1904, Dutton, Kasongo, re: 1903 questionnaire; 846.22, 5 May 1903, VGG, circular and example of questionnaire.
17 Todd, 'The distribution', p. 28; LSTM TM/14/DUJ 10, 1 February 1904. During their sea voyage to West Africa, the researchers learned an important fact they had not known previously – that Europeans also suffered sleeping sickness. In a few years, this presented a delicate problem in public health administration. Sleeping sickness had come to be considered an 'African disease' by most Europeans early this century, but as the government wished to screen *all* victims, it was placed in an awkward situation. For instance, in 1907, the doctor at Leopoldville saw twenty-three Europeans returning from service in the Upper Congo and according to their medical certificates, four of them (or 17 per cent) were infected with trypanosomes. Some health authorities now felt that *all* Europeans should be examined at the end of their tours in the Congo State, but how to do this without causing alarm. The vice governor-general believed that state agents should consent voluntarily to the medical examinations in order 'to avoid the European element exaggerating the importance of the epidemic and avoiding panic'.
18 MAEAA 846.22 for an example of the questionnaire; MAEAA 861.54, 14 November 1904, VGG to SS.

19 MAEAA 846.27, 20 July 1903, W. Holman Bentley to GG enclosing responses to questionnaire.
20 MRAC 58.20.46, 10 December 1903, Commandant Bouillot, Camp Luki, Bas Congo.
21 MAEAA 846 . . . , 13 February 1904, Dutton, Kasongo, to GG, Boma.
22 Todd, *Letters*, 12 July 1904, aboard *Roi des Belges*, River Congo.
23 WIHM, Western Manuscripts Collection, Ms. 2268, 10 July 1904.
24 J. L. Todd, 'Concerning the sex and age of Africans suffering from trypanosomiasis', *Annals of Tropical Medicine and Parasitology*, 7 (1913), 309–19; WIHM, Autograph Letters Collection, Ms. 31452, 14 October 1904, Dutton to his family; most observations of African 'natives' were either made while travelling past their settlements or based upon secondary accounts.
25 WIHM, Western Manuscripts Collection, Ms. 4801, J. L. Todd, 'Congo Free State as a political unit', typescript, n.d. [*c.* 1910], presented to the Association for the Defence of Belgian Interests Abroad.
26 WIHM, Western Manuscripts Collection, Ms. 2268, 21 July 1904. At Bamania mission, Pères Laurent and Théodore told the researchers that around 1899–1900 many of the twenty-five boys transferred there from the mission at Berghe Ste Marie had died of a disease later recognised to have been sleeping sickness. Those boys had come from Equateur, Lolol Bokatala and Ikelemba.
27 WIHM, Western Manuscripts Collection, Ms. 2268, 7 July 1904.
28 WIHM, Western Manuscripts Collection, Ms. 314522, 5 October 1904, Ponthierville, Dutton to 'sisters and brothers'.
29 WIHM, Western Manuscripts Collection, Ms. 4794, J. L. Todd, 'Congo Native and Cattle Examination', 29 November 1904–3 March 1905; MAEAA 861.180, 13 July 1908, MacDonald College, Quebec, Todd to SS Liebrechts. Todd was making further enquiries about former victims.
30 MAEAA 861.180, 13 July 1908, MacDonald College, Quebec, Todd to Ss Liebrechts. MAEAA 861 . . . , 20 December 1907. Secretary of State, re: Dr Trolli's response to Todd's enquiry about victims seen in 1904.
31 Todd, *Letters*, 8 November 1903, Matadi, Todd to family.
32 Todd, *Letters*, 19 June 1904, Leopoldville, Todd to family.
33 Todd, *Letters*, 14 April 1903, Kasongo, Todd to family.
34 Todd, *Letters*, 29 October 1904, Lokandu, Todd to family.
35 Todd, *Letters*, 14 October 1903, Boma; 24 December 1903, Leopoldville; 19 June 1904, Leopoldville, Todd to family.
36 WIHM, Western Manuscripts Collection, Ms. 2268, 12 July 1904, Lukolela Mission.
37 Todd, 'The distribution", p. 4; Ford, 'Ideas', p. 271.
38 LSTM, TM/14/DUJ 10, 1 February 1904, Dutton to Professor Ross.
39 For Liverpool researchers on symptomless carriers, see MAEAA 841.3, Dr Vedy, Bambili Post, 1 May 1907. He reported that the Liverpool researchers had been struck by the number of trypanosomes found among people who had been declared well. See also: Todd, 'Sex and age'. The

scientists issued five 'Reports of the trypanosomiasis expedition to the Congo Free State', which were published in the School's *Memoir* series in August 1904 and March 1906.

40 In the north, sleeping sickness had been referred to in reports as being present at Basoko between 1889 and 1896; at Ibembo on the Itimbiri river in 1894; at Van Kerckhovenville in the north-eastern corner of Uele in 1902; and at Loka in 1904 according to map IV drawn by the expedition. Dutton and Todd, 'Distribution of sleeping sickness in Congo Free State'; J. E. Dutton and J. L. Todd, 'Gland palpation in human trypanosomiasis: being the third progress report of the expedition of the Liverpool School of Tropical Medicine to the Congo, 1903–04–05', *Memoir XVIII* (Liverpool School of Tropical Medicine, 1906). After Basoko, up to the Falls, the researchers believed that all except two sleeping sickness cases they saw were 'imported' from elsewhere. Report of 20 September 1904 sent to LSTM and published as 'The Liverpool Expedition to the Congo', *British Medical Journal*, 2 (26 November 1904), pp. 1481–2.

41 I stress that this was Todd's history, which was incorrect in many respects. Its importance lies in the fact that public health policies were based upon the advice of experts like Todd.

42 Todd's history of the epidemiology is contained in 'The distribution'.

43 MAEAA 846.16, 4 February 1903, A. H. Milne to SS Liebrechts, enclosing 4 February, Ross to Milne; MAEAA 846.22, 5 May 1903, VGG to all administrators, doctors and commandants.

44 Dutton and Todd, 'Distribution and spread', p. 36; MAEAA 847.143, 23 April 1906, Todd to Dr Van Campenhout; J. R. Baker, 'Epidemiology of African sleeping sickness', in *Symposium on Trypanosomiasis and Leishmaniasis with Special Reference to Chaga's Disease* (Ciba Symposium 20) (London, Associated Scientific Publishers, 1974). The key to understanding Gambian sleeping sickness is its chronicity. Baker points out that it can be maintained only in areas where man–fly contact is close and repeated and that it is a 'peridomestic' disease.

45 WIHM, Western Manuscripts Collection, Ms. 2268, 17 September 1904, Stanley Falls. Van der Broeck explained that the present epidemic of sleeping sickness had begun in the region of Kabambare and spread towards Kivu following the passage of these troops.

46 WIHM, Western Manuscripts Collection, Ms 4801. Todd noted thirty-six steamers on the Upper Congo in 1903–5; WIHM, Western Manuscripts Collection, Ms 2268, 16 March 1903 and MAEAA 846.20, 5 May 1903.

47 A. Dubois, 'Le développement', p. 96. Todd showed the necessity of the specialisation of tropical medicine. In Belgium, Charles Firket was propounding the same.

48 LSHTM, Balfour Papers, Box 1 (12), Ms. FC: D1, A. Balfour, 'Some tropical lacunae', notes of a lecture presented to the Universities of Leiden, Utrecht and Amsterdam, March 1927, pp. 6–7. Much later Balfour, Director of the London School, became very interested in the then new area of specialisation, human nutrition. He explained:

'the susceptibility of native tribes to sleeping sickness is undoubtedly determined in large measure by food conditions and the course of the disease can certainly be modified by improving the dietary'.

7 The campaign. Part one: sleeping sickness and social medicine

1 J. Schwetz, *L'Evolution de la Médecine au Congo Belge* (Brussels, Université Libre de Bruxelles, 1946), pp. 13–15; MAEAA 4389.1090, 19 November 1943, Dr A. Duren to Leemans, Régie des Distributions d'Eau, Brussels, 'Etat sanitaire des populations du Congo avant sa colonisation par la Belgique'.
2 D. J. Bradley, 'The situation and the response', in E. E. Sabben-Clare, D. J. Bradley and K. Kirkwood, eds., *Health in Tropical Africa During the Colonial Period* (Oxford, Clarendon Press, 1980), p. 9.
3 F. M. J. C. Nevens, 'Projet de plan général de l'organisation da la lutte contre les trypanosomiases en Afrique', *Bulletin de l'Académie Royale des Sciences d'Outre-Mer* , 17 (1965), 12–13.
4 Schwetz, 'L'Evolution', p. 86.
5 See chapter 4, section on 'ecological disaster', page 54.
6 MAEAA 4389.1090, 19 November 1943, Duren to Leemans.
7 Ford, *The Role*, pp. 473–4. The Belgians certainly did not waste their time concentrating upon mass sterilisation. Ford believed that, in time, the Belgians would have moved from 'prophylaxis of the population' to 'agricultural prophylaxis', or, in other words, they would have eventually moved towards an ecological solution.
8 Victims in the first stage of the disease when the parasites frequent the peripheral circulatory system are particularly infectious as the vector flies can then transmit to new victims. Clearing a victim's blood of the parasites is referred to as 'sterilisation'; for an example of the British campaign, see M. C. Musambachime, 'The social and economic effects of sleeping sickness in Mweru-Luapula, 1906–1922', *African Economic History*, 10 (1981), 151–73.
9 In 1885, there were only two doctors in the Congo Free State although there were forty-five posts and ninety Europeans. By 1891 there were 8 doctors, and, in 1903, 25 for 215 posts and 1,272 Europeans; by 1908 the number of doctors had increased to 30. C. Stasser, 'Etude d'un milieu professionnel: les médecins au service de la colonie entre 1910 et 1918'. Mémoire, Université Catholique de Louvain, 1986–7.
10 MAEAA 855.25, 20 December 1911, A. Bertrand to GG.
11 MAEAA 846.19, 4 April 1903, A. Broden to GG; MAEAA 846.18, 22 February 1903, SS to GG; MAEAA 846.20, 5 May 1903, GG Fuchs, circular; MAEAA 846.9, 20 January 1903, Dr C. Low, Superintendent of London School of Tropical Medicine to Ministry; MAEAA 846.12, 28 January 1903, Low to Ministry. The list of notifiable diseases comprised: cholera, typhus, typhoid fever, smallpox, diphtheria, leprosy, yellow fever, bovine pleuropneumonia and sleeping sickness.
12 MAEAA 846.1, 24 October 1902, Dr Rossignon.

13 MAEAA 846.19, 22 February 1903, SS to GG; MAEAA 846.19, 4 April 1903, Broden to GG.

14 MAEAA 846.22, 5 May 1903, VGG Fuchs, Boma, circular, 'Maladie du sommeil, mesures preventives'.

15 MRAC Fuchs Papers 114, 7 December 1905, Vice Governor-General Lantonnois to all administrators, camp commanders, doctors, missionaries and companies.

16 MRAC Fuchs Papers 114, 4 December 1905.

17 J. Rodhain, 'Documents pour servir à l'histoire de la maladie du sommeil au Congo Belge. III: La période 1907 à 1911. Les premiers lazarets et les débuts de l'expérimentation de l'atoxyl et de l'émétique', *Bulletin de l'Institut Royal Colonial Belge*, 19 (1948), 943–55; Nevens, 'Projet de plan', p. 11. Rodhain conducted the first trials on man with the arsenicals prepared by the great German researcher, Paul Ehrlich; MAEAA 847.356, 12 January 1908, Rupert Boyce, Liverpool School to Sir Alfred Jones, Elder Dempster & Co.; MAEAA 843.126, 5 April 1906, Ronald Ross, Liverpool School to J. L. Todd and 6 April 1906, J. L. Todd to Secretary-General, Congo Free State, Brussels; MAEAA 847.357, 14 January 1908, A. L. Jones, Liverpool to SS Liebrechts, Brussels; MAEAA 847.372, 25 January 1908, VGG to SS, re: Dr Zerbini.

18 MAEAA 847.372, 25 January 1908, Dr Zerbini; MAEAA 838.3, 19 June 1908, VGG to SS. On Zerbini's recommendations, he advised that no agents should administer atoxyl injections.

19 From the beginning of the sleeping sickness campaign, the central government continually stressed the importance of gaining the cooperation of African chiefs and authority figures. The 2 May 1910 decree had included articles specifying the duties of such figures in relation to public health. MRAC 50.30.221, 16 October 1912, ZC Landeghem to all TAs; MRAC 50.30.372, 11 August 1914, S'Heeren, Bili, 'Rapport sur l'examination systematique'; MRAC 50.30.12, 31 December 1914, monthly reports of TA, Likati; TA Liaudet, Titule; TA, Semio; TA, Zobia; MAEAA 855.63, 18 November 1921, Sleeping Sickness Mission report.

20 MAEAA 847.112, 28 November 1905, Dr Zerbini, Boma, to GG.

21 MAEAA 845.8, 24 October 1907, Director of Justice, de Meulemeester to Director of the Medical Service; 4 September 1907, note for GG.

22 MAEAA 4420.20, 25 September 1912, notes for the 1913 Annual Report.

23 Dr Verroni reported in July 1910 that the English Baptist Missionary Society at Yakusu had such a magnificent medical facility that the state should take note, as it would not do to be 'outdone'. MAEAA 837.19, July 1910, Dr Verroni report.

24 WIHM, Western Manuscript Collection, Ms. 2268, 15 July 1904; Ibembo training camp took in 1,200 Africans and dependants every eight to twelve months and most of the internees at Ibembo lazaret were from the army or in state employment.

25 MAEAA 843.20, 14 February 1910, Dr Heiberg, 'Rapport et propositions de lazaret d'Ibembo'.

26 In June 1907 there were twenty-two patients, increasing to eighty-four by August, and during the first year 323 patients passed *through* the lazaret. By January 1910 there were 470 patients on the register. Between June 1907 and July 1910, about 600 patients had been interned although nearly 200 had been sent on to other lazarets and 159 had died, leaving 193 patients isolated at Ibembo in December 1910. The registers list 179 soldiers, 45 paddlers, 69 women, 27 'miscellaneous' occupations and only 8 non-State-employees. MAEAA 843, Ibembo statistics between 1907 and 1910; MAEAA 843.63, 2nd semester 1910; MAEAA 843.11, 15 March 1909, Ibembo lazaret report of 1907–8; MAEAA 843,34, 29 September 1910, VGG Malfeyt, report of a visit to Ibembo lazaret in 1910.

27 MAEAA 843.20, 14 February 1910, Heiberg, 'Rapport'.

28 MAEAA 842.26, 9 June 1908, SS to GG; MAEAA 843,3, 11 November 1907, SS to GG.

29 MAEAA 843.11, 15 March 1909, Ibembo lazaret report; MAEAA 843.11, 2 July 1909, VGG to Min.

30 MAEAA 843.36, 22 June 1910, Dr Bottalico report contained in GG to Min. of 24 September 1910; Dr Heiberg reported in the same year that inside the lazaret one heard the repeated cry, 'n'zala, n'zala' meaning 'hunger, hunger'. MAEAA 843.20, 14 February 1910, Heibert 'Rapport'; MAEAA 843.34, 29 September 1910, VGG Malfeyt, report of a visit to Ibembo lazaret.

31 For discussion of this widespread African practice, see: J. M. Janzen, *The Quest for Therapy in Lower Zaire* (Berkeley, University of California Press, 1978), pp. 3–11.

32 MAEAA 843.1, 19 July 1907, ZC Landeghem to GG.

33 MRAC, Fuchs Papers 114, Dr Trolli, 1907.

34 MAEAA 843.35, 28 September 1910, ZC Landeghem to GG.

35 MAEAA 842.81, 14 December 1910, VGG to Min; MAEAA 842.82, January 1911, Min. to GG; for labour problems, see: MAEAA 845.36, 10 January 1910 [*sic* 1911], Dr Grossule, report on Stanleyville lazaret; MAEAA 844.1, 20 March 1910, Dr A. Zerbini, report on Yakoma lazaret; MAEAA 842.12, 14 October 1910, Dr Van Goidtsnoven, report on Barumbu lazaret; MAEAA 842.89, 1 March 1911, VGG to Min. He complained he could find only four African clerks; MAEAA 842.81, 14 December 1910, VGG to Min.; MRAC 50.30.384, 25 February 1911. Pharmacien Passaniti, Ibembo, found the following staff at Ibembo: twenty-six permanent labourers, thirty sanitary brigade men, two meat provisioners (hunters), one *infirmier* and five *aides-infirmiers*, and one *infirmier* at the post.

36 MAEAA 855.45, 16 February 1911, Dr Grossule report; MAEAA 4419.602, 25 June 1909, Rodhain's note on sleeping sickness campaign.

37 MAEAA 845.20, 16 December 1908, VGG Lantonnois to Min.; MAEAA 843.34, 29 September 1910, VGG Malfeyt to GG.

38 MAEAA 842.1, 17 July 1908, SS Liebrechts to GG; MAEAA 842.3; 15 December 1908, Dr Grossule to DC; MAEAA 842.6, 23 May 1909, DC Lund to GG.

39 MAEAA 842.70, 4 January 1910. VGG Malfeyt's report; MAEAA 842.10, 21 September 1910, VGG Malfeyt to GG.

40 MAEAA 842.12, 14 October 1910, Van Goidtsnoven to GG; MAEAA 842.17, 15 March 1911, Barumbu report.

41 MAEAA 842.51, 22 March 1909, Kervyn report; MAEAA 842.52, 30 March 1909, Minister Renkin.

42 MAEAA 842.8, 2nd semester 1909, lazaret report; MAEAA 842.8, 12 May 1909, Dr Errera to Bertrand.

43 MAEAA 842.15, 31 December 1910, 2nd semester 1910, lazaret report.

44 MAEAA 842.20, 1911, lazaret report; MAEAA 842.16, 19 June 1911, Dr Vincent Rosas to Bertrand.

45 MAEAA 842.15, 31 December 1910, Dr Errera. Concerning sleeping sickness in the region of the Yei river, of what was by then the southern Sudan, and around the Belgian territory of Aba, Dr Errera pointed out that the British authorities were carefully watching how the Belgians responded. Soon after their take-over of the Lado enclave from the Belgians in June 1910, the British sent medical specialists to survey for sleeping sickness which had been known to exist in the region since at least 1907. In the spring of 1909 the recently formed Sudan Sleeping Sickness Commission discovered the disease to exist in the Lado enclave and there were fears it would spread along the Yei river because of the great amount of trade and other movements of Africans in that region. Capt. Colin MacKenzie and Dr Yusef Derwish of the Egyptian Army Medical Corps found fifteen cases of sleeping sickness at Yei on 8 June 1910 and by 1911 the Sudanese authorities were treating 268 cases in the Yei region alone. By 1914 the official statistic for sleeping sickness in Yei was twenty-three new cases; by 1924 the epidemic was considered to be over.

'The Anglo-Egyptian Sudan and sleeping sickness', *Sleeping Sickness Bulletin*, 9 (1909), 345–7; B. H. H. Spence, 'Annual Report on Sleeping Sickness in the Sudan", in *Interim Report on Tuberculosis and Sleeping Sickness in Equatorial Africa* (Geneva, League of Nations, 1923); Mathias, 'Sleeping Sickness in the Anglo-Egyptian Sudan', in A. Balfour, *Fourth Report of the Wellcome Tropical Research Laboratories*, London, Balliere, Tindall & Cox, 1911, vol. I, p. 94; G. K. Maurice, 'The history of sleeping sickness in the Sudan', *Journal of the Royal Army Medical Corps*, 55 (1930), 161–241.

46 A. J. Rodhain, 'Trypanosomiases humaines et animales dans l'Ubangi', *Archiv für Schiffs- und Tropen-Hygiene*, 11 (1907), 283–97; see also R. Headrick 'Sleeping sickness at Nola (Central African Republic)', collected papers of the African Studies Association meeting, Bloomington, Ind., October 1981.

47 MAEAA 844.1, 20 March 1910, Dr Zerbini; MAEAA 844.3, February 1912, Min. to GG.

48 MAEAA 844.4, 31 December 1910, Dr Zerbini to GG.

49 MAEAA 844.8, 9 April 1912, Min. to GG regarding a letter in a Capuchin mission review.

50 MAEAA 845.8, letter of Préfet Apostolique de l'Ubangi which appeared in *Revue de l'Ordre de Capuchins* on 4 April 1912.

51 MAEAA 844.6, 5 April 1911, Dr Zerbini to GG.
52 Rodhain, 'Documents III', p. 950.
53 Schwetz, *L'Evolution*, p. 100. Schwetz reported the rumour, widespread among Africans, that the sick were inoculated with the illness by Europeans who then placed them inside lazarets to await their death. The bodies, it was believed, were then 'cut into bits and put into containers sold in the shops under the names "corned beef", "carbonnade flammands", etc.'; MAEAA 846.1, 24 October 1902, Dr Rossignon to GG.
54 MAEAA 843.20, 14 February 1910, Heiberg, 'Rapport'.
55 MAEAA 843.35, 29 September 1910, ZC Landeghem to GG.
56 MAEAA 843.20, 14 February 1910, Heiberg, 'Rapport'.
57 *Ibid.*
58 MAEAA 4419.4, *c.* 1909, A. J. Rodhain, 'Notes et propositions'; Schwetz, *L'Expedition*, p. 90.
59 MAEAA 4419.602, 25 June 1909, A. Broden to Min. enclosing 'La lutte contre la trypanose humaine', by Broden and A. J. Rodhain.
60 MAEAA 843.20, 14 February 1910, Heiberg, 'Rapport'; MAEAA 847.143, 23 April 1906, J. L. Todd to Van Campenhout.
61 MAEAA 850.9, 10 May 1918, GG to all VGGs and DCs.
62 F. O. Stohr, in *Bulletin of the Sleeping Sickness Bureau*, 4 (1912), 302.
63 W. B. Johnson, *Notes on a Journey Through Certain Belgian, French and British African Dependencies to Observe General Medical Organisation and Methods of Trypanosomiasis Control* (Lagos, Government printer, 1929), p. 3; see also: S. Kivilu, 'Population et santé au Zaire à l'époque colonial de la fin de XIX siècle à 1960', *Transafrican Journal of History*, 13 (1984), 74–91, 93.
64 See appendix B for examples; MRAC 50.30.215, 24 September 1910, Fuchs' circular reprimanding TAs and doctors for lax attitude re: passports; MRAC 50.30, *feuillet matricule* (Lucien Kumu, *infirmier*); MRAC 50.30, *livret d'identité* form; MRAC 50.30.179, *feuille de route* and *passeport médical*; MAEAA 850.260, 30 April 1910, Fuchs' circular re: new passports.
65 MAEAA 847.143, 23 April 1906, J. L. Todd to Van Campenhout; MAEAA 831, 10 June 1910, 'Mesures complementaires prisés en 1910 pour enrayer le développement de la maladie du sommeil'; MAEAA 848.114, 17 January 1910; MAEAA 848.115, 17 January 1910; MAEAA 849.206, 30 April 1910, Fuchs' instruction on medical passports; 8 September 1910. *Receuil Mensuel*, 9 (new sleeping sickness regulations which replaced those of 5 December 1906).
66 On paper war, see J. Burke, 'Historique de la lutte contre la maladie du sommeil au Congo', *Annales de la Société Belge de Médecine*, 51 (1971), p. 468; MAEAA 849.291, 18 May 1911, Dr Van der Sloten to GG. This doctor at Buta complained that issuing medical passports took up half of each day; MAEAA R/CB 150.1, 12 May 1929, J. Schwetz, 1928 report of medical service in Province Orientale, explained that the sleeping sickness programme was too '*paperassières*'; Bakonzi, 'Gold mines', p. 154.
67 MAEAA 847.330, 7 November 1907. For instance, Sacré Coeur Mission at Stanley Falls requested medicines for sleeping sickness work as they

intended to establish their own lazaret; MAEAA R/CB 149/3, April 1923. The state doctor, Van Goidtsnoven, in great contrast, reported in 1922 that many missions in the province avoided sleeping sickness work because 'the battle is slow, without dramatic visible effects, routine and fastidious'. Africans did not come voluntarily; most often they refused this help. He added that 'from the point of view of recruiting Christians, sleeping sickness work is harmful! In contrast, yaws, etc., with short cures is acceptable to missionaries.'

68 MAEAA 850.411, Van Campenhout note on GG's request to missions; MRAC 58.20.46, 27 March 1908, SS to GG, re: missionaries.

69 MAEAA 847.259, 18 February 1907. Heiberg to Secretary-General, 'Rapport sur la maladie du sommeil', 34 pp.; MAEAA 855.25, 20 December 1911, Heiberg to GG; MAEAA 849.333, 30 August 1912. In 1912, Heiberg made the following budgetary calculations for a brigade consisting of one *capita* and thirty-six labourers for each sector: *capita*, 15 francs per month plus 0.24 francs per day for food; labourers, 8 francs and 0.12 francs; a cover for each man at 4 francs each; four loin-cloths at 1.50 francs for each man over a two-year period. The total annual cost per brigade was calculated at 6,000–6,500 francs.

70 MAEAA 4420.20, 25 September 1912, Note for 1913 annual report.

71 MRAC 50.30.372, 1 December 1913, Rodhain report of Uere-Bili sleeping sickness tour; MAEAA 4408.2, 12 June 1912, Grenade to DC; MAEAA 4408.12, 12 June 1912, DC Meulemaere, Bambili to GG, re: Grenade's report. He established a cordon sanitaire around the Uere river (Api) from its source to Uere post at the mouth of the Ango river and along a straight line to Bili post, then along the Bili river to Bomu, and he ordered the evacuation of all troops; MAEAA 4408.2, 2 August 1912, GG to Min. re: sleeping sickness in northern Uele. He urgently requested three medical specialists and a new observation post in the contaminated zones discovered in northern Uele. The Semio observation post was moved south; there were now four observation points: Doruma, Uere, Bili and Monga.

72 MRAC 50.30.216, 3 July 1912, PC Jenssen, Sasa, to Lt. Beck; MRAC 50.30.128, 24 July 1912, ZC Landeghem, Uere-Bilio to PC, Limbala; a Protestant mission bulletin reported that the Belgians had collected together 1,000 soldiers to 'subdue' Sasa and that there was 'plenty of sleeping sickness in the Sasa district'. 'Notes from C. T. Studd . . . ', *Heart of Africa* (Heart of Africa Missionary Society), 2 (May 1914).

73 MRAC 50.30.222, 4 August 1912, DC Meulemaere decree; MAEAA 4420.22, 'Rapport à presenter aux Chambres, 1912'.

74 MAEAA 833, 21 April 1913, GG, re: annual report of Uere-Bili for 1912.

75 A. de Calonne-Beaufaict, *Azande* (Brussels, M. Lamertin, 1921), Appendix VII, pp. 237–40.

76 MAEAA 855.53, 27 May 1914, A. J. Rodhain, Preliminary report of Uere-Bili tour; MRAC 58.20.55, 15 March 1915, A. J. Rodhain, Final report of the sleeping sickness tour of Uele.

77 A. J. Rodhain, 'Documents pour servir à l'histoire de la maladie du

sommeil au Congo Belge. I: la maladie du sommeil dans l'Ubangi en 1905 et 1906', *Bulletin de l'Institut Royal Colonial Belge*, 16 (1945), p. 112.

78 See B. Fetter, *Colonial Rule and Regional Imbalance in Central Africa* (Boulder, Colo., Westview Press, 1983); MAEAA AI 1422.3, 27 August 1929, TA Gregoire, 'Rapport politique, 1929. District de l'Uele-Nepoko'. He said that it was a shame that the administrative policy of regrouping Africans was not further along because sleeping sickness was being spread through the incessant travel among the Azande; MAEAA R/CB 151.1, 21 May 1932, Dr L. Fontana complained bitterly that territorial and medical administrators did not cooperate in the resiting of Africans for public health purposes; see also: M. L. Nkamba, 'Histoire de la maladie du sommeil au Kwango (1933–1957)', *Zaire-Afrique*, 160 (1981), 645–54. The initial policy of regrouping scattered hamlets, in this writer's opinion, *spread* sleeping sickness to healthy populations. It was called '*prophylaxie agronomique*'.

79 Dominican House, Louvain, Belgium, Library Archives. R.-C. Lagae, Vicaire Apostolique de Niangara, 18 July 1927, 'Rapport extraordinaire sur le vicarat de Niangara Congo belge confié aux Dominicains de la Province Belge de Sainte Rose', t.s.

80 MAEAA 4429.20, 25 September 1912, Note for 1913 annual report.

81 MAEAA 848.118, 29 October 1909. For instance, Dr Heiberg suggested to the GG that special 'sanitary police' should be based at Aba and frequently patrol the frontier.

82 MAEAA 855, 5 September 1913, Substitut Neve, Bambili to Rodhain; MRAC 50.30.293, 9 June 1914, Substitut, Buta to DC, Buta.

8 The campaign. Part two: the surveys and tensions

1 Bakonzi, 'Gold mines', p. 127.

2 MRAC 50.30.156, 23 July 1915, VGG Malfeyt, circular to administrators in Province Orientale instructing them to promote rubber production.

3 MRAC 50.30.16, DC Landeghem, 'Rapport annuel, Bas-Uele 1915'.

4 MRAC 50.30.156, 26 October 1915, GC Mertens for the VGG to DC, Buta; MRAC 50.30.167, 9 March 1916, TA Brugger, Bambili to DC, Buta; MRAC 50.30.167, 3 June 1916, Brugger to DC; MRAC 26 August 1916, TA Hurlet, Zobia to DC.

5 MRAC 58.20.48, 2 January 1909, Min. to GG. Writing about the sleeping sickness campaign reforms, he explained: 'we cannot dream of Belgian doctors . . . we could address medical candidates, mostly Italian . . . ' and from the beginning of the Congo Free State there were many Italian doctors; MRAC 50.30.91, 2 April 1915, DC Landeghem to VGG; MRAC 50.30.158, 19 July 1915, GC to DC, Buta.

6 MRAC 50.30.91, 26 July 1915, Nyblom to DC Landeghem.

7 MRAC 50.30.90, 4 August 1915, TA, Dakwa to DC.

8 MRAC 50.30.91, 22 August 1916, DC Landeghem to VGG.

9 MRAC 50.30.91, 19 September 1915, Dr Dubois, Buta to DC, Buta; MRAC 50.30.164, 11 January 1916, Dubois, Bili to DC, Buta.

10 MRAC 50.30.16, May 1916, DC Landeghem, 'Rapport annuel, Bas-Uele, 1915'.

11 MRAC 50.30.91, 19 September 1916, Dubois, Buta to DC, Buta.

12 A. J. Duggan, 'Tropical medicine: a submerging art?', *Transactions of the Royal Society of Tropical Hygiene and Medicine*, 76 (1982), p. 569.

13 MAEAA 850.9, 10 May 1918, GG to VGG and DCs. These ideas parallel those implemented in neighbouring French territories a year earlier. There in 1916, Colonel Jamot had created the first *équipes mobiles* to survey and treat sleeping sickness in the Oubangui-Chari region of French Congo. It was a new idea of 'mobile prevention'. M. B. Eyidi, *Le Vainquer de la Maladie du Sommeil: le Docteur Eugene Jamot (1879–1937)* (Paris, The Author, 1950), p. 45.

14 League of Nations. Health Organisation. *Interim Report on Tuberculosis and Sleeping Sickness in Equatorial Africa* by A. Balfour, E. Van Campenhout, Gustave Martin and A. G. Bagshawe (Geneva, 26 May 1923); MAEAA 4420.31, 'Report of hygiene measures since 1920', 1925.

15 MAEAA R/CB 150.1, 5 February 1932, Dr Marone, 'Mission prophylactique maladie du sommeil Uele: travail accompli pendant l'année 1931.'

16 MRAC 50.30.26, 30 September 1918, TA de Wilder, Gwane, Report for 4th quarter; MRAC 50.30.30, 31 December 1922, 'Rapport annuel, Bas-Uele, 1922'.

17 MAEAA 855.63, 18 November 1921, GG Lippens to Min., containing Rodhain, 16 October, 'Avis et considérations' on S'Heeren's thirty-two-page report of the survey. For an impression of the British policy of forced removals see: Musambachime, 'Social and economic effects'. Around 1910 some 12,000 to 25,000 people were 'herded' thirty, sometimes one hundred, miles in forced moves which were chaotic.

18 In fact, until very recently, chemotherapy for this disease has remained relatively undeveloped. Some explain that the pharmaceutical firms have not been highly motivated to work on sleeping sickness. Dr Leonard Goodwin, Acting Director of the Wellcome Museum for Medical Science, interview, 15 October 1984. Dr Goodwin explained that the World Health Organisation had tried unsuccessfully to get pharmaceutical firms to produce new sleeping sickness drugs. (One-day meeting on African trypanosomiasis held at London School of Hygiene and Tropical Medicine on 11 April 1986; *World Health Chronicle*, 5 (1985), 179.) At the moment, clinical trials are underway with a promising new drug, DFMO (DL-a-dicluoromethylornithene), one of the very few new ones in almost half a century. Report of the UNDP/World Bank/WHO Special Programme for Research and Training in Tropical Disease, 'Round table discussion on current leads in research relevant to the development of potential new chemotherapeutic agents for African trypanosomiases' (Geneva, 10 March 1986). UNDP/World Bank/WHO Special Programme for Research and Training in Tropical Diseases, Seventh Programme Report, 1 January 1983–31 December 1984 (19 pp., Geneva, 1985), chapter 5: 'African trypanosomiases'.

19 Atoxyl was developed by the 'father of bacteriology", Robert Koch, who

quickly discovered the unfortunate side-effect of too much atoxyl and regulated the dose to half a gram every ten days. This was not perfectly effective against trypanosomes, but it was a low enough dose to avoid blinding victims; it became the standard treatment for years. The problem remained, however, of achieving just the correct dose of the trypanocide. Too much blinded the victim, while too little permitted the parasite to adapt to the drug, that is to become drug-resistant. Through the years, many efforts were made to find safer, more effective trypanocides. In 1906, King Leopold II had established a 200,000 franc (£8,000) prize for the discovery of a cure, but half a century later the prize remained unawarded. A. Duren, 'Prix institué pour la découverte de remède contre la trypanosomiase', *Bulletin de l'Institut Royal Colonial Belge* (1952), 1106–9; *British Medical Journal*, 30 June 1906, p. 1547.

20 Dr Cammermeyer, 'Notes de pratique médicale africaine', *Archiv für Schiffs-und Tropen-Hygiene*, 16 (1912), 84; R. Mouchet, 'Notes anatomiques et médicales sur la pathologie du Moyen Congo', *Archiv für Schiffs- und Tropen-Hygiene*, 17 (1913), 659.

21 C. C. C. Chesterman, 'Some results of tryparsamide and combined treatment of Gambian sleeping sickness', *Transactions of the Royal Society of Tropical Medicine and Hygiene*, 25 (1932), 433; MAEAA 4404.170, 10 December 1925, Dr A. Broden; J. Williamson, 'Review of chemotherapeutic and chemoprophylactic agents', in H. Mulligan, ed., *The African Trypanosomiases* (London, Allen & Unwin, 1970), p. 128; C. Singer and E. A. Underwood, *A Short History of Medicine* (1962), p. 484. A recent recommendation for treatment suggests that first-stage Gambian sleeping sickness be treated with suramin or pentamadine, while the advanced, or second stage, formerly treated with tryparsamide, should be treted with melarsoprol, 'a toxic drug often with side-effects such as nausea, diarrhoea, vomiting and abdominal pain'. WIHM, Museum, Trypanosomiasis Bay; 7 June 1924; A. J. Rodhain, Médecin en Chef, Boma, Note re: Dr Strada's report of 1923 sleeping sickness survey.

22 MAEAA R/CB 150.1, 5 February 1932. Marone's report of the sleeping sickness survey for 1931.

23 MAEAA R/CB 151.1, 21 May 1932, Dr L. Fontana, 'Rapport annuel du Service Médical, Province Orientale, 1931'.

24 These statistics were derived from the following: MAEAA 4419.604, 12 March 1923, Dr Van Campenhout, Director of the Medical Service; MAEAA R/CB 149.3, April, 1923, Dr Van Goidtsnoven, 'Rapport sur l'hygiène publique, Province Orientale, 1922'; MAEAA 4419.604, 16 January 1925, Van Campenhout; MAEAA 4462.300, 'Rapport sur l'hygiène publique pendant l'année 1927'; MAEAA 4404.264, 30 June 1928, Dr Infante; MAEAA AI 1422.1, political report for Uele-Nepoko district 1928; MAEAA R/CB 156.1, political report for Uele-Nepoko 1930; MAEAA R/CB 151.1, 21 May 1932, Dr Fontana, 'Rapport annuel du Service Médical, Province Orientale, 1931'; MAEAA 4420.32, 15 April 1926, Van Campenhout's talk on sleeping sickness in 1923; MAEAA 4453.19, 13 January 1925, note on general hygiene in the

Congo; MAEAA 4405.155, 15 January 1925, Director of Hygiene to Min.; MAEAA 4389.1090, 19 November 1943, A. Duren to M. Leemans, Régie des Distributions d'Eau, Brussels.
25 A. Duren, 'Le service médicale de la colonie et ses problèmes d'avenir', *Le Materiel Colonial*, 2 (1936), 38–50, p. 45.
26 MAEAA R/CB 150.1, 5 February 1932, Marone's report of the sleeping sickness survey for 1931; A. Bertrand, *Le Problème de la Main d'Oeuvre au Congo Belge* (Brussels, Ministère des Colonies, 1931), p. 54; MAEAA 4389.930, 31 July 1930, GG Tilkens, circular.
27 MAEAA 4461.58, 3 September 1924, Van Campenhout, London. 'Rapport au Société des Nations re: campagne contre la maladie du sommeil en Afrique equatoriale'.
28 A. Dubois, 'Alphonse-Hubert-Jerome Rodhain', in *Biographie Belge d'Outre-Mer*, vol. VI (Brussels, Académie Royale des Sciences d'Outre-Mer, 1968); A. Dubois, 'Jerome Rodhain (1876–1956), Membre de la Classe des Sciences Naturelles et Médicales', *Bulletin de l'Académie Royale des Sciences Coloniales*, 1 (1957), 159–90.
29 A. Dubois, 'Campenhout (Van), Jean-Emile', *Biographie Belge d'Outre-Mer*, vol. VI (Brussels, Académie Royale des Sciences d'Outre-Mer, 1968).
30 MAEAA 4419.4, *c.* 1909, A. J. Rodhain, 'Notes et propositions'.
31 MAEAA R/CB 150.1, 12 April 1929, Schwetz report on sleeping sickness in Province Orientale.

9 The African response

1 MAEAA 838.19, 25 January 1905. Dr Zerbini to GG. Appendix A contains a lengthy list of directives in the form of decrees, *arrêtés* and circulars issues by the administration during the campaign.
2 See, for instance, O. Ransford, *Bid the Sickness Cease: Disease in the History of Black Africa* (London, John Murray, 1983).
3 *Documents pour servir à la connaissance des populations du Congo Belge, Archives de Congo Belge* (Léopoldville, Government Printer, 1959).
4 For instance, see C. A. Lemaire, 'Les Mangbetu', *Belgique Coloniale*, 4 (1898), 4–5 and 'Notes pour servir à l'histoire des races congolaises', *Belgique Coloniale*, 4 (1898); J.-A. A. Hutereau, *Notes sur la Vie Familiale et Juridique de Quelques Populations du Congo Belge* (Tervuren, Annales du Musée Royal du Congo Belge, 1909); and *Histoire des Peuplades de l'Uele et de l'Ubangi* (Brussels, Goemaere, Falk Fils, 1922); J. Czekanowski, *Forschungen im Nil-Kongo Zwischengebiet*, vol. II (Leipzig, Klinkhardt & Biermann, 1924); A. Calonne-Beaufaict, *Azande: Introduction à une Ethnographie Générale des Bassins de l'Ubangi-Uele et de l'Aruwimi* (Brussels, M. Lamertin, 1921); M. H. Lelong, *Mes Frères du Congo* (2 vols., Algiers, Editions Baconnier, 1946); R. P. L. Lotar, 'Souvenirs de l'Uele', *Congo* (Brussels), 1925, vol. II, p. 367; 1927, vol. II, p. 405; 1932, vol. II, p. 1; R. P. L. Lotar, *La Grande Chronique de l'Uele* (Brussels, Institut Royal Colonial Belge, 1946); R. P. L. Lotar, *La Grande Chronique du Bomu* (Brussels, Institut Royal Colonial Belge, 1940); R. P. L. Lotar, *La Grande*

Chronique de l'Ubangi (Brussels, Institut Royal Colonial Belge, 1937); *Redjaf* (Brussels, Jean Dewit, 1937); P. Denis, *Histoire des Mangbetu et des Matshaga jusqu'à l'Arrivé des Belges* (Tervuren, Musée Royal de l'Afrique Central, 1961).

5 B. Fetter, *Colonial Rule and Regional Imbalance in Central Africa* (Boulder, Colo., Westview Press, 1983), p. 145; MAEAA 850.9, 3 February 1917, Landeghem, political report for 1916; L. de Saint Moulin, 'Histoire de l'Organisation administrative du Zaire', *Zaire-Afrique*, 224 (April 1988), 197–222.

6 MRAC 50.30.12, 18 August 1914, DC, Buta, 'Rapport trimestrielle sur l'administration générale de la district Bas-Uele'.

7 See appendix B for example of *procès-verbal d'investiture*; MRAC 50.30, 26 April 1918, VGG Meulemeester, Stanleyville to DC, Bas-Uele, Buta; MRAC 50.30, 31 December 1924, TA Gregoire, Niangara; MRAC 50.30, 31 May 1929, TA Mox, Niangara, 'Renseignements politiques', re: Chiefs Kereboro and Datule.

8 MRAC 50.30.11, 28 February 1914, TA Daelmar, Ibembo, 'Rapport politique'.

9 P. Curtin, S. Feierman, L. Thompson and J. Vansina, *African History* (London, Longman, 1978), p. 554.

10 Janzen, *Quest for Therapy*, pp. 34, 9.

11 R. Horton, 'African traditional thought and Western Science', *Africa*, 37 (1967), 50–72; V. W. Turner, *The Drums of Affliction* (Oxford University Press, 1968), p. 46; A. B. Chilivumbu, 'Social basis of illness: a search for therapeutic meaning', in F. X. Grollig and H. B. Haley, eds., *Medical Anthropology* (The Hague, Mouton, 1976), p. 67; Janzen, *Quest for Therapy*; R. Packard, 'Social change and history of misfortune among the Bashu of eastern Zaire', in I. Karp and C. S. Bird, eds., *Explorations in African Systems of Thought* (1980), pp. 237–40; G. Bibeau *et al.*, International Development Research Centre, Ottawa, *Traditional Medicine in Zaire* (1980).

12 Bibeau *et al.*, p. 28.

13 A major contribution to Azande studies was made by the British anthropologist, Edward E. Evans-Pritchard. Works of his I found useful for this study include: *Wtichcraft, Oracles and Magic Among the Azande* (Oxford, Clarendon Press, 1937); *The Zande Trickster* (Oxford, Clarendon Press, 1967); *The Azande: History and Political Institutions* (Oxford, Clarendon Press, 1971); *Man and Woman Among the Azande* (London, Faber and Faber, 1974); 'Zande theology', *Sudan Notes and Records*, 19 (1936), 5–46; 'Zande therapeutics', in E. E. Evans-Pritchard, R. Firth, B. Malinowski and I. Schapera, eds., *Essays Presented to C. G. Seligman* (London, Kegan Paul, 1934); 'The Zande corporation of witchdoctors', *Journal of the Royal Anthropological Institute*, 62 (1932), 291–336; 63 (1933), 63–100; 'A history of the kingdom of Gbudwe', *Zaire*, 10 (1956), 451–91; 675–710' 815–80; 'A further contribution to the study of Zande culture', *Africa*, 33 (1963), 183–97; 'Zande notions about Death, Soul and Ghost', *Sudan Notes and Records*, 50 (1969), 41–52; 'A note on some Zande physiological notions', *Sudan Notes and Records*, 51 (1970), 162–5.

Other sources include: A Bertrand, 'Introduction', in A. de Calonne-Beaufaict, *Azande. Introduction à une Ethnographie Générale des Bassins de l'Ubangi-Uele et de l'Aruwimi* (Brussels, M. Lamertin, 1921); C.-R. Lagae and V. H. Vanden Plas, *La Langue des Azande: Introduction Historico-Géographique* (2 vols., Ghent, Editions Dominicaines 'Veritas', 1921–2); C.-R. Lagae, *Les Azande ou Niam-Niam* (Brussels, Vromant and Co., 1926); P. M. Larken, 'Zande background: notes on the Azande of Tambura and Yambio, 1911-1912' (typescript, *c.* 1954); P. T. W. Baxter and A. Butt, *The Azande and Related Peoples of the Anglo-Egyptian Sudan and Belgian Congo* (London, International Africa Institute, 1953); A. Thuriaux-Hennebert, *Les Azande dans l'Histoire du Bahr el Ghazal et de l'Equatoria* (Brussels, Institut de Sociologie, 1964); M. McLeod, 'Oracles and accusation among the Azande", in A. Singer and B. V. Street, eds., *Zande Themes* (Oxford, Blackwell, 1972), 158–78.

14 Evans-Pritchard, 'Zande therapeutics', p. 49; Evans-Pritchard, *The Zande Trickster*, p. 11; Evans-Pritchard, *Witchcraft, Oracles and Magic*, p. 479; Lagae and Vanden Plas, *La Langue*, vol. I, p. 167; P. A.-M. de Graer, 'L'art de guérir chez les Azande', *Congo*, 1 (1929), 220–51; 361–408.

15 Evans-Pritchard, *The Zande Trickster*, p. 12; Evans-Pritchard, 'Zande theology', p. 170.

16 Evans-Pritchard, *Witchcraft, Oracles and Magic*, p. 9; Evans-Pritchard, 'Zande therapeutics', p. 57;E. E. Evans-Pritchard, 'Sorcery and native opinion', *Africa*, 4 (1931), p. 26; Lagae and Vanden Plas, *La Langue*, p. 167. These experts defined 'medicine' as *ziga* which means 'antidote'. For Azande, since most illness was provoked by an evil cause, the medicine took the form of an antidote. The term, *ngwa*, used on its own denotes a suspicious quality, and *ira ngwa*, master of drugs, is a poisoner. The term for European medicine is *ngwa kaza*.

17 De Graer, 'L'art de guérir'; Evans-Pritchard, *Witchcraft, Oracles and Magic*, p. 494; Evans-Pritchard, 'Zande therapeutics', p. 51.

18 Dr Mokassa, Budu informant (Wamba District, Haut-Zaire), interview, Brussels, 23 August 1982.

19 *Ngwa* according to Calonne-Beaufaict is tree, root or plant. *Azande*, p. 179. It is significant that medicine and tree are designated by the same word in several languages: *amaga* for the Akare, Ambaga and Amadi. See also: W. Z. Conco, 'The African Bantu traditional practice of medicine and the problems of communication' (unpublished typescript, WIHM, 1970). 'In Africa medicine is never separated from philosophy, religion, magic, politics or economics. Medicine became elevated to dominate all spheres of life. All successes in life could *only* come through the use of good medicine', p. 34.

20 Calonne-Beaufaict, *Azande*, p. 176.

21 Evans-Pritchard, 'A further contribution", p. 196; Khartoum, Sudan, Historical Archives. Native Societies, Archive X. Subject: Native societies and Cults, 17 October 1916, Dungu, TA Torissen to Inspector, Meridi District (Sudan).

22 FO 367.69/27004, 24 June 1907, G. B. Michell to Cromie. In another report Michell wrote: 'a Mobali tells me that their medicine is efficacious only for those who have observed strict continence . . . ', FO 367.69/29312, 12 August 1907, Michell to Cromie.
23 Janzen, *Quest for Therapy*, pp. 8–9.
24 It was believed that leprosy was caused by a disruption of social relations or by breaking clan taboos; thus, it was regarded as a *sino* disease (*sino*-taboo in form of a totemic animal). Lagae, *Les Azande*, pp. 39–40. Evans-Pritchard, *Witchcraft, Oracles and Magic*, p. 479; Evans-Pritchard, 'Zande theology', p. 301.
25 Lagae, *Zande*, pp. 206–7
26 Interviews with Mboli André (Azande) and Ngbato Gilbert (Babua) at Tongerloo Abbey, Belgium, 20–1 August 1982; Larken, 'Azande background', p. 32; Hutereau, *Histoire des Peuplades*, p. 74, relates an Abandyia tradition.
27 Ethnographic film by André Singer, anthropologist and film-maker. Interview, London, 29 February 1984.
28 Two species of *benge* were known: (1) *nawada* – the red root of a vine which after being made into a paste quickly lost its strength; thus it was usable for only one day; (2) *benge andehe*, which was made from birds which had died after eating certain flowers. The birds were called *andehe*. This substance was more powerful and lasted for two to three days. Lagae, *Les Azande*, p. 85. See also: A. M. Vergiat, *Les Rites Secrets des Primitifs de l'Oubangui* (Paris, Payot, 1936), p. 60.
29 McLeod, 'Oracles and accusation'; Lagae, *Les Azande*, p. 84; D. T. Lloyd, 'The Precolonial economic history of the Agongara-Azande, *c.* 1750–1916', Ph.D. dissertation, University of California, Los Angeles, 1978, p. 280.
30 E. E. Evans-Pritchard, 'Azande kings and princes', in *Essays in Social Anthropology* (London, Faber & Faber, 1969), pp. 95–7; De Graer, 'L'art de guérir'; A.-M. de Graer, 'L'état actuel des recherches sur la médecine en territoire de Doruma', in *Compte Rendu de la 13ème Semaine Missiologie à Louvain*, Louvain, 1935.
31 Calonne-Beaufaict, *Azande*, p. 22.
32 South of the Ubangi-Uele rivers (23–26½° E. and 2–3½° N: just west of Ibembo and south of the Uele river and east of Bambili through to south of the Aruwimi river) reside the numerous Babua who will represent the Bantu linguistic family in this study. M. A. McMaster, 'Patterns of interaction: a comparative ethnographic perspective on the Uele region of Zaire, *ca.* 500 B.C. to 1900 A.D.', Ph.D. dissertation, University of California, Los Angeles, 1988; A. de Calonne-Beaufaict, *Les Ababua* (Brussels, Mouvement Sociologique Internationale, 1909); A. Landeghem, 'Etude preparatoire sur les Babua', Prevince Oriental, District de l'Uele (ms.).
33 Calonne-Beaufaict, *Les Ababua*, p. 106; Hutereau, *Notes sur la Vie*, pp. 91–2; Dr Vedy, 'Les Ababuas', *Bulletin de la Société Royal Belge de Géographie*, 28 (1904), pp. 267–8.

34 A. de Calonne-Beaufaict, 'Les Ababua', in J. Halkin, *Les Ababua* (Brussels, A. Dewit, 1910), pp. 342–5.

35 MRAC 50.30.26, 30 June 1918, TA Hurlet, Zobia, 'Rapport général'.

36 Hutereau, *Notes sur la Vie*, p. 98; Calonne-Beaufaict, *Les Ababua*, pp. 107–9.

37 More accurately, these people are one clan (*nebasadjo*) among those who form the more numerous Makere-speaking population. I shall, however, use the appellation, Mangbetu, to refer to the larger population. C. A. Keim, 'Precolonial Mangbetu rule: political and economic factors in 19th-century Mangbetu history (northeast Zaire)', Ph.D. dissertation, Indiana University, 1979, p. 21; C.Ehret *et al.*, 'Some thoughts on the early history of the Nile–Congo watershed', *Ufahamu*, 5 (1974), 85–112.

38 Schweinfurth, *Heart of Africa*, vol. II, pp. 43, 81, 85.

39 Commandant Renier, *Héroisme et Patriotisme des Belges: l'Oeuvre Civilisatrice au Congo* (Ghent, Heckenrath, 1913), p. 288.

40 Hutereau, *Notes sur la Vie*, p. 76.

41 *Mapingo* consisted of a horizontally arranged, smooth banana stalk upon which were balanced a certain number of short, well-polished or oiled cylindrical sticks in groups of threes. The *namapingombi*, or consultant, circled the oracle, speaking to it and clapping his hands until some sticks moved or fell. Predictions were then read from their configurations. Castai, *Ten Years*, p. 92; G. Burrows, 'On the natives of the Upper-Welle District of the Belgian Congo', *Journal of the Anthropological Institute*, 28 (1898), p. 45; Keim explained that the power of the oracle resided in the *elinga* leaves used to prepare the palm kernel oil with which the sticks were rubbed. Half of them represented 'yes' and half 'no'. 'Precolonial Mangbetu rule', p. 88.

42 V.-H. Van den Plas, *Les Missions Dominicaines* (1925), 50–4; De Graer, 'L'art de guérir'.

43 Keim, 'Precolonial Mangbetu rule', p. 86.

44 T. H. Parke, *My Personal Experiences in Equatorial Africa* (London, Sampson, Low, Marston & Co., 1891), p. 307; MRAC 50.30.27, 12 November 1918, DC, Buta to TA, Zobia, 'Rapport général, 1918'.

45 P. G. Janssens, 'Le climat social: la mortalité infantile aux Mines de Kilo', *Bulletin de l'Académie Royale des Sciences d'Outre-Mer*, 20 (1952), 105–19. Professor Janssens (formerly Chief of Medicine and Public Health, Kilo-Moto Gold Mines, northern Zaire) explained that, in his experience, in spite of long contact with European ideas regarding illness and death, the Africans in the region of the mines clearly believed that the paramount task was to discover *who*, not what, had caused their misfortunes.

46 Evans-Pritchard, *Witchcraft, Oracles and Magic*, p. 316.

47 De Graer, 'L'art de guérir', p. 44.

48 Lelong, *Mes Frères du Congo*, vol. II, p. 187.

49 MAEAA 846.34, 11 August 1903, Dr Sims; MAEAA 846.34, September 1903, Rev. Peder Frederickson, American Baptist Missionary Union, Stanley Pool; MAEAA 846.19, 4 April 1903, Dr Broden.

50 MAEAA 847.338, 2 June 1907, Dr Borzini, Lado.

51 MAEAA 4403.435, 16 February 1914, GG to Min., re: circular to all DCs.
52 De Graer, 'L'art de guérir', pp. 42–5. He believed the disease had been introduced in the Azande region of his study within the previous thirty years (which would have been since 1890–1). He believed that during the wars of colonial conquest during which many Azande sought refuge north of the Bomu river, sleeping sickness had been introduced from the French Congo.
53 Janzen, *Quest for Therapy*, p. 43.
54 Rodhain, 'Documents pour servir', p. 950. During this period, the official mortality rate in Ibembo lazaret was 28 per cent while in *all* lazarets (Stanleyville, Leopoldville and Ibembo) it was roughly 20 per cent and we must recall the great probability that numbers of non-infected people were isolated.
55 Elephantiasis is hyperendemic in Uele, southern Sudan and the Central African Republic. Rodhain in 1913–14 identified a focus of *filaria volvulus* between Bambili and Bondo. A. W. Wodruff, eds., *Medicine in the Tropics* (London, Churchill and Livingstone, 1974), p. 238; Rodhain, 'Quelques aspects', p. 742; 'The doctor', *Inland Africa*, 4 (April 1921), 7; MAEAA 841.8, 30 November 1909, Dr Haavik Rubi, 'Rapport sanitaire'; MAEAA 839.7, 16 July 1909, Dr Neri, Gurba-Dungu, 'Rapport sanitaire'.
56 MAEAA 841.2, December 1906, Dr Moscioni, Buta, 'Rapport sanitaire'. He visited the military camp where he performed circumcisions, one hundred for free, and he boasted that this was attractive to the men as the native specialists were expensive. In this way, he helped to prevent long absence from work, and he believed the circumcisions were an excellent introduction to Western medicine. Free, or at least cheap, European services in contrast to the generally quite costly African specialists were occasionally given as the reason for the popularity of the former. Yet, it must be recalled that the Azande, for example, tended to reserve their trust in the authority of their own specialists for the precise reason that those specialists were costly. Here, perhaps, cheap and accessible was questionable? De Graer, 'L'art de guérir', p. 2.
57 R. Dumont, 'Le conflit des conceptions médicales au Congo", *l'Avenir Colonial Belge* (1934); Lelong, *Mes Frères du Congo*, vol. I, p. 232. Refers to H. Labouret's article, 'Le ballet de la maladie du sommeil', *Monde Colonial Illustré* (1935), 246–87, which describes an African dance in which lumbar punctures were mimed.
58 Many societies were quite familiar with one form of physical examination – autopsies. Throughout the colonial period, there were occasional confrontations as state officials attempted to end this African practice because they did not approve its function. Many groups of people in northern Congo found it necessary from time to time to examine a body for signs of *likundu*, witchcraft substance, in order to carry out the necessary rituals for its eradication. In 1915, for instance, Kabu was arrested and charged by the authorities with the 'mutilation of a corpse' and, in 1926, Bawe was similarly charged. MRAC 50.30.155, 4 September 1915, Buta, Judicial Police Officer Heinzmann, *Procès-verbal* against Kabu of Amboma

chefferie; MRAC 50.30.307, 2 April 1926, Bambili, TA F. Payen, *Procès-verbal* against Bawe; C.-R. Lagae, 'Le mauvais oeil chez les Azande', *Les Missions Dominicaines* (1923), 53–4.

59 A missionary explained that among the Azande, slaves were not cared for when ill nor mourned upon death. They were, he added, buried without the least ceremony. Lagae, *Les Azande*, p. 49.

60 MAEAA 847.338, 2 June 1907, Dr Borzini, Lado enclave, 'Rapport sanitaire'.

61 In Calonne-Beaufaict, *Azande*, annexe, p. 239.

62 MRAC 50.30.13, 31 December 1914, TA Frederickssen, Gwane, report.

63 MRAC 50.30.4, 10 August 1914, Dr Fauconnier, Buta to DC.

64 MRAC 50.30.30, 17 September 1923, Dr Strada to DC, Buta.

65 MAEAA 855.63, 18 November 1921, Dr S'Heeren, report on mission; De Graer, 'L'état actuel'; MAEAA R/CB 149.4, 3 January 1924, Dr Bonferroni, Doruma, report; MRAC 58.20.51, 7 May 1914, Vanden Plas to Rodhain.

66 MRAC 50.30.13, 31 December 1914, TA Frederickssen, Gwane; MAEAA R/CB 149.4, 3 January 1924, Dr Bonferroni, Doruma.

67 MRAC 50.30.173, 8 July 1909, ZC to all TAs, Likati sector; MRAC 50.30.221, 16 October 1912, Landeghem to TAs; MRAC 50.30.320, 30 November 1912, PC Angodia, Rubi zone; MRAC 50.30.372, 11 August 1914, Dr S'Heeren; MRAC 58.20.55, 15 December 1915, A. J. Rodhain; MAEAA 4404.264, 15 July 1928, Dr Infante, 'Notes sur le travail effectué au cours de Ière semestre'.

68 MRAC, 31 December 1924, TA Gregoire, Niangara, 'Renseignements politiques'; 15 May 1929, 31 May 1929 and 1 October 1930, TA Mox, Niangara, 'Renseignements politiques'.

69 MAEAA 855.67, 1914, Rodhain's fourth report; MAEAA 755.55, 27 April 1914, Rodhain's third report; MRAC 50.30.372, 1 December 1913, A. J. Rodhain, report of sleeping sickness inspection of Uere-Bili district.

70 MRAC 58.20.51, 7 May 1914, V.-H. Van den Plas, Amadis mission to Rodhain; Lagae, *Les Azande*, p. 154.

71 MRAC 50.30.381, 3 May 1918, DC, Buta.

72 Dr D. Breyne, Note, in *Aide Médical aux Missions*, 2 (April 1939), 26–9.

73 Lelong, *Mes Frères du Congo*, vol. II, pp. 44–5.

74 League of Nations, Health Organisation, *Interim Report on Tuberculosis and Sleeping Sickness in Equatorial Africa*, Geneva, May 1923, p. 63.

75 Todd, *Letters*, 14 October and 24 December 1903.

76 MAEAA 843.53, 6 February 1912, Ibembo lazaret director.

77 MAEAA 845.2, 17 August 1907, Federspeil to GG, re: Trolli's report of 15 August 1907; MAEAA 845.3, 21 August 1907, SS to GG; MAEAA 842.17, 15 January 1911, Dr Van Goidtsnoven.

78 MRAC 50.30.372, 11 August 1914, S'Heeren; J. Schwetz, 'A propos du diagnostique le plus expéditif de la maladie du sommeil dans la pratique ambulatoire de la brousse', *Bulletin de la Société de Pathologie Exotique*, 12 (1919), 726–30.

79 MRAC 50.30.373, 10 April 1915, Ph. Piton, Ango.
80 Schwetz, 'A propos'.
81 MAEAA AI 1422.2, 1930, Uele-Nepoko report on general administration.
82 MAEAA R/CB 156.1, 1930, Uele-Nepoko, 'Rapport politique annuel';
MAEAA 4388.50, 14 August 1928, VGG Moeller, notes on Dr Trolli's
1928 report.
83 MAEAA 841.35, 28 March 1905, Dr Verroni *et al*, Stanley Falls; MAEAA
841.1, 13 December 1905, Dr Moscioni, Buta, 'Rapport sanitaire';
MAEAA 841.2, December 1906, Dr Moscioni, Buta, 'Rapport sanitaire';
MAEAA 839.7, 10 July 1909, Dr Neri, Gurba-Dungu zone, 'Rapport
sanitaire'; MAEAA 841.8, 30 November 1909, Dr Haavik, Rubi zone,
'Rapport sanitaire'.
84 De Graer, 'L'état actuel', p. 222.
85 Mboli André and Ngbato Gilbert. Interviews at Tongerloo Abbey,
Belgium, 20 and 21 August 1982.
86 'La maladie du sommeil', *Les Missions Dominicaines* (1924), 262.
87 Dr Eugène Jamot, an eminent authority on the disease in French
Equatorial Africa, calculated that diagnosis by palpation alone carried an
error rate between 50 and 75 per cent. During a study in Cameroon, he
discovered only 18,000 victims of the disease among 60,000 who had been
diagnosed by means of enlarged glands only. In spite of efforts like this, the
Belgian, Dr Dumont, was amazed that in parts of the Congo as late as 1928
(for example, Aruwimi district), palpation alone was still used for diagnosis. R. Dumont, 'Le conflit'.
88 Schwetz, 'L'Evolution', p. 90.
89 MAEAA 855.63, S'Heeren, report of sleeping sickness campaign in Uele
district, contained in 18 November 1921, GG to MAEAA 4420.21, July
1912, containing A. Broden note of 17 July 1912.
90 MRAC 50.30.310, 30 October 1911, ZC Landeghem to Substitut;
MRAC 50.30.308, 24 November 1911, ZC Landeghem to Substitut.
91 MRAC 50.30.91, 18 March 1915, DC Landeghem, Buta to DC,
Niangara; MRAC 50.30.273, 9 June 1909, GC Tombeur, Niangara to
ZC, Rubi; MRAC 50.30.273, 8 July 1909, SC, Go to TAs in Likati
sector; MRAC 50.30.114, 24 February 1912, ZC Heinzmann, Rubi to
PC, Bima; MRAC 50.30.221, 14 May 1912, ZC, Buta, circular; MRAC
50.30.154, 7 April 1914, PC, Semio to DC, Buta; MRAC 30.30.154,
12 June 1914, PC Lt. Defoin, Semio to DC, Buta; MRAC 50.30.148,
31 August 1914, TA de Wilder, Monga to DC, Buta; MRAC 50.30.148,
1 September 1914, TA Lavorel, Ibembo to DC, Buta; MRAC 50.30.373,
5 February 1915, Dr Olivier to DC; MAEAA 843.20, 14 February 1910,
Heiberg, 'Rapport'.
92 MAEAA 843.20, 14 February 1910, Heiberg, 'Rapport'.
93 MAEAA 843.18, 22 January 1910, ZC Millo Ribotti to GG.
94 MAEAA 843.18, 16 March 1910, VGG to Min.
95 MAEAA 836.16, Yei, first semester 1910, report of the Hygiene Commission.

96 MAEAA 842.10, 21 September 1910; MAEAA 842.70, 4 January 1910.
97 MAEAA 844.4, 31 December 1910, Dr A. Zerbini, Yakoma to GG; MAEAA 844.8, 9 April 1912, Min. to GG.
98 MAEAA 844.6, 5 July 1911, Dr A. Zerbini to GG.
99 MAEAA 855.3, 20 November 1912, Dr G. Bomstein, Yakoma lazaret report; MAEAA 855.3, 29 November 1911, Adjoint Supérieure, Millo Ribotti, Yakoma; MAEAA 855.5, 2 January 1913, Dr Bomstein.
100 MAEAA R/CB 149.4, 7 June 1924, Médecin en Chef Rodhain, Boma, note to GG concerning 1923 medical report.
101 MAEAA 855.63, S'Heeren, report contained in 18 November 1921, Médecin-Inspecteur Rodhain to Min.
102 MRAC 58.20.51, 7 May 1914, Vanden Plas, Amadi to Rodhain; MAEAA 841.35, Dr N. Veroni, Stanley Falls.
103 MAEAA 838.5, 26 November 1909, S'Heeren, 'Rapport médical', Aruwimi district.
104 MAEAA 838.6, 18 May 1910, S'Heeren, 'Rapport médical', Aruwimi district.
105 Edgar Coles, note of 19 December 1914 quoted by C. T. Studd, *Heart of Africa*, 2 (April 1915), p. 17.
106 MRAC 50.30.373, 12 January 1915, Mgr Van den Broele, Bondo to DC.
107 Van den Plas, quoted in *Les Missions Dominicaines* (14 July 1924), p. 50.

10 Public health, social engineering and African lives

1 See chapter 7.
2 MAEAA 849.355, 23 November 1911, Dr Puleri, Coquilhatville to GG; and 7 December 1912, GG to Min.; MAEAA 850.1, 12 April 1914, VGG Malfeyt to GG.
3 MRAC 50.30.91, 2 August 1915, Acting DC Nyblom to GG.
4 MRAC 50.30.373, 24 April 1915, Dr Wille, Ango to DC; MRAC 50.30.373, 5 April 1915, Stagini, Bili to TA, Bili.
5 MRAC 50.30.161, 23 July 1916, Fredrickssen report on medical passports.
6 MRAC 50.30.381, 7 October 1918, Chief of observation post at Bili to Chief, Medical Service, Buta; MRAC 50.30.88, 1 October 1914, DC, Buta to DC, Bangala.
7 MAEAA 855.55, 27 April 1914, Rodhain, third report on sleeping sickness survey in Uele; MRAC 50.30.4, 1 October 1914, Landeghem, Buta to DC, Bangala; MRAC 50.30.4, 1 October 1914, Landeghem to Dr Olivier, Buta.
8 Royal Commonwealth Society, Archives, Cuthbert Christy Papers. C. Christy, 'Final Report to the Sudan Sleeping Sickness Commission', typescript, October 1916.
9 C. Christy, 'Final Report'; in 1912–14, Rodhain had noticed heavy trade in iron and rubber in the region of Yakoma. He also commented on intense trade in ironwork between the Bira-Gembele and people from the region of Bondo-Likati. He added that this trade had been equally intense

during his first visit to the region in 1905. MRAC 50.20.55, 15 March 1915, Rodhain's report.

10 MAEAA 855.63, 18 November 1921, Dr S'Heeren, report.
11 MRAC 58.20.59, 5 December 1914, A. J. Rodhain to DC.
12 MRAC 50.30.156, 23 January 1915, GC Moulaert to GG; see also: MRAC 50.30, 30 April 1915, Adnet, Ibembo to DC, Buta.
13 MRAC 50.30.90, 8 May 1915, TA, Ibembo to DC.
14 MAEAA 855.45, 16 February 1911, Dr Grossule, Stanleyville lazaret. Notes on Pharmacien Marcoz' report of 15 February 1911, MRAC 50.30.372, 11 August 1915, Dr S'Heeren, 'Rapport sur l'examination systematique'.
15 Dr Vedy, 'Les Ababuas', *Bulletin de la Société Royale Belge de Géographie* (1904), 191–205, 265–91; MRAC 50.30.25, 31 December 1916, AT Leroy, Titule, 'Rapport Général Annuel'.
16 Hutereau, *Notes sur la Vie*, pp. 65–7.
17 Lloyd, 'Precolonial economic history", p. 364; Larken, 'Zande background'; Lagae, *Les Azande*, pp. 153–4.
18 Lagae, *Les Azande*, pp. 188–96.
19 MRAC 50.30.44, October 1908. Landeghem, Rubi, October report.
20 MRAC 50.30.120, 12 June 1912, ZC, Buta to PC, Titule; MRAC 50.30.119, 12 June 1912, ZC, Buta, to PC, Likati; MRAC 50.30.148, 7 May 1914, TA Barisi; MRAC 50.30.163, 7 July 1916, Nyblom, Go to DC, Buta.
21 MRAC 58.20.55, 13 March 1915, Rodhain, sleeping sickness survey report.
22 C. Christy, 'Final Report'.
23 Rhodes House, Oxford. Sir John Hobbis Harris Papers. J. C. McLaren, 7 March 1907, 'Congo Atrocities', *Western Daily Mercury*, Plymouth.
24 MAEAA 847.354, 10 September 1907, Landeghem, Buta to GG.
25 MRAC 50.30.381, Pharmacien Corillon, Bagidi-Dakwa, report of first semester, 1908.
26 MAEAA 848.113, 15 October 1909, ZC Millo Ribotti to GG.
27 MAEAA 841.11, 20 December 1910, Dr Van den Sloten, 'Rapport sanitaire', second semester, 1910.
28 MAEAA 843.47, 12 December 1910, Landeghem, report.
29 MAEAA 4408.6, 17 May 1913, Brussels, Administrateur-Délégué du Société Commerciale et Minière du Congo to Minister.
30 MAEAA 850.9, 16 April 1917, Bertrand to VGG; see also: MAEAA 847.354, 10 September 1907, ZC Landeghem, Buta to GG; MRAC 50.30.372, 11 August 1914, Dr S'Heeren, report.
31 MRAC 50.30.90, 1 April 1915, DC Landeghem to TA, Dakwa.
32 Several administrators of Gwane territory complained about the pressures upon Africans in the south of the region. One administrator suggested lowering the tax rate for southerners. Nevertheless, rubber-buyers continued to ignore the cordon sanitaire while local administrators pressured Africans to collect rubber. MRAC 50.30.11, 31 May 1914, TA Fredrickssen, Gwane, 'Proposition for tax, 1915'. MRAC 50.30.91,

13 September 1915, Landeghem to VGG; MRAC 50.30.374, 19 July 1916, TA Fredrickssen, Gwane; MRAC 50.30.23, 6 January 1917, TA De Wilder, Gwane.

33 MRAC 50.30.381, 18 September 1918, DC Landeghem, Buta to VGG.

34 MAEAA 840.9, 11 October 1918, GC Tombeur for the absent VGG to GG.

35 MAEAA 855.63, 1921 sleeping sickness survey report, contained in 18 November 1921, GG to Min. In December 1922, the administrator of Gwane, who happened to be the medical representative of the sleeping sickness mission in Uele, explained that in the region 'conditions for existence are more painful for the people who are decimated by sleeping sickness – they are forbidden to hunt elephants or collect rubber, which are their *only* resources'. The tax had been lowered to two francs fifteen centimes in the light of the 'double prohibition' in effect. MRAC 50.30.30, 31 December 1922, TA Corillon, 'Rapport annuel', Gwane, 1922.

36 MRAC 50.30.18, 10 August 1917, Landeghem, circular.

37 MAEAA 849.273, 1 April 1911, Deuxième Direction-Général. Première Direction. Deuxième Division to Secrétariat-Général. Text for a brochure for the London Exposition.

38 MRAC 58.20.55, 15 March 1915, Rodhain, sleeping sickness survey report.

39 MRAC, Felix Fuchs papers, RG 765.114. 'Règlement coordonnant les mesures prises pour enrayer la maladie du sommeil', Brussels, 1913.

40 MRAC 50.30.117, ZC, Buta to PC, Ibembo.

41 Again, in January, the state agent at Limbala on the Uere river reported that during his reconnaissance along the river he had found only one canoe, which he had seized, and he had also destroyed two rope or vine bridges which had been thrown across the river by the natives. MRAC 50.30.153, 30 January 1914, TA, Limbala to DC, Buta.

42 MRAC 50.30.133, 14 November 1912, ZC, Bondo, Uere-Bili zone to PC, Lebo.

43 MRAC 50.30.293, 7 May 1914, Substitut Philippe Nève, Bili (Paquet de Bambili) to DC, Buta.

44 MRAC 50.30.13, 30 September 1914, TA Fredrickssen, Gwane, 'Rapport'.

45 MRAC 50.30.61, 3 November 1914, DC Landeghem, Titule to GG; MRAC 50.30.293, 9 October 1914, Juge Ch. Smets and Greffier Henin, 'Tribunal de première instance de Niangara. Audience Publique du dix-neuf Octobre 1914. En cause Ministère Publique, Onga'.

46 MRAC 50.30.379, 5 September 1916, DC Landeghem, Buta, decision.

47 MRAC 50.30.374, 5 October 1916, TA, Dakwa to DC, Buta.

48 MRAC 50.30.380, 27 December 1917, DC Landeghem to VGG. Five years later, the district commissioner forbade fishing on the Ango river and proposed extending the prohibition to the Uere because fishermen from the Uere were travelling north of Api to fish and he considered them to

constitute a real danger. MRAC 50.30.30, 17 September 1923, DC Liaudet to TA, Gwane.
49 MRAC 54.95.75, Emmanuel Muller Papers. Containing papers of Emile Christiaens, a member of the Van Kerckhoven expedition. Letters addressed to 'Felix', Djabbir, 2 November 1892. In October 1892, along the Itimbiri river, Christiaens observed the local method of manufacturing salt. 'There are grasses of a certain species that the natives burn in order to extract potassium salt ash.'
50 MAEAA 843.46, Dr Bottalico, 1910 Annual Report of Ibembo lazaret.
51 MAEAA 855.25, 17 January 1912, VGG to Min.
52 MAEAA 4420.20, September 1912. Notes for the annual report for 1913.
53 MAEAA 4403.386, 14 May 1913, Min. to GG; MAEAA 4403.387, 9 May 1913, Min. to GG.
54 Lagae, *Les Azande*, p. 156; Calonne-Beaufaict, *Azande*, pp. xxii–xxiii.
55 C. G. Seligman and B. Seligman, *Pagan Tribes of the Nilotic Sudan* (London, Routledge and Kegan Paul, 1932), p. 504; MAEAA 831.383, 20 February 1912, ZC Ermingen, Uere, 'Rapport Annuel Service Médical et Hygiène'; MRAC 50.30.25, 30 December 1916, De Wilder, Gwane, 'Rapport Annuel'. He explained that as in all Azandeised areas one saw agglomerations of people around chiefs and notables whereas all other Azande lived in dispersed family units or even alone.
56 Rhodes House, Oxford, A. Boyd ms. diary, 30 June 1906 entry; MAEAA 855.63, 1921, Dr S'Heeren, report on sleeping sickness survey; Evans-Pritchard, *The Zande Trickster*, pp. 2, 5.
57 MAEAA, R/CB 150.1, 5 February 1932, Dr Marone, 1931 Sleeping Sickness Report.
58 MAEAA 855.50, 12 December 1913, GC Bertrand, Zobia to GG.
59 MRAC 50.30.372, 10 October 1913, SC Fredrickssen to PC.
60 MRAC 50.30.379, 12 November 1913, SC Fredrickssen to PC.
61 MRAC 50.30.153, 29 November 1913, TA Liteca, Limbala to GC, Bambili.
62 MRAC 50.30.11, 31 January 1914, TA, Buta, Monthly report.
63 MRAC 50.30.12, 31 December 1914, TA Liaudet, Titule.
64 MRAC 50.30.91, 24 March 1915, TA Heinzemann, Buta to DC.
65 MRAC 50.30.379, 3 May 1918, DC, Buta, decision.
66 MRAC 50.30.30. 17 September 1923, PC Liaudet, Buta to TA, Gwane. It is interesting that as recently as 1923 such a view could obtain; by then there were fairly clear ideas about the epidemiology of the disease and one of the essential features of a potentially grave epidemic situation was contiguous settlement.
67 MAEAA 855, 14 September 1927. Inspecteur-Général, note to Min., 'Prophylaxie de trypanosomiase dans le Haut-Uele'.
68 MAEAA R/CB 151.1, 23 May 1932, Dr L. Fontana, 'Rapport annuel, technique et administrative du service médical du Province Orientale, 1931'; MAEAA R/CB 150.1, 5 February 1932, Dr Marone, Niangara, 'Rapport de la mission maladie du sommeil, 1931'.

69 The 2 May 1910 decree concerning 'Native Districts, *Chefferies* and *Messagers*' created a new category of intermediary between chiefs, sub-chiefs and the colonial administration. They were the *messagers* whose roles were similar to bailiffs' in the *chefferies*. The 1910 decree had listed chiefs' duties which included: relating all legislation to the people; assisting with the census; policing their regions; notifying the administration of 'all important news including contagious disease, epidemics' and isolating victims; implementing public health regulations; ensuring public works; and supervising the collection of taxes. Congo Free State, Local Government, Boma, *Bulletin Officiel* (1910), 433–71.

70 MAEAA 4408.6, 7 August 1913, Van Ermingen, Bili, 'Rapport politique, 1913' enclosed in 18 September 1913, letter to GG.

71 MRAC 50.30.372, 16 April 1914, Dr Wille, 'Report of tour through *chefferies* Dungara, Zemio-bio (Alias Zemoi) and Gugwa'.

72 MRAC 50.30.11, 30 November 1913, PC, Angu, political report.

73 MAEAA 855.50, 12 December 1913, GC Bertrand, Zobia to GG.

74 MAEAA R/CB 149.4, 3 January 1924, Dr Bonferroni, Doruma.

75 MRAC, 15 May 1929, 31 May 1929; 1 October 1919, TA Mox, Niangara, 'Renseignements politiques'; MRAC, 31 December 1924, TA Gregoire, Niangara, 'Renseignements politiques'. Chief Kereboro was specifically cited for not having obliged all his subjects to present themselves for sleeping sickness examinations. Chief Datule was charged, among other things, for 'having set a bad example to his subjects by escaping sleeping sickness treatment'.

76 MRAC 50.30, 26 April 1918, VGG de Meulemeester to DC, Buta; MRAC 50.30, 16 February 1918, GC Tombeur to all DCs and VGG; MRAC 50.30, 6 March 1918, DC, Buta to VGG.

77 MAEAA 842.70, 4 January 1910, VGG Malfeyt, report of lazaret tour; MAEAA 842.10, 21 September 1910, VGG Malfeyt to GG; MAEAA 842.17, 15 January 1911, Médecin-directeur, Van Goidtsnoven, Barumbu, 'Exposition de la situation du lazaret, considérations et désiderata'.

11 Conclusion and legacy

1 G. Brausch, *Belgian Administration in the Congo* (Oxford University Press, 1961), p. 8. American University, Foreign Area Studies Division, *Area Handbook for the Republic of the Congo (Léopoldville)*, Washington, D.C., 1962, p. 238.

2 M. F. Shapiro, 'Medicine in the service of colonialism', Ph.D. dissertation, University of California, Los Angeles, 1983; F. Fanon, 'Medicine and colonialism', in J. Ehrenreich, ed., *The Cultural Crisis of Modern Medicine* (New York, Monthly Review Press, 1978), 229–51. See also: R. MacLeod and M. Lewis, eds., *Disease, Medicine and Empire* (London, Routledge, 1988); D. Arnold, ed., *Imperial Medicine and Indigenous Societies* (Manchester University Press, 1988).

3 M. Turshen, *The Political Ecology of Disease in Tanzania* (New Brunswick, N.J., Rutgers University Press, 1984), p. 5.

4 J. Paul, 'Medicine and imperialism in Morocco', *Middle East Research Information Project (MERIP)*, 60 (1977), 3–12.

5 MAEAA 4389.1090, 19 November 1943, Dr A. Duren to M. Leemans, Régie des Distributions d'Eau, Brussels.

6 Shapiro, 'Medicine'.

7 MRAC 50.30.372, 1 December 1912, Dr Russo.

8 MAEAA 855.40, 20 May 1912, DC de Meulemaere to GG; MRAC 50.30.13, 31 December 1914, Fredrickssen, Gwane, 'Rapport tri-mestrielle, 4ème'.

9 T. McKeown, *The Role of Medicine: Dream, Mirage or Nemesis?* (Oxford, Blackwell, 1979); M. Muller, *The Health of Nations: A North–South Investigation* (London, Faber and Faber, 1982).

10 A treponemal infection, yaws is transmitted non-venereally among children by contact and earlier this century most of a population was infected before adolescence. Childhood yaws protected against infection with other treponemal diseases; thus affected children did not contract venereal syphilis in adulthood.

11 C. J. Hackett, 'Yaws', in E. E. Sabben-Clare, D. J. Bradley and K. Kirkwood, eds. *Health in Tropical Africa During the Colonial Period* (Oxford, Clarendon Press, 1980), p. 84.

12 R. Yeager, 'Historical and ecological ramifications for AIDS in Eastern and Central Africa', in N. Miller and R. c. Rockwell, eds., *AIDS in Africa: the Social and Policy Impact* (Washington, D.C. and Hanover, N.H., National Council for International Health and African Caribbean Institute, 1988), p. 71.

13 This may be a reflection of the earlier research paradigms. Focusing on urban areas, where facilities allow some systematic survey and analysis of the situation, Western scientists have assumed AIDS to be more a problem for urban individuals.

Select bibliography

Secondary sources: medical, ecological, geographical

Académie Royale des Sciences d'Outre-Mer, *Livre Blanc. Rapport Scientifique de la Belgique au Développement de l'Afrique Centrale*, 3 vols. Brussels, Académie Royale des Sciences d'Outre-mer, 1962–3.

Anderson, R. G., 'Final report of the Sudan Sleeping Sickness Commission, 1908–09', *Journal of the Royal Army Medical Corps*, 16 (1911): 200–7.

Anon., 'Waking to the threat', *Sudanow* (November 1984): 29–30.

Apted, F. I. C., Letter to editor, *East African Medical Journal*, 38 (May 1961): 266–7.

Arnold, David, ed., *Imperial Medicine and Indigenous Societies*. Manchester University Press, 1988.

Ashcroft, M. T., 'A critical review of the epidemiology of human trypanosomiasis in Africa', *Tropical Diseases Bulletin*, 56 (1959): 1073–93.

'The importance of wild animals as reservoirs of trypanosomiasis', *East African Medical Journal*, 36 (1959): 289–97.

Baker, J. R., 'Epidemiology of African sleeping sickness', in *Symposium on Trypanosomiasis and Leishmaniasis with Special Reference to Chaga's Disease*. London, Ciba symposium 20, 1974, pp. 29–42.

Balfour, Andrew, *First Report of the Wellcome Research Laboratories*. Khartoum, Sudan Government, Department of Education, 1904.

Second Report of the Wellcome Research Laboratories. Khartoum, Sudan Government, Department of Education, 1906.

'Trypanosomiases in the Anglo-Egyptian Sudan', *Journal of Tropical Medicine*, 9 (1906): 84–92.

Third Report of the Wellcome Research Laboratories. Published for the Department of Education, Sudan Government. London, Balliere, Tindall & Cox, 1908.

Fourth Report of the Wellcome Tropical Research Laboratories, 2 vols. Published for the Department of Education, Sudan Government. London, Balliere, Tindall & Cox, 1911.

War Against Tropical Disease: Being Seven Sanitary Sermons Addressed to All Interested in Tropical Hygiene and Administration. London, Balliere, Tindall & Cox, 1920.

Balfour, A., Van Campenhout, E., Martin, G. and Bagshawe, A. G., 'Interim

Report on tuberculosis and sleeping sickness in Equatorial Africa', League of Nations, Health Organisation, May 1923.

'Further report on tuberculosis and sleeping sickness in Equatorial Africa', League of Nations, Health Organisation, April 1925.

Bayoumi, A., *The History of the Sudan Health Services*. Nairobi, Kenya Literature Bureau, 1979.

Beck, Ann, *A History of the British Medical Administration of East Africa, 1900–1950*. Cambridge, Mass., Harvard University Press, 1970.

Bibeau, G. *et al.*, *Traditional Medicine in Zaire*, Ottawa, International Development Research Centre, 1980.

Boothroyd, J. C., 'Antigenic variation in African trypanosomiasis', *Annual Review of Microbiology*, 39 (1985): 475–502.

Bourguignon, A., Cornet, J., Dryepondt, G., Firket, Ch., Lancaster, A. and Meuleman, E., *Rapport sur le Climat, la Constitution du Sol et l'Hygiène de l'Etat Indépendant du Congo*, Report of Congrès National d'Hygiène et de Climatologie Médicale de la Belgique et du Congo. Brussels, 1897.

Bradley, D. J. 'The situation and the response', in E. E. Sabben-Clare, D. J. Bradley and K. Kirkwood, eds., *Health in Tropical Africa During the Colonial Period*. Oxford, Clarendon Press, 1980, pp. 6–12.

Breinl, A. and Todd, J. L., 'Atoxyl in the treatment of trypanosomiasis', *British Medical Journal* (19 January 1907): 132–4.

Breyne, D., Note, in *Aide Médical aux Missions*, 2 (Brussels, April 1939): 26–9.

Briggs, A., 'Cholera and society in the nineteenth century', *Past and Present*, 19 (April 1961): 76–96.

Broden, A., 'The sleeping sickness', *Journal of the African Society*, 5 (1906): 409–17.

L'Hygiène Coloniale et les Principales Maladies Tropicales. Ghent, Congrès International Colonial, [1913].

L'Organisation Médicale et Hygiènique au Congo-Belge. Rapport à la Session de Bruxelles de l'Institut Colonial International, vol. I, Brussels, Bibliothèque Coloniale Internationale, 1923.

Broden, A. and Rodhain, J., 'Traitement de la trypanosomiase humaine', *Archiv für Schiffs- und Tropen-Hygiene*, 10 (1906): 693–707; 11 (1907): 73–9; 12 (1908), 443–55; 12 (1908), 743–50; 13 (1909), 269–83.

'Atoxyl dans le traitement de la trypanose humaine', *Annales de la Société Belge de Médecine Tropicale*, 1 (1921): 179–226.

Broden, A., Rodhain, J. and Corin, G., 'Le salvarsan et la trypanose humaine', *Archiv für Schiffs- und Tropen-Hygiene*, 16 (1912): 749–79.

Bruce, David, 'Sleeping sickness in Uganda', *Journal of the Royal Army Medical Corps*, 3 (1904): 17–41.

'Sleeping sickness in Africa', *Journal of the African Society*, 7 (1908): 249–59.

Bruce-Chwatt, L. J., 'Movements of populations in relation to communicable disease in Africa', *East African Medical Journal*, 45 (1968): 266–75.

Brumpt, Emile, 'Maladie du sommeil et mouche tsé-tsé', *Comptes Rendus de la Société de Biologie*, 4 (1903): 839–40.

Buell, Raymond L., *The Native Problem in Africa*, 2 vols. New York, Macmillan, 1928.

Burke, J., 'Historique de la lutte contre la maladie du sommeil au Congo', *Annales de la Société Belge de Médecine Tropicale*, 51 (1971): 465–82.

'Aperçu de la situation de la trypanosomiase au Congo-Kinshasa', *Bulletin de l'Information de la Coopération au Développement*, 25 (Brussels, March–April 1969): 1–6.

Calonne-Beaufaict, Adolphe de, 'Extraits d'un rapport établi par de Calonne, à la suite d'un voyage d'études (été 1913) en territoire Anunga (ex-chefferie Sasa) avec le docteur Rodhain', Appendix 7 in A. de Calonne-Beaufaict, *Azande*. Brussels, Institut Solvay, Maurice Lamertin, 1921.

Commermeyer, Dr, 'Notes de pratique médicale africaine', *Archiv für Schiffs- und Tropen-Hygiene*, 16 (1912): 84.

Carpenter, G. D. Hale, 'Sleeping Sickness', *Kenya and East African Medical Journal*, 6 (1929): 131–48.

A Naturalist on Lake Victoria with an Account of Sleeping Sickness and the Tsetse Fly. London, T. Fisher Unwin, 1920.

Cartwright, F. F., *Disease and History*. London, Hart-Davis, 1972.

A Social History of Medicine. London, Longman, 1977.

Castellani, Aldo, 'Etiology of sleeping sickness', *British Medical Journal*, 1 (14 March 1903): 617–18.

Chalmers, Albert J. and O'Farrell, W. R., 'Sleeping sickness in the Lado of the Anglo-Egyptian Sudan', *Journal of Tropical Medicine and Hygiene*, 17 (1914): 273–84.

Chesterman, C. C. C., 'Some results of tryparsamide and combined treatment of Gambian sleeping sickness', *Transactions of the Royal Society of Tropical Medicine and Hygiene*, 25 (1932): 433.

Chilivumbu, A. B., 'Social basis of illness: a search for therapeutic meaning', in F. X. Grollig and H. B. Haley, eds., *Medical Anthropology*. The Hague, Mouton, 1976.

Chorley, C. W., 'The effects of cloud on the behaviour of tsetse fly', *Uganda Journal*, 5 (1938): 245–51.

Christy, Cuthbert, 'Sleeping Sickness', *Journal of the African Society*, 3 (1903): 1–11.

'The epidemiology and etiology of sleeping sickness in Equatorial East Africa, with clinical observations', *Reports of the Sleeping Sickness Commission* [The Royal Society], 3 (November 1903): 3–32.

'Sleeping sickness (trypanosomiasis): the prevention of its spread, and the prophylaxis', *British Medical Journal*, 2 (1904): 1456–7.

Ciba Foundation, *Trypanosomiasis and Leishmaniasis with Special Reference to Chaga's Disease*. London, Scientific Publication, 1974.

Cipolla, C. M., *Christofano and the Plague: a Study in the History of Public Health in the Age of Galileo*. London, Collins, 1973.

Faith, Reason and the Plague: A Tuscan Story of the Seventeenth Century. Brighton, The Harvester Press, 1977.

Cloudsley-Thompson, J. L., *Insects and History*. London, Weidenfeld & Nicolson, 1976.

Clyde, D. F., *History of Medical Services in Tanganyika*. Dar-es-Salaam, Government Printer, 1962.

Comité Mixte FAO/OMS de la Trypanosomiase Africaine, *Situation Démocratique du Congo*. World Health Organisation, Geneva, 25–30 November 1978.

Congrès Internationale d'Hygiène et Démographie, *Proceedings*, 8 vols. Brussels, P. Weissenbruch, 1903.

Cook, Albert, 'How sleeping sickness came to Uganda', *East African Medical Journal*, 17 (1941): 408–13.

'On sleeping sickness as met with in Uganda, especially with regard to its treatment', *Transactions of the Society of Tropical Medicine and Hygiene*, 1 (1907–8): 25–43.

Curtin, Philip, 'Epidemiology and the slave trade', *Political Science Quarterly*, 83 (1968): 190–216.

Daco, Dr, 'Situation sanitaire et organisation du Service Médicale aux Mines de Kilo-Moto', *Bruxelles-Médical*, 9 (1926): 273–90.

Davies, J. N. P., 'The cause of sleeping sickness? Entebbe, 1902–03. Part I', *East African Medical Journal*, 39 (1962): 81–99.

'Informed speculation on the cause of sleeping sickness, 1898–1903', *Medical History*, 12 (1968): 200–4.

Pestilence and Disease in the History of Africa. Johannesburg, Witwatersrand University Press, 1979.

De Graer, Albertus-M., O. P., 'La maladie du sommeil', *Les Missions Dominicaines*, 3 (Amiens, 1924): 257–67.

'L'art de guérir chez les Azandes', *Congo* (1929): 220–54; 361–408.

'Etat actuel des recherches sur la médecine indigène en territoire de Doruma', in *Compte Rendu de la 13ème Semaine Missiologie à Louvain* (Louvain, 1935), pp. 101–9.

Deshler, W., 'Livestock, trypanosomiasis and human settlement in northeastern Uganda', *Geographical Review*, 50 (1960): 541–55.

De Wildeman, Emile, *A Propos de Médicaments Indigènes Congolais*. Brussels, Institut Royal Colonial Belge, 1935.

Dols, M. W., *The Black Death in the Middle East*, Princeton University Press, 1977.

Doyal, Lesley and Pennel, Imogene, 'Pox Britannica: health, medicine and underdevelopment', *Race and Class*, 2 (1976): 155–76.

The Political Economy of Health. London, Pluto Press, 1979.

Dubois, A., 'La médecine au Congo Belge en fin du XIX siècle', *Bulletin de l'Institut Royal Colonial Belge*, 2 (1944): 350–9.

'Note pour servir à l'histoire du service médicale au Congo Belge', *Bulletin de l'Institut Royal Colonial Belge*, 3 (1945): 388–9.

'Le développement de la médecine expérimentale au Congo Belge', in *Deuxième Rapport Annuel, IRSAC*, Brussels, M. Hayez, 1949, pp. 82–148.

'Jerome Rodhain (1876–1956), Membre de la Classe des Sciences Naturelles et Médicales', in *Bulletin de l'Academie Royale des Sciences Coloniales*, 1 (1957): 159–90.

'Médecine–Introduction', in *Livre Blanc*, vol. II. Brussels, Académie Royale des Sciences d'Outre-Mer, 1962, pp. 873–4.

'Médecine clinique', in *Livre Blanc*, vol. II. Brussels, Académie Royale des Sciences d'Outre-Mer, 1962, pp. 935–40.

'Campenhout (van), Jean-Emile', in *Biographie Belge d'Outre-Mer*, vol. VI. Brussels, Académie Royale des Sciences d'Outre-Mer, 1968, pp. 167–74.

'Rodhain (Alphonse-Hubert-Jerome)', in *Biographie Belge d'Outre-Mer*, vol. VI. Brussels, Académie Royale des Sciences d'Outre-Mer, 1968, pp. 159–90.

Dubois, A. and Duren, A., 'Soixante ans d'organisation médicale au Congo Belge', in *Liber Jubilaris*. Brussels, Société Belge de Médecine Tropicale, 1947, pp. 1–36.

Duggan, A. J., 'An historical perspective', in H. W. Mulligan, ed., *The African Trypanosomiases*. London, Allen & Unwin, 1970.

'Tropical medicine: a submerging art?' *Transactions of the Royal Society of Tropical Hygiene and Medicine*, 76 (1982): 569–74.

Duke, H. Lyndhurst, 'Tsetse flies and trypanosomiasis. Some questions suggested by the late history of the sleeping sickness epidemic in Uganda Protectorate', *Parasitology*, 11 (1919): 415–29.

Duke, H. Lyndhurst and Van Hoof, L., 'Epidemiology of sleeping sickness in the Upper Uele (Belgian Congo)', *Final Report of The League of Nations International Commission on Human Trypanosomiasis*. Geneva, League of Nations, 1928.

Dukes, P. 'Arsenic and old taxa: subspeciation and drug sensitivity in *Trypanosoma brucei*', *Transactions of the Royal Society of Tropical Medicine and Hygiene*, 78 (1984): 711–25.

Dumont, Robert, 'Le conflit des conceptions médicales au Congo', *L'Avenir Colonial Belge* (Leopoldville), 26 November and 4 December 1934.

Duren, A., 'Le service médical de la colonie et ses problèmes d'avenir', *Le Material Colonial*, 2 (1936): 38–50.

'Prix institué pour la découverte du remède contre la trypanosomiase', *Bulletin de l'Institut Royal Colonial Belge* (Brussels, 1952): 1106–9.

Dutton, Joseph Everett, 'Preliminary note upon a trypanosoma occurring in the blood of a man', *Thompson Yates Laboratories' Reports*, 4 (1902): 455–68.

Dutton, J. E. and Todd, J. L., 'First report of the trypanosomiasis expedition to Senegambia (1902) of the Liverpool School of Tropical Medicine and Medical Parasitology', in *Memoir XI*, Liverpool School of Tropical Medicine, 1903.

'Human trypanosomiasis and its relation to Congo sleeping sickness: being the second progress report of the expedition of the Liverpool School of Tropical Medicine to the Congo, 1903', in *Memoir XIII*, Liverpool School of Tropical Medicine, August 1904, pp. 13–48.

'Gland puncture in trypanosomiasis: compared with other methods of demonstrating the presence of the parasite', in *Memoir XVI*, Liverpool School of Tropical Medicine, October 1905, pp. 1–21.

'Gland palpation in human trypanosomiasis: being the third progress report of the expedition of the Liverpool School of Tropical Medicine to the Congo, 1903–04–05', in *Memoir XVIII*, Liverpool School of Tropical Medicine, March 1906, pp. 1–21.

'The distribution and spread of "sleeping sickness" in the Congo Free State with suggestions on prophylaxis: being the fourth progress report of the expedition of the Liverpool School of Tropical Medicine to the Congo, 1903–05', in *Memoir XVIII*, Liverpool School of Tropical Medicine, March 1906, pp. 25–38.

'Prophylaxie de la malaria dans les principaux postes de l'Etat Indépendant du Congo', in *Memoir XX*, Liverpool School of Tropical Medicine, 1906, pp. 1–58.

Dutton, J. E., Todd, John Lancelot and Christy, Cuthbert, 'Human trypanosomiasis on the Congo: being the first progress report of the expedition of the Liverpool School of Tropical Medicine to the Congo, 1903', in *Memoir XIII. Reports of the Trypanosomiasis Expedition to the Congo, 1903–1904 of the Liverpool School of Tropical Medicine and Medical Parasitology*, Liverpool School of Tropical Medicine, August 1904, pp. 1–10.

Ehrenreich, J., ed., *The Cultural Crisis of Modern Medicine*. New York, Monthly Review Press, 1978.

Evans, J., 'Rinderpest and trypanosomiasis', *Sudan Wildlife*, 1 (1949): 7–9.

Evens, F. M. J. C., 'Projet de plan général de l'organisation de la lutte contre les trypanosomiases en Afrique', *Bulletin de l'Académie Royale des Sciences d'Outre-Mer*, Classe des Sciences Naturelles et Médicales, 17–2 (1965): 1–55.

'Recherches Médicales', in *Livre Blanc*, vol. II. Brussels, Académie Royale des Sciences d'Outre-Mer, 1982, pp. 875–94.

Eyidi, Marcel Bebey, *Le Vainquer de la Maladie du Sommeil: le Docteur Eugène Jamot (1879–1937)*. Paris, The Author, 1950.

Fanon, Frantz, 'Medicine and colonialism', in J. Ehrenreich, ed., *The Cultural Crisis of Modern Medicine*. New York, Monthly Review Press, 1978, pp. 229–51.

Feierman, Steven, 'The social origins of health and healing in Africa', African Studies Meeting, Los Angeles, California, 23–28 October 1984.

Fendall, N. R. E., Southgate, B. A. and Berrie, J. R. H., 'Trypanosomiasis control in relation to other public health services', *Bulletin of the World Health Organisation*, 28 (1963): 787–95.

Ferguson, H., 'Equatoria Province', in J. D. Tothill, ed., *Agriculture in the Sudan*. Oxford University Press, 1948, pp. 875–918.

Fialkowski, Bridget T., *John L. Todd 1876–1949. Letters*. Senneville, Quebec, Canada, The Author, 1977.

Fiske, W. F., 'A history of sleeping sickness and reclamation in Uganda', Entebbe, Government Printer, 1926.

Ford, John, 'The control of African trypanosomiases with special reference to land use", *Bulletin of the World Health Organisation*, 40 (1969): 879–92.

The Role of the Trypanosomiases in African Ecology: A Study of the Tsetse Fly Problem. Oxford, Clarendon Press, 1971.

'Ideas which have influenced attempts to solve the problem of African trypanosomiasis', *Social Science and Medicine*, 13B (1979): 269–76.

'Early ideas about sleeping sickness and their influence on research and control', in E. E. Sabben-Clare, D. J. Bradley and K. Kirkwood, eds.,

Health in Tropical Africa During the Colonial Period. Oxford, Clarendon Press, 1980, pp. 30–6.

'Interactions between human societies and various trypanosome–tsetse–wild fauna complexes', in J. P. Garlick and R. W. J. Keay, eds., *Human Ecology in the Tropics,* Oxford, Pergaman, 1970, pp. 81–97.

Garnham, P. C. C., 'Arthropods and disease', in J. Leniham and W. W. Fletcher, eds., *Health and Environment.* London, Blackie, 1976.

Gelfand, M., *Tropical Victory: An Account of the Influence of Medicine on the History of Southern Rhodesia, 1900–1923.* Cape Town, Juta, 1953.

Gero, F., *Death Among the Azande of the Sudan,* trans. W. H. Paxman. Bologna, Editrice Nigrizia, 1968.

Gevaerts, N., *Tussel Uele en Itimbiri.* Antwerp, Tongerloo Abbey, 1948.

Goodwin, L. G., 'Chemotherapy and tropical disease: the problem and the challenge', in M. Hooper, ed., *Chemotherapy of Tropical Diseases.* Chichester, Wiley, 1987.

Harrison, G., *Mosquitoes, Malaria and Man: A History of the Hostilities since 1880.* London, John Murray, 1978.

Hartwig, Gerald Walter and Patterson, K. David, *Disease in African History: an Introductory Survey and Case Studies.* Durham, N.C., Duke University Press, 1978.

Headrick, Rita, 'French health services and African health in French Equatorial Africa, 1918–1939', seminar paper, University of Chicago, 8 June 1977.

'Sleeping sickness at Nola (Central African Republic)', in collected papers of the African Studies Association, Bloomington, Ind., 1981.

Hissette, J., 'Considérations pratiques sur des accidents oculaires de la trypanosomiase ou de son traitement', *Annales de la Société Belge de Médecine Tropicale,* 12 (1932): 531–8.

Hodges, A. D. P., 'Report on sleeping sickness in Uganda', *Reports of the Sleeping Sickness Commission* [The Royal Society], 9 (1908): 3–62.

Hoepli, R. and Lucasse, C., 'Old ideas regarding cause and treatment of sleeping sickness held in West Africa', *Journal of Tropical Medicine and Hygiene,* 67 (1964): 60–8.

Horton, Robin, 'African traditional thought and Western science', *Africa,* 37 (1967): 50–71; 155–87.

Hutchinson, M. P., 'The epidemiology of human trypanosomiasis in British West Africa', *Annals of Tropical Medicine and Parasitology,* 48 (March 1954): 75–94.

International Development Research Centre, *Traditional Medicine in Zaire: Present and Potential Contribution to the Health Services.* Ottawa, Canada, IDRC, 1980.

Jamot, Eugène, 'Essai de prophylaxie médicale de la maladie du sommeil dans l'Oubangui-Chari', *Bulletin de la Société de Pathologie Exotique et de ses Filales,* 13 (12 May 1920): 348–76.

Janssens, P. G., 'La mortalité infantile aux Mines de Kilo', *Bulletin de l'Académie Royale des Sciences d'Outre-Mer,* 20 (1952): 105–19.

'Old and new dimensions in medical aid', *Transactions of the Royal Society of Tropical Medicine and Hygiene,* 65 (1971): 2–15.

'Quatre decennies de maladie du sommeil', *Annales de la Société Belge de Médecine Tropicale*, 57 (1977): 191–200.

'Comparative aspects. I: The Belgian Congo', in E. E. Sabben-Clare, D. J. Bradley and K. Kirkwood, eds., *Health in Tropical Africa During the Colonial Period*. Oxford, Clarendon Press, 1980, pp. 209–27.

'The Congo legacy: health and medicine in the Belgian Congo', *Tropical Doctor*, 11 (1981): 132–40.

'Parasitism, parasites and disease', *Annales de la Société Belge de Médecine Tropicale*, 62 (1982): 183–212.

Janzen, J. M. with Arkinstall, Dr W., *The Quest for Therapy in Lower Zaire*. Berkeley, University of California Press, 1978.

Janzen, J. M. and Feierman, S., eds., 'The social history of disease and medicine in Africa', *Social Science and Medicine*, 13b (December 1979).

Janzen, J. M. and Prins, G., eds., 'Causality and classification in African medicine and health', *Social Science and Medicine*, 15b (July 1981).

Johnson, W. B., *Notes on a Journey Through Certain Belgian, French and British African Dependencies to Observe General Medical Organisation and Methods of Trypanosomiasis Control*. Lagos, Government Printer, 1929.

Johnston, Harry H., 'A few notes on sleeping sickness', *Transactions of the Society of Tropical Medicine and Hygieie*, 1 (1907–8): 22–3.

Jones, Norman Howard, *The Scientific Background of the International Sanitary Conferences, 1851–1938*. Geneva, World Health Organisation, 1975.

Jordan, A. M., *Trypanosomiasis Control and African Rural Development*. London, Longman, 1986.

Kazyumba, G. L., 'L'epidémie sommeileuse en République du Zaire au cours des 25 derniers années', *Médecine d'Afrique Noire*, 26 (1979): 47–52.

Kermorgant, A., 'Notes sur la maladie du sommeil au Congo état approximatif de sa diffusion au mois de juillet 1905', *Annales d'Hygiène et de Médecine Coloniales*, 9 (1906): 126–31.

Kivilu, Sabakinu, 'Notes sur l'histoire de la maladie du sommeil dans la région de Kisantu, 1900–1912', *Likundoli*, 2 (1974): 151–63.

'Population et santé au Zaire à l'époque coloniale de la fin du XIX siècle à 1960', *Transafrican Journal of History*, 13 (1984): 74–91.

Kjekshus, Helge, *Ecology Control and Economic Development in East African History: The Case of Tanganyika, 1850–1950*. London, Heinemann, 1977.

Kuborn, Hyac, *Aperçu Historique sur l'Hygiène Publique en Belgique depuis 1830*. Brussels, Hayez, 1897.

Ladurie, Emmanuel Le Roy, *Times of Feast, Times of Famine: A History of Climate Since the Year 1000*. London, Allen & Unwin, 1972.

Lambrecht, Frank L., 'Aspects of evolution and ecology of tsetse flies and trypanosomiasis in prehistoric African environment', *Journal of African History*, 5 (1964): 1–24.

'Trypanosomiasis in prehistoric and late human populations: a tentative reconstruction', in D. Brothwell and A. T. Sandison, eds., *Diseases in Antiquity: a Survey of the Diseases, Injuries and Surgery of Early Populations*. Springfield, Ill., Charles C. Thomas, 1967, pp. 1–24.

Langlands, Brian W., 'The sleeping sickness epidemic of Uganda, 1900–1920: a study in historical geography', WHO course in parasitology at Makerere University College, May 1967.

Laveran, Charles L. A. and Mesnil, Felix, *Trypanosomes et Trypanosomiases*. Paris, Masson et Cie, 1904.

League of Nations, Health Organisation. *Interim Report on Tuberculosis and Sleeping Sickness in Equatorial Africa.* Geneva, 1923.

Final Report of the League of Nations International Commission on Human Trypanosomiasis, Geneva, 1928.

Learmonth, Andrew, 'Geography and health in the tropical forest zone', in R. Miller and J. W. Watson, eds., *Geographical Essays in Memory of A. E. Ogilvie*. London, Nelson, 1959, pp. 195–220.

Patterns of Disease and Hunger. Newton Abbot, David and Charles, 1978.

Lechat, M. F., 'L'expédition Dutton–Todd au Congo 1903–05. De Boma à Coquilhatville, Septembre 1903–Juillet 1904', *Annales des Sociétés Belges de Médecine Tropicale, de Parasitologie et de Mycologie*, 44 (1964): 493–512.

Lejeune, E., 'La prophylaxie de la maladie du sommeil: son organisation au Congo Belge', *Revista Medica de Angola*, 4 (August 1923): 180–99.

Liverpool School of Tropical Medicine, *Historical Record 1898–1920*. Liverpool University Press, 1920.

Livingstone, David, *Missionary Travels and Researches in South Africa*. London, Ward, Lock & Co., 1857.

'Arsenic as a remedy for the tsetse bite', *British Medical Journal*, 1 (1 May 1858): 360–1.

Lucasse, C., 'Present control of human sleeping sickness', *Annales de la Société Belge de Médecine Tropicale*, 44 (1964): 285–94.

Lumsden, W. H. and Hutt, M. S. R., 'Some episodes in the history of African trypanosomiasis', *Proceedings of the Royal Society of Medicine*, 67 (1974): 789–96.

Lyons, Maryinez, 'From "death camps" to cordon sanitaire: the development of sleeping sickness policy in the Uele district of the Belgian Congo, 1903–1914', *Journal of African History*, 26 (1985): 69–91.

'Sleeping sickness epidemics and public health in the Belgian Congo', in D. Arnold, ed., *Imperial Medicine and Indigenous Societies*. Manchester University Press, 1988, pp. 105–24.

'Sleeping sickness, colonial medicine and imperialism: some connections in the Belgian Congo', in R. MacLeod and M. Lewis, eds., *Disease, Medicine and Empire*. London, Routledge, 1988, pp. 242–56.

'Human trypanosomiases in the history of Africa', in K. F. Kiple, ed., *The History and Geography of Human Disease*. Cambridge University Press, forthcoming.

'Disease in sub-Saharan Africa since 1860', in K. F. Kiple, ed., *The History and Geography of Human Disease*. Cambridge University Press, forthcoming.

'Politics and funding in medical research: the case of African sleeping sickness', in Michael Twaddle, ed., *Imperialism and the State in the Third World: A Festschrift in Honour of Professor Kenneth Robinson*. London, Lester Crook, forthcoming.

McGlashan, Neil D. and Blunden, John R., eds., *Geographical Aspects of Health: Essays in Honour of Andrew Learmonth*. London, Academic Press, 1983.

McKelvey Jr, John J., *Man Against Tsetse: Struggle for Africa*. Ithaca, Cornell University Press, 1973.

MacKenzie, C., 'Report on the existence of sleeping sickness in the Lado enclave on taking over the country from the Belgian Government, June 16, 1910', *Bulletin of the Sleeping Sickness Commission*, 3 (1911): 89.

McKeown, Thomas, *The Role of Medicine: Dream, Mirage or Nemesis?* Oxford, Blackwell, 1979.

McLeod, M., 'Oracles and accusation among the Azande', in A. Singer and B. C. Street, eds., *Zande Themes*. Oxford, Blackwell, 1972, pp. 158–78.

MacLeod, Roy and Milton Lewis, eds., *Disease, Medicine, and Empire: Perspectives on Western Medicine and the Experience of European Expansion*. London, Routledge, 1988.

MacMahon, B. and Pugh, T. F., *Epidemiology: Principles and Methods*. Boston, Little, Browne & Co., 1970.

McNeill, W., *Plagues and People*. Oxford, Basil Blackwell, 1977.

Mack, R., 'The great African cattle plague epidemic of the 1890s', *Tropical Animal Health and Production*, 2 (1970): 210–19.

Maegraith, B. G., 'History of the Liverpool School of Tropical Medicine', *Medical History*, 16 (1972): 354–68.

Mansell-Prothero, R., 'Population mobility and trypanosomiasis in Africa', *Bulletin of the World Health Organisation*, 28 (1963): 615–26.

People and Land in Africa South of the Sahara: Readings in Social Geography. Oxford University Press, 1972.

'Disease and human mobility: a neglected factor in epidemiology', *International Journal of Epidemiology*, 6 (1977): 259–67.

'Medical geography in tropical Africa', in N. D. McGlashen and J. R. Blunden, eds., *Geographical Aspects of Health*. London, Academic Press, 1983, pp. 137–53.

Manson, Patrick, 'Trypanosomiasis on the Congo', *British Medical Journal*, 1 (28 March 1903): 720.

Manson-Bahr, Philip E. C., *History of the School of Tropical Medicine in London (1899–1949)*. London, K. K. Lewis, 1956.

Manson's Tropical Diseases, 18th edn, London, Balliere Tindall, 1982.

Marti-Ibanez, Felix, 'Medical geography and history', in J. M. May, *The Ecology of Human Disease*. New York, MD Publications, 1958.

Maurice, G. K., 'The history of sleeping sickness in the Sudan', *Journal of the Royal Army Medical Corps*, 55 (1930): 161–241.

Mausner, J. S. and Bahn, A. K., *Epidemiology: An Introductory Text*. Philadelphia, W. B. Saunders, 1974.

May, Jacques M., *The Ecology of Human Disease*. New York, MD Publications, 1958.

Meldon, Major J. A., 'Notes on the Sudanese in Uganda', *Journal of the African Society*, 7 (1907–8): 123–48.

Mettam, R., 'A short history of rinderpest with special reference to Africa, *Uganda Journal*, 5 (1937): 22–6.

Molyneux, D. H. and Ashford, R. W., *The Biology of Trypanosoma and Leishmania, Parasites of Man and Domestic Animals*. London, Taylor and Francis, 1983.

Morris, K. R. S., 'The ecology of epidemic sleeping sickness. I: The significance of location', *Bulletin of Entomological Research*, 42 (1951): 427–43.

'The ecology of epidemic sleeping sickness. II: The effects of an epidemic', *Bulletin of Entomological Research*, 43 (1952): 375–96.

'Studies on the epidemiology of sleeping sickness in East Africa. III: The endemic area of Lakes Edward and George in Uganda', *Transactions of the Royal Society of Tropical Medicine and Hygiene*, 54 (1960): 213–14.

'Eradication of sleeping sickness in the Sudan', *Journal of Tropical Medicine and Hygiene*, 64 (1961): 217–24.

'The epidemiology of sleeping sickness in East Africa. V: Epidemics on the Albert Nile', *Transactions of the Royal Society of Tropical Medicine and Hygiene*, 56 (1962): 316–38.

'The movement of sleeping sickness across Central Africa', *Journal of Tropical Medicine and Hygiene*, 66 (March 1963): 159–76.

Morris, R. J., *Cholera 1832: The Social Response to an Epidemic*. London, Croom Helm, 1976.

Mouchet, R., 'Notes anatomiques et médicales sur la pathologie du Moyen Congo', *Archiv für Schiffs- und Tropen-Hygiene*, 17 (1913): 659.

Mulambu, Mvuluya, 'Cultures obligatoires et colonisation dans l'ex-Congo Belge', *Cahiers de CEDAF*, 6–7 (1974).

Muller, Mike, *The Health of Nations: A North–South Investigation*. London, Faber and Faber, 1982.

Mulligan, Hugh W., *The African Trypanosomiases*. London, Allen & Unwin, 1970.

Musambachime, Mwelwa C., 'The social and economic effects of sleeping sickness in Mweru-Luapula 1906–1922', *African Economic History*, 10 (1981): 151–73.

Nash, Thomas A. M., *Africa's Bane: the Tsetse Fly*. London, Collins, 1969.

'The ecology of the West African riverine species of tsetse in relation to man–fly contact', in H. W. Mulligan, ed., *The African Trypanosomiases*. London, Allen and Unwin, 1970, pp. 602–13.

Neujean, G., 'Aspects pratiques de la lutte contre la trypanosomiase humaine dans la République du Congo (Léopoldville)', *Bulletin of the World Health Organisation*, 28 (1963): 797–810.

Nevens, F. M. J. C., 'Projet de Plan Général de l'Organisation de la lutte contre les trypanosomiases en Afrique', *Bulletin de l'Académie Royale des Sciences d'Outre-Mer*, 17 (1965): 12–13.

Nkamba, M. L., 'Histoire de la maladie du sommeil au Kwango (1933–1957)', *Zaire-Afrique*, 160 (1981): 645–54.

Ofcansky, Thomas P., 'The 1889–97 rinderpest epidemic and the rise of British and German colonialism in eastern and southern Africa', *Journal of African Studies*, 8 (1981): 31–8.

'The great rinderpest epidemic of 1889–97', *Historicus*, 2 (1981): 28–54.

Palmberg, Albert, *A Treatise on Public Health and its Applications in Different*

European Countries, translated by Arthur Newsholme. London, Swan Sonnenschein & Co., 1893.

Paul, Jim, 'Medicine and imperialism in Morocco', *Middle East Research Information Project*, 60 (1977): 3–12.

Pearce, Louise, 'Tryparsamide treatment of African sleeping sickness', *Science*, 61 (23 January 1925): 90–2.

Philips, Gladys, Historical Record, 1920–47, Liverpool School of Tropical Medicine, typescript, n.d.

Post, J., 'Famine, mortality and epidemic disease in the process of modernisation', *Economic History Review*, 21 (1976): 14–37.

Prothero, R. M., *see* Mansell-Prothero, R.

Ranger, Terence O., 'Healing in the history of colonial south central Africa', *Bulletin of the Society for the Social History of Medicine*, 23 (1978): 9–10.

'Medical science and Pentecost: the dilemma of Anglicanism in Africa', offprint.

'Godly medicine: the ambiguities of mission medicine in southeast Tanzania, 1900–45', *Social Science and Medicine*, 15B (1981): 261–78.

Ransford, Oliver, *Bid the Sickness Cease: Disease in the History of Black Africa*. London, John Murray, 1983.

Richards, Paul, 'Ecological change and the politics of African land use', *African Studies Review*, 26 (1983): 1–72.

Robert, Maurice, 'Le climat du Congo Belge', in *Encyclopédie du Congo Belge*, 3 vols. Brussels, Editions Bieleveld, 1952, vol. I, pp. 269–304.

Rodhain, Alphonse Jerome, 'Trypanosomiases humaines et animales dans l'Ubangi', *Archiv für Schiffs- und Tropen-Hygiene*, 11 (1907): 283–97.

'Quelques aspects de la pathologie indigène dans l'Ouellé', *Bulletin de la Société de Pathologie Exotique*, 8 (1915): 734–45,

'La maladie du sommeil dans l'Uélé (Congo Belge)', *Bulletin de la Société de Pathologie Exotique*, 9 (1916): 38–72.

'Rapport sur la tuberculose humaine au Congo Belge', *Revista Médica de Angola*, 4 (August 1923): 203–14.

'Les grands problèmes de l'hygiène et l'organisation du service médical au Congo Belge', *Congo*, 2 (June 1926): 1–20.

'Documents pour servir à l'histoire de la maladie du sommeil au Congo Belge. I: La maladie du sommeil dans l'Ubangi en 1905 et 1906', *Bulletin de l'Institut Royal Colonial Belge*, 16 (Brussels, 1945): 112–22.

'Documents pour servir à l'histoire de la maladie du sommeil au Congo Belge. II: La trypanosomiase humaine dans le district de l'Aruwimi en 1907 et en 1908', *Bulletin de l'Institut Royal Colonial Belge*, 17 (Brussels, 1946): 368–79.

'Documents pour servir à l'histoire de la maladie du sommeil au Congo Belge. III: La période 1907 à 1911. Les premiers lazarets et les débuts de l'expérimentation de l'atoxyl et de l'émétique', *Bulletin de l'Institut Royal Colonial Belge*, 19 (Brussels, 1948): 943–55.

'Historique de la recherche scientifique médicale et vétérinaire dans les territoires de l'Afrique au sud du Sahara', *Annales de la Société Belge de Médecine Tropicale*, 34 (1954): 535–54.

Royal Society of London. Sleeping Sickness Commission. *Reports*, 1–17, 1903–1919.

Ruppol, J. F. and Kazyumba, Libala, 'Situation actuelle de la lutte contre la maladie du sommeil au Zaire', *Annales de la Société Belge de Médecine Tropicale*, 57 (1977): 299–314.

'L'endémie sommeileuse en République du Zaire au cours des 25 années (1952–1978)', *Médecine en Afrique Noire*, 26 (1979): 47.

Sabakinu, Kivilu, 'Les sources de l'histoire démographique du Zaire', *Etudes d'Histoire Africaine*, 6 (1974): 119–36.

'Notes sur l'histoire de la maladie du sommeil dans la région de Kisantu, 1900–1912', *Likundoli*, 2 (1974): 151–63.

Sabben-Clare, E. E., Bradley, D. J. and Kirkwood, K., eds., *Health in Tropical Africa During the Colonial Period*. Oxford, Clarendon Press, 1980.

Sand, René, *La Belgique Sociale*. Brussels, J. Lebègue et Cie, 1933.

Schwetz, J., 'A propos du diagnostique le plus expéditif de la maladie du sommeil dans la pratique amublatoire de la brousse', *Bulletin de la Société de Pathologie Exotique*, 12 (1919): 726–30.

'Un voyage médical et paramédical dans la forêt de l'Ituri', *Congo*, 2 (1934): 20–34.

L'Evolution de la Médecine au Congo Belge. Brussels, Université Libre de Bruxelles, 1946.

'Problèmes médicaux actuels au Congo Belge', *Zaire*, 1 (1948): 4–5.

S'Heeren, Dr, 'Rapport sur la Mission de la Maladie du Sommeil dans l'Uele', *Annales de la Société Belge de Médecine Tropicale*, 2 (1922): 83–110.

Scott, D., 'The epidemiology of Gambian sleeping sickness', in H. W. Mulligan, ed., *The African Trypanosomiases*. London, Allen and Unwin, 1970, pp. 614–44.

Scott, H., *A History of Tropical Medicine*, 2 vols. London, Edward Arnold, 1939.

Singer, C. and Underwood, E. A., *A Short History of Medicine*. Oxford University Press, 1962.

Smith, G. Joan, 'The work of the Liverpool School of Tropical Medicine expedition to the Congo, 1903–05, as revealed in the letters of Dr J. L. Todd', *Annals of Tropical Medicine and Parasitology*, 72 (August 1978): 305–22.

Soff, Harvey G., 'Sleeping sickness in the Lake Victoria region', *African Historical Studies*, 2 (1969): 264.

Stark, Evan, 'The epidemic as a social event', *International Journal of Health Services*, 7 (1977): 681–705.

Susser, Mervyn, *Causal Thinking in the Health Sciences: Concepts and Strategies of Epidemiology*. Oxford University Press, 1973.

Thomas, H. Wolferstan and Breinl, Anton, 'Trypanosomes, trypanosomiasis and sleeping sickness: pathology and treatment', in *Memoir XVI*. Liverpool School of Tropical Medicine, October 1905, pp. 1–64 and 66–94.

Thompson, W. E. F., 'Historical fragments on trypanosomiases and the spread of sleeping sickness to British East Africa', *East African Medical Journal*, 38 (1960): 55–6; 90–2; 266–7; 432–4; 466.

Todd, John Lancelot, 'The distribution, spread and prophylaxis of "sleeping sickness" in the Congo Free State', *Transactions of the Epidemiological Society of London*, 25 (1905–6): 1–30.
'Notes re: Congo Expedition', *British Medical Journal* (25 November 1905): 1401.
'Sleeping sickness', *British Medical Journal*, 1 (1906): 943.
'The spread of sleeping sickness in Africa: address by Dr J. L. Todd', *Lancet*, 1 (21 April 1906): 1141.
'The treatment of human trypanosomiasis by atoxyl', *British Medical Journal*, 1 (June 1906): 1037.
'The prevention of sleeping sickness', *British Medical Journal*, 2 (October 1908): 1061–3.
'Parasitology', *Montreal Medical Journal*, 38 (October 1909): 654.
'A review of the recent advances in our knowledge of tropical disease', *The Johns Hopkins Hospital Bulletin*, 21 (July 1910): 1–18.
'Concerning the sex and age of Africans suffering from trypanosomiasis', *Annals of Tropical Medicine and Parasitology*, 7 (1913): 309–19.
'After-history of African trypanosomiasis, 1911-24', *British Medical Journal*, 2 (1924): 298.
'Tropical medicine, 1898–1924', paper presented at International Conference on Health Problems in Tropical Africa, Boston, 1924.
Tothill, J. D., ed., *Agriculture in the Sudan*. Oxford University Press (1948), 1952.
Trolli, G., *Rapport sur l'Hygiène Publique du Congo Belge en 1925*. Brussels, Van Gaufel, 1925.
'Le service médical du Congo Belge depuis sa création jusqu'en 1925', *Congo*, 1 (1927): 187–204.
Historique de l'Assistance Médicale aux Indigènes du Congo Belge. Mont-St. Amand, Van Doolselaere, 1935.
Exposé de la Législation Sanitaire du Congo Belge et du Ruanda-Urundi. Brussels, Ferd, Larcier, 1938.
Turshen, Meredeth, *The Political Ecology of Disease in Tanzania*. New Brunswick, N.J., Rutgers University Press, 1984.
UNDP/World Bank/WHO Special Programme for Research and Training in Tropical Diseases, 'Informal meeting on the pathology of African trypanosomiases', Abidjan, Ivory Coast, 12–16 September 1983.
'Seventh Programme Report. 1 January 1983–31 December 1984'. Excerpted from *Tropical Disease Research*, ch. 5, 'African trypanosomiases'. Geneva, 1985.
'Geographical distribution and prevalence of human African trypanosomiasis and its vectors', Geneva, 16–23 October 1985.
'Round-table discussion on current leads in research relevant to the development of potential new chemotherapeutic agents for African trypanosomiases', Geneva, 10 March 1986.
Van Hoof, L. M. J. J., 'Observations on trypanosomiasis in the Belgian Congo', *Transactions of the Royal Society of Tropical Medicine and Hygiene*, 40 (1947): 728–61.
Van Hoof, L., Henrard, C. and Peel, E., 'Contribution à l'epidémiologie de la

maladie du sommeil au Congo Belge', *Annales de la Société Belge de la Médecine Tropicale*, 18 (1938): 143–201.

Van Riel, J. and Janssens, P. G., 'Lutte contre les endémo-epidémies', *Livre Blanc*, vol. II. Brussels, Académie Royale des Sciences d'Outre-Mer, 1962, pp. 917–28.

Vedy, Dr, 'La vie d'un médecin dans l'Uele il y a cinquante ans. Extraits du journal du docteur Vedy", *Revue Congolaise Illustrée*, 25, no. 9 (1953): 27–9; 25, no. 10 (1953): 15–16; 25, no. 11 (1953): 11; 25, no. 12 (1953): 7–10; 26, no. 3 (1954): 25; 26, no. 8 (1954): 21; 26, no. 9 (1954): 25–8; 26, no. 10 (1954): 27–30; 26, no. 12 (1954): 31–3.

Verleyen, Emile, *Congo: Patrimoine de la Belgique*. Brussels, 1950.

Warren, Kenneth S. and Bowers, John Z., *Parasitology: A Global Perspective*. New York, Springer Verlag, 1983.

Wijers, J. B., 'The history of sleeping sickness in Yimbo location (Central Nyanza, Kenya) as told by the oldest inhabitants of the location', *Tropical and Geographical Medicine*, 21 (1969): 323–37.

Wilcocks, C. and Corson, J. F., *A Survey of Recent Work on Trypanosomiasis and Tsetse-Flies*. London, Bureau of Hygiene and Tropical Diseases, 1946.

Willett, K. C., 'Some principles of the epidemiology of human trypanosomiasis in Africa', *Bulletin of the World Health Organisation*, 28 (1963): 645–52.

Williamson, J., 'Review of Chemotherapeutic and Chemoprophylactic Agents', in H. W. Mulligan, ed., *The African Trypanosomiases*. London, Allen and Unwin, 1970.

Wohl, A. S., *Endangered Lives: Public Health in Victorian Britain*. London, Methuen, 1984.

Woodruff, A. W., ed., *Medicine in the Tropics*. London, Churchill and Livingstone, 1974.

Worboys, Michael, 'The emergence and early development of parasitology', in K. S. Warren and J. Z. Bowers, eds., *Parasitology: A Global Perspective*. New York, Springer Verlag, 1983, pp. 1–18.

World Health Organisation, 'Health in the Congo', *World Health Chronicle*, 15 (1961).

'The African trypanosomiases'. Report of the Joint WHO and FAO Expert Consultation. Technical Report Series, 635 (1979).

'Control of sleeping sickness due to *Trypanosoma brucei gambiense*, *Bulletin of the World Health Organisation*, 60 (1982): 821–5.

Trypanosomiasis Control Manual. Geneva, 1982.

'Report on special programme for research and training in tropical diseases', *World Health Chronicle*, 39 (1985): 179.

Yeager, R., 'Historical and ecological ramifications for AIDS in Eastern and Central Africa', in N. Miller and R. C. Rockwell, eds., *AIDS in Africa: the Social and Policy Impact*. Washington, D.C. and Hanover, N.H., National Council for International Health and African Caribbean Institute, 1988.

Yoder, P. S., ed., *African Health and Healing Systems: Proceedings of a Symposium*. Los Angeles, Crossroads Press, 1982.

Secondary sources: general works

Alexander, Lt Boyd, *From the Niger to the Nile*, 2 vols. London, Edward Arnold, 1908.

Anstey, Roger, *King Leopold's Legacy: the Congo under Belgian Rule, 1908–60*. Oxford University Press, 1966.

Asiwaju, A. I., *Partitioned Africans: Ethnic Relations Across Africa's International Boundaries 1884–1984*. London, Hurst, 1985.

Atkins, John, *The Navy-Surgeon: or, A Practical System of Surgery*. London, Caesar Ward and Richard Chandler, 1734.

   Voyage to Guinea, Brasil, and the West-Indies: In His Majesty's Ships, the Swallow and Weymouth. London, Caesar Ward and Richard Chandler, 1735.

Austin, Ralph A. and Headrick, Rita, 'Equatorial Africa under colonial rule', in *History of Central Africa*, vol. II. London, Longman, 1983, pp. 27–94.

Autrique *et al.*, *Vocabulaire Français–Mangbetu et Mangbetu–Français*. Brussels, Monnom, 1912.

Bates, Darrell, *The Fashoda Incident of 1898: Encounter on the Nile*. Oxford University Press, 1984.

Baxter, P. T. W. and Butt, A., *The Azande and Related Peoples of the Anglo-Egyptian Sudan and Belgian Congo*. London, International Africa Institute, 1953.

Bentley, William Holman, *Pioneering on the Congo*, 2 vols. London, Religious Tract Society, 1900.

Bertrand, A., 'Introduction', in A. de Calonne-Beaufaict, *Azande. Introduction à une Ethnographie Générale des Bassins de l'Ubangi-Uele et de l'Aruwimi*. Brussels, M. Lamertin, 1921.

   Le Problème de la Main d'Oeuvre au Congo Belge (Rapport de la Commission de la Main d'Oeuvre Indigène 1930-31. Province Orientale). Brussels, Ministère des Colonies, 1931.

   'La fin de la puissance Azande', *Bulletin de l'Institut Royal Colonial Belge* (1943): 264–83.

Boulger, D. C., *The Congo State, or the Growth of Civilisation in Central Africa 1860–98*. London, W. Thacker & Co., 1898.

Bozas, Robert du Bourg de, *Mission Scientifique du Bourg de Bozas de la Mer Rouge à l'Atlantique à Travers l'Afrique Tropicale (Octobre 1900–Mai 1903)*. Paris, F. R. de Rudeval, 1906.

Brausch, Georges, *Belgian Administration in the Congo*. Oxford University Press, 1961.

Burrows, Guy, *The Land of the Pigmies*. London, C. Arthur Pearson, 1898.

   'On the natives of the Upper-Welle district of the Belgian Congo', *Journal of the Royal Anthropological Institute*, 28 (1898): 35–47.

   The Curse of Central Africa. London, R. A. Everett & Co., 1903.

Calonne-Beaufaict, Adolphe de, *Les Ababua: Observations Sociologiques*. Brussels, Mouvement Sociologique Internationale, 1909.

   La pénétration de la civilisation au Congo Belge et les Bases d'une Politique Coloniale. Brussels, Institut de Sociologie Solvay, 1912.

312   Select bibliography

Azande. Introduction à une Ethnographie Générale des Bassins de l'Ubangi-Uele et de l'Aruwimi. Brussels, M. Lamertin, 1921.

Casati, Gaetano, *Ten Years in Equatoria and the Return of Emin Pasha*. London, Frederick Warne & Co., 1891; reprint edn, New York, Negro Universities Press, 1969.

Cattier, Felicien, *Etude sur la Situation de l'Etat Indépendant du Congo*, 2nd edn. Brussels, F. Larcier, 1906.

Ceulemans, R. P. P., 'Les tentatives de Leopold II pour engager le Colonel Charles Gordon au service de l'Association Internationale Africaine (1880)', *Zaire*, 12 (1958): 251–74.

La Question Arabe et le Congo (1883–1892). Brussels, Académie Royale des Sciences d'Outre-Mer, 1959.

Chateleux, Roger de ['Chalux'], *Un An au Congo Belge*. Brussels, Albert Dewit, 1925.

Christiaens, Emile, *Le Pays des Mangbettus*. Brussels, Cercle Africain de Bruxelles, Van Campenhout Frères & Soeur, 1896.

Christy, Cuthbert, 'The Nile–Congo Divide', *The Geographical Journal*, 50 (1917): 199–218.

Big Game and Pygmies. London, Macmillan, 1924.

Cohen, David W., *The Historical Tradition of Busoga: Mukama and Kintu*. Oxford, Clarendon Press, 1972.

Collins, Robert O., 'The transfer of the Lado enclave to the Anglo-Egyptian Sudan, 1910', *Zaire*, 2–3 (1960): 193–210.

The Southern Sudan 1883–1898: A Struggle for Control. New Haven, Yale University Press, 1962.

King Leopold, England and the Upper Nile, 1899–1909. New Haven, Yale University Press, 1968.

'Sudanese factors in the history of the Congo and central West Africa in the nineteenth century', in Yusuf Fadl Hasan, ed., *Sudan in Africa*. Khartoum University Press, 1971.

Land Beyond the Rivers: The Southern Sudan, 1898–1918. New Haven, Yale University Press, 1971.

Conco, W. Z., 'The African Bantu traditional practice of medicine and the problems of communication'. Unpublished typescript, WIHM, 1970.

Cookey, Sylvanus J. S., 'West African immigrants in the Congo, 1885–1896', *Journal of the Historical Society of Nigeria*, 3 (1965): 261–70.

Britain and the Congo Question: 1885–1913. New York, Humanities Press, 1968.

Cornet, R. J., *Bwana Muganga: Hommes en Blanc en Afrique Noire*. Brussels, Académie Royale des Sciences d'Outre-Mer, 1971.

Curtin, Philip, Feierman, Steven, Thompson, Leonard and Vansina, Jan, *African History*. London, Longman, 1978.

Czekanowski, Jan, *Forschungen im Nil-Kongo Zwischengebiet*, vol. II: *Ethnographie, Uele Nil-Lander*. Leipzig, Klinkhardt & Biermann, 1924.

De Bauw, A., ed., *Trente Années de Culture Cotonnière au Congo Belge, 1918–48*. Brussels, Compagnie Cotonnière Congolaise, c. 1945.

De Cort, Laudet et Van Goethem, *Vocabulaire Française-Ababua et Ababua-Français*. Brussels, Monnom, 1912.

Delhaise-Arnould, C., 'Les associations secrètes au Congo Belge: le Nébili ou Negbo', *Bulletin de la Société Etudes Coloniales*, 26 (1919): 283–90.

'Dans l'antre du "Nébili"', *Illustration Congolaise*, 114 (1931): 3422; 115 (1931): 3464.

Denis, P., *Histoire des Mangbetu et des Matshaga jusqu'à l'Arrivée des Belges*. Tervuren, Musée Royal de l'Afrique Central, 1961.

De Schlippe, Pierre, *Shifting Cultivation in Africa. The Zande System of Agriculture*. London, Routledge & Kegan Paul, 1956.

du Plessis, J., *Thrice Through the Dark Continent: a Record of Journeyings Across Africa During the Years 1913–1916*. London, Longmans, Green & Co., 1917.

Ehret, Christopher, *et al.*, 'Some thoughts on the early history of the Nile–Congo watershed', *Ufahamu*, 5 (1974): 85–112.

Ehret, C. and Posnansky, M., *The Archaeological and Linguistic Reconstruction of African History*. Berkeley, University of California Press, 1982.

Evans-Pritchard, Edward E., 'Sorcery and native opinion', *Africa*, 4 (1931): 23–8.

'The Zande corporation of witchdoctors', *Journal of the Royal Anthropological Institute*, 62 (1932): 291–336; 63 (1933): 63–100.

'Zande therapeutics', in E. E. Evans-Pritchard *et al.*, eds., *Essays Presented to C. G. Seligman*. London, Kegan Paul, 1934.

'Zande theology', *Sudan Notes and Records*, 19 (1936): 5–46.

Witchcraft, Oracles and Magic Among the Azande. Oxford, Clarendon Press, 1937.

'A history of the kingdom of Gbudwe', *Zaire*, 10 (1956): 451–91; 675–710; 815–60.

'Zande kings and princes', in *Essays in Social Anthropology*. London, Faber and Faber, 1969.

'A contribution to the study of Zande culture', *Africa*, 30 (1960): 309–24.

'A further contribution to the study of Zande culture', *Africa*, 33 (1963): 183–97.

The Zande Trickster. Oxford, Clarendon Press, 1967.

'Zande notions about Death, Soul and Ghost', *Sudan Notes and Records*, 50 (1969): 41–52.

'A note on some Zande physiological notions', *Sudan Notes and Records*, 51 (1970): 162–5.

The Azande: History and Political Institutions. Oxford, Clarendon Press, 1971.

Man and Woman Among the Azande. London, Faber and Faber, 1974.

Fetter, Bruce, *Colonial Rule and Regional Imbalance in Central Africa*. Boulder, Colo., Westview Press, 1983.

Flament, F., ed., *La Force Publique de sa Naissance à 1914*. Brussels, Académie Royale des Sciences d'Outre-Mer, 1952.

Flandrau, Grace, *Then I Saw the Congo*. New York, Harcourt, Brace & Co., 1929.

Franck, Louis, *Le Congo Belge*, 2 vols. Brussels, La Renaissance du Livre, 1930.

Galbraith, J. S., 'Gordon, MacKinnon and Leopold: the scramble for Africa, 1876–84', *Victorian Studies*, 14 (1971): 369–88.

Gann, L. H. and Duignan, P. J., *The Rulers of Belgian Africa, 1885–1914*. Princeton University Press, 1979.

Giorgetti, Filiberto, *La Superstizione Zande*. Bologna, Editrice Nigrizia, 1966.

Gore, Rev. Canon and Gore, E. C., *Zande and English Dictionary*. London, The Sheldon Press, 1952.

Gourou, Pierre, *L'Afrique*. Paris, Hachette, 1970.

Gray, J. Richard, *A History of the Southern Sudan, 1839–1889*. Oxford University Press, 1961.

Guebels, Leon M. J., *Relation Complète des Travaux de la Commission Permanente pour la Protection des Indigènes, 1911–1951*. Gembloux, J. Duculot, 1952.

Halkin, Joseph, *Les Ababua*. Brussels, A. Dewit, 1910.

Headrick, Rita, 'French health services and African health in French Equatorial Africa, 1918–1939', unpublished Seminar paper, University of Chicago, 8 June 1977.

Holt, P. P., 'Egypt and the Nile Valley', in J. E. Flint, ed., *The Cambridge History of Africa*, vol. V: 1790–1870. Cambridge University Press, 1976.

Horton, Robin, 'African traditional thought and Western science', *Africa*, 37 (1967): 50–71; 155–87.

Hutereau, J.-A. Armand, *Notes sur la Vie Familiale et Juridique de Quelques Populations du Congo Belge*. Tervuren, Annales du Musée Royal du Congo Belge, 1909.

  Histoire des Peuplades de l'Uele et de l'Ubangi. Brussels, Goemaere, Falk Fils, 1922.

Jewsiewicki, Benoit, 'Notes sur l'histoire socio-economique du Congo 1880–1969', *Etudes d'Histoire Africaine*, 3 (1972): 209–41.

  'Modernisation ou destruction du village africaine: l'économie politique de la "modernisation agricole" au Congo Belge', *Les Cahiers du Cedaf*, 5 (1983).

Johnston, Harry H., *The River Congo*. London, Sampson Low, Marston, Searle and Rivington, 1884.

  George Grenfell and the Congo, 2 vols. London, Hutchinson & Co., 1908.

Junker, Wilhelm, *Travels in Africa, 1879–1889*, 3 vols., trans. A. H. Keane. London, Chapman and Hall, 1890–2.

Keim, Curtis A., 'Long-distance trade and the Mangbetu', *Journal of African History*, 24 (1983): 1–22.

Kirk, R., 'Sir Henry Wellcome and the Sudan', *Sudan Notes and Records*, 37 (1956): 79–87.

Lagae, C.-R., *Les Azande ou Niam-Niam: l'Organisation Zande, Croyances Religieuses et Magiques, Coutumes Familiales*. Brussels, Vromant and Co., 1926.

Lagae, C.-R. and Vanden Plas, V. H., *La Langue des Azande: Introduction Historico-Géographique*, 2 vols. Ghent, Editions Dominicaines 'Veritas', 1921 and 1922.

Larken, P. M., 'Zande background: notes on the Azande of Tambura and Yambio, 1911–1932', foreword by T. A. T. Leitch (typescript, *c.* 1954).

Larochette, J., *Grammaire des Dialects Mangbetu et Medje Suivie d'un Manuel de Conversation et d'un Lexique*. Tervuren, Musée Royal du Congo Belge, 1958.

Lelong, Maurice Hyacinthe, *Mes Frères du Congo*, 2 vols. Algiers, Editions Baconnier, 1946.

Lemaire, Charles, *Au Congo: Comment les Noirs Travaillent*. Brussels, Bulens, 1895.

'Les Mangbetu", *Belgique Coloniale*, 4 (1898): 4–5.

'Notes pour servir à l'histoire des races congolaises', *Belgique Coloniale*, 4 (1898): 42–3.

Leplae, Edmund, 'Histoire et développement des cultures obligatoires de coton et de riz au Congo Belge de 1917 à 1933', *Congo*, 14 (1933): 645–753.

Livingstone, David, *Missionary Travels and Researches in South Africa*. London, John Murray, 1857.

Lotar, R. P. Leon, 'Souvenirs de l'Uele', *Congo*, 1 (1930): 607–11; 771–81; 2 (1930): 1–8; 149–65; 635–61; 1 (1931): 671–86; 2 (1931): 481–502; 2 (1932): 1–32; 342–61; 498–503; 1 (1933): 199–213; 333–50; 2 (1933): 658–82; 1 (1934): 1–12; 1 (1935): 641–67; 2 (1935): 665–84.

La Grande Chronique de l'Ubangi. Brussels, Institut Royal Colonial Belge, 1937.

La Grande Chronique du Bomu. Brussels, Institut Royal Colonial Belge, 1940.

La Grande Chronique de l'Uele. Brussels, Institut Royal Colonial Belge, 1946.

Louis, William Roger, 'Roger Casement and the Congo', *Journal of African History*, 5 (1964): 99–120.

Louis, William Roger and Stengers, Jean, eds., *E. D. Morel's History of the Congo Reform Movement*. Oxford, Clarendon Press, 1968.

Lugard, Frederick D., *The Rise of our East African Empire*, 2 vols. London, W. Blackwood and Sons, 1893.

McMaster, Mary, 'Linguistic evidence for the history of Bua Mangbetu interactions', unpublished paper, University of California, June 1978.

Mecklenburg-Schwerin, Adolph Friedrich, *From the Congo to the Niger and the Nile*, 2 vols. London, Duckworth & Co., 1913.

Meldon, J. A., 'Notes on the Sudanese in Uganda', *Journal of the African Society*, 7 (1907–8): 123–46.

Meyers, Dr, *Le Prix d'un Empire*. Brussels, Charles Dessart, 1943.

Meoller de Laddersous, A., 'L'adaptation des sociétés indigènes de la Province Orientale à la situation créée par la colonisation', *Bulletin de l'Institut Royal Colonial Belge* (1931): 52–66.

'Les origines et l'introduction de la culture de coton au Congo Belge', in A. de Bauw, ed., *Trente Années*. Brussels, Compagnie Cotonnière Congolaise, *c.* 1945, pp. 14–18.

Morel, Edmund Denille, 'The Congo State and the Bahr el-Ghazal', *Nineteenth Century* (August 1901): 202–13.

Red Rubber: The Story of the Rubber Slave Trade Flourishing in the Congo in the Year of Grace 1906. London, T. Fisher Unwin, 1906.

Great Britain and the Congo: The Pillage of the Congo Basin. London, Smith, Elder & Co., 1909.

Moulaert, G., 'Les exploitations minières de Kilo Moto et de la Province Orientale', *Congo* (January 1935), 31 pp.

Vingt Années à Kilo Moto. Brussels, Charles Dessart, 1950.

Mulambu, Mvuluya, 'Cultures obligatoires et colonisation dans l'ex–Congo Belge', *Cahiers de CEDAF*, 6–7 (1974), 99 pp.

Muller, Emmanuel, *Ouellé, Terre d'Héroisme*. Brussels, Editions l'Essor, 1941.

Murdock, George P., *Africa: Its Peoples and Their Culture History*. New York, McGraw-Hill, 1959.

Parke, T. H., *My Personal Experiences in Equatorial Africa*. London, Sampson, Low, Marston & Co., 1891.

Reining, Conrad C., *The Zande Scheme: An Anthropological Case Study of Economic Development in Africa*. Evanston, Ill., Northwestern University Press, 1966.

Renier, Commandant, *Héroisme et Patriotisme des Belges: l'Oeuvre Civilisatrice au Congo*. Ghent, Heckenrath, 1913.

Robert, M., *Le Congo Physique*. Liège, H. Vaillaut-Carmanne, 1946.

Roget, L., 'Le district de l'Arouwimi-et-Ouellé', *Bulletin de la Société Royale Belge de Géographie*, 15 (1891): 97–128.

Saint Moulin, Léon de, 'Histoire de l'organisation administrative du Zaire', *Zaire-Afrique*, 224 (April 1988): 197–222.

Salmon, Pierre, *Le Reconnaissance Graziani Chez les sultans du Nord de l'Uele, 1908*. Brussels, Centre Scientifique et Médical de l'Université Libre de Bruxelles en Afrique Centrale [Cemubac], 1963.

La Dernière Insurrection de Mopoie Bangezegino (1916). Brussels, Académie Royale des Sciences d'Outre-Mer, 1969.

'Les Zande sous l'administration Belge (1908–1960), *Comptes Rendus Séances de l'Académie des Sciences d'outre-Mer* (Paris), 31 (1971): 90–137.

'Sectes secrètes Zande (Republique du Zaire)', in *Etudes de Géographie Tropicale Offertes à Pierre Gourou*. Paris, Mouton, 1972, pp. 427–40.

Le Voyage de Van Kerckhoven aux Stanley Falls et au Camp de Yambuya (1888). Brussels, Académie Royale des Sciences d'Outre-Mer, 1978.

'L'Etat Indépendant au Congo et la question arabe (1885–1892)', in *Le Centenaire de l'Etat Indépendant du Congo*. Brussels, Académie Royale des Sciences d'Outre-Mer, 1988, pp. 437–60.

Saxon, Douglas, 'Linguistic evidence for the eastward spread of Ubangian peoples', in C. Ehret and M. Posnansky, eds., *The Archaeological and Linguistic Reconstruction of African History*. Berkeley, University of California Press, 1982.

Schweinfurth, Georg, *The Heart of Africa* (1868–71), 2 vols. New York, Harper & Brothers, 1874.

Schweinfurth, G., Ratzel, R., Felkin, R. W. and Hartlaub, G., *Emin Pasha in Central Africa: Being a Collection of His Letters and Journals*. London, George Philip & Son, 1888.

Seligman, C. G. and Seligman, Brenda, *Pagan Tribes of the Nilotic Sudan*. London, Routledge and Kegan Paul, 1932.

Singer, André and Street, Brian V., *Zande Themes: Essays Presented to Sir E. E. Evans-Pritchard*. Oxford, Blackwell, 1972.

Slade, Ruth, *King Leopold's Congo*. Oxford University Press, 1962.

Stanley, Henry Morton, *The Congo and the Founding of its Free State*, 2 vols. London, Sampson Low, Marston, Searle & Rivington, 1885.

In Darkest Africa, 2 vols. London, Sampson Low, Marston, Searle & Rivington, 1890.

Stengers, J., 'The Congo Free State and Belgian Congo before 1914', in L. H. Gann and P. Duignan, eds., *Colonialism in Africa, 1870–1960*, vol. I. Cambridge University Press, 1969.

Stengers, J. and Vansina, J., 'King Léopold's Congo 1886–1908', in R. O. Oliver and G. N. Sanderson, eds., *The Cambridge History of Africa*, vol. VI. Cambridge University Press, 1985.

Thuriaux-Hennebert, Arlette, *Les Azande dans l'Histoire du Bahr el Ghazal et de l'Equatoria*. Brussels, Institut de Sociologie, 1964.

Tilkins, E., 'Les Ababua', *Belgique Coloniale*, 6 (1900): 220a–221b; 231b–233b; 245b–246b; 255a–256d; 267a–269a.

Turner, Victor, *The Drums of Affliction*. Oxford, Clarendon, 1968.

Vanden Bergh, Leonard John, *On the Trail of the Pigmies*. London, T. Fisher Unwin, 1922.

Van den Plas, V.-H., *Les Missions Dominicaines* (1925): 50–4.

Van den Plas, V.-H. and Lagae, C.-R., *La Langue des Azande*, 2 vols. Ghent, Editions Dominicaines 'Veritas'', 1921.

Vander Kerken, G., *Notes sur les Mangbetus*. Antwerp, Université Coloniale de Belgique, 1932.

Vangroenweghe, Daniel, *Du Sang sur les Lianes: Léopold II et son Congo*. Brussels, Didier Hatier, 1986.

Vangroenweghe, D. and Vellut, J. L., eds., 'Le rapport Casement', *Enquêtes et Documents d'Histoire Africaine*, 6 (1985): 1–174.

Van Overbergh, C. and de Jonghe, J., *Les Mangbetu*. Brussels, Albert Dewit, 1909.

Vansina, Jan, *Introduction à l'Ethnographie du Congo*. Kinshasa, Université Lovanium, 1966.

'L'Afrique Centrale vers 1875', in *La Conférence de Géographie de 1876: Recueil d'Etudes*. Brussels, Académie Royale des Sciences d'Outre-Mer, 1976.

Vedy, Dr, 'Les Ababuas', *Bulletin de la Société Royale Belge de Géographie*, 28 (1904): 191–203; 265–94.

Vekens, A., *La Langue des Makere, des Medje et des Mangbetu*. Ghent and Brussels, Editions Dominicaines 'Veritas', 1921.

Vellut, Jean-Luc, 'The "classical" age of Belgian colonialism: outline for a social history (1910–40)', seminar paper presented at School of Oriental and African Studies, 1978.

'Les bassins miniers de l'ancien Congo Belge. Essai d'histoire économique et sociale (1900–1960)', *Les Cahiers du Cedaf*, 7 (November 1981): 2–70.

'La misère rurale dans l'expérience coloniale du Zaire, du Rwanda, et du Burundi', unpublished paper presented to African Studies Association Conference, Boston, December 1983.

'Mining in the Belgian Congo', in D. Birmingham and P. M. Martin, eds., *History of Central Africa*. Harlow, Longman, 1983.

'La violence armée dans l'Etat Indépendant du Congo. Ombres et clartés dans l'histoire d'un état conquerant', unpublished paper given to Colloque International sur les Relations Africaines à la Colonisation en Afrique Centrale, Kigali, 6–10 May 1985.

Vergiat, A. M., *Les Rites Secrets des Primitifs de l'Oubangui*. Paris, Payout, 1936.

Wauters, Joseph, *Le Congo au Travail*. Brussels, l'Eglantine, 1924.

Wingate, F. R., *Mahdism and the Egyptian Sudan*. London, Macmillan, 1891.

Winterbottom, T., *An Account of the Native Africans in the Neighbourhood of Sierra Leone to Which is Added an Account of the Present State of Medicine Among Them*. London, John Hatchard and J. Mawman, 1803.

Witterwulghe, Georges F., *Vocabulaire à l'Usage des Fonctionnaires se rendant dans les territoires du district de l'Uele et de l'Enclave Redja-Lado*. Brussels, l'Etat Indépendant du Congo, 1904.

Wundu, Lutumba-Lu-Vilu Na, *Histoire du Zaire: l'Administration Centrale du Ministère Belge des Colonies (1908–1940)*. Kinshasa, Editions Okapi, 1972.

Government publications

Belgium. Chambre des Représentants, *Rapport Annuel sur l'Activité de la Colonie du Congo Belge pendant l'Année*. Brussels, 1921, 1922, 1924.

Colonie du Congo Belge, *Rapport sur l'Hygiène Publique pendant l'Année 1925*. Brussels, 1925 [and 1926–33].

Ministère des Affaires Africaines, *Guide Médical Abrégé à l'Usage du Voyageur au Congo*. Brussels, 1929.

Ministère des Colonies, *Annuaire Officiel du Congo Belge*. Brussels, 1910–14; 1921–60.

Ministère des Colonies, *Recueil à l'Usage des Fonctionnaires et des Agents du Service Territorial au Congo Belge*, 4th edn, Brussels, 1925; 5th edn, Brussels, 1930.

Ministère des Colonies, *Vade-Mecum, à l'Usage des Infirmiers et des Assistants Médicaux Indigènes* by Dr David. Brussels, 1922.

Ministère du Congo Belge, Inspection Générale de l'Hygiène, *La Santé en Afrique Belge*. Brussels, InforCongo, 1958.

Service de l'Hygiène, *Ordonnance du 6 Mars 1929 Portant Nouveau Règlement de Police Sanitaire des Frontières et Ports de Mer et des Frontieres et Ports des Lacs*. Boma, 1929.

Congo Free State, Local Government, Boma. *Recueil Mensuel des Ordonnances, Arrêtés, Circulaires, Instructions et Ordres de Service*. January 1896.

Recueil Administratif. 1903.

Bulletin Officiel. 1885– .

Great Britain, Colonial Office, Departmental Committee on Sleeping Sickness. *Report of the Inter-Departmental Committee: Minutes of Evidence*, 2 parts,

Cd 7349–50. London, 1914. (Written statement from Professor J. L. Todd at McGill University.)

Colonial Office, *Proceedings of the First International Conference held at the Colonial Office*, Cd 3778. London, 1907. ('Report on the Sanitary Police measures enforced by the government of the Independent Congo State' by Dr Emile Van Campenhout.)

Foreign Office. *Africa*, no. 4. London, 1890. 'Correspondence respecting Mr Stanley's expedition for relief of Emin Pasha'.

Parliamentary Papers. *Africa*, no. 1, London, 1904. 'Correspondence and reports from H.M. Consul at Boma respecting the administration of the Independent State of the Congo.'

Parliamentary Papers. 'Correspondence respecting the expedition for the relief of Emin Pasha, 1886–87', C 5601. London, 1888.

Naval Intelligence Division. *Manual of Belgian Congo*. London, 1920.

Naval Intelligence Division. *The Belgian Congo*. London, 1944.

USA, American University. *Area Handbook for the Democratic Republic of the Congo (Congo-Kinshasa)*. Washington, D.C., US Government Printing Office, 1971.

Zaire, Département de la Santé Publique, Bureau Central de la Trypano-somiase. 'Rapport d'Activités 1981', May 1982.

Primary sources: Belgium

Ministère des Affaires Etrangères. Archives Africaines, Brussels

Service de l'Inspecteur-Général de l'Hygiène, Administration, 1910–1950

1–33 Administration du Service. Généralités et administration du Service, 1910–50

Service de l'Hygiène, 1889–1946

34–53 Correspondance générale, 1907–44
54–78 Correspondance avec les districts du Congo Belge, 1910–1914
83–110 Commissions d'hygiène des districts, 1903–13
111–39 Rapports sanitaires des districts, de la Compagnie des Chemins de Fer du Congo Supérieur aux Grands Lacs Africains, des Mines de Kilo-Moto et du Comité Spécial du Katanga, 1905–14
140–77 Fonctionnement des lazarets, 1907–14
178–217 Fonctionnement des hôpitaux, 1894–1947
275–379 Maladie du sommeil, 1902–46
601–3 Missions d'études, 1903–31
604–6 Rapports et notes, 1911–28
695–6 Conseil Supérieur d'Hygiène Coloniale, 1933–45
697–706 Ecoles médicales indigènes, 1921–51
707–56 Ecole de Médecine Tropicale de l'Etat à Bruxelles, 1906–49
845–911 Office International d'Hygiène Publique (Paris), 1928–46
937–41 *Varia*, 1927–43

Service de l'Inspecteur-Général de l'Hygiène, 1946–62

1152 Organisations, institutions et commissions belges (1901–1945); 1946–
Papiers Dr A. Duren, Directeur de Service de l'Hygiène, 1929–45

Première Direction: Droit Public, Institutions Politiques et Administratives

1–12 Arrêtés et decrêts de l'Etat Indépendant du Congo, 1887–1908
532– Hygiène, 1908–

Fonds Annexe-Rapports Officiels de Congo Belge
49– Conseil de Province de la Province Orientale, 1929–
80– Hygiène, 1908–
137– Hygiène, 1922–

Deuxième Section, Affaires Etrangères

Première Partie: 1885–1914 (1918)
428–33 Conférences médicales, 1899–1908
489–507 Voyages, missions et explorations au Congo, 1885–1905
555 Voies de communication vers le Nil, 1918–1922

Deuxième Partie: 1914–1962
504– Conférences et conventions relatives à l'Hygiène, 1921–
898– La Société des Nations, 1920–
1680– Hygiène, 1928–

Première Direction, Affaires Indigènes

1368–9, 1391–7 Protection des indigènes, 1885–
1370–1, 1407–13 Etudes des populations, 1888–
1414 Missions scientifiques, 1911–

Première Direction, Domaine et Cadastre

Collection des cartes et plans. Cartes sanitaires, 1910–

Musée Royal de l'Afrique Centrale, Section Historique, Tervuren

Documents Provenant de la Mission Franz Cornet au Congo, 1948–9
(656 documents)

Uele administration (50.30.1–56)
Gouverneur-Général et Vice-Gouverneur-Général: Correspondance expediée
(50.30.57–62)
Gouverneur-Général et Vice-Gouverneur-Général: Correspondance reçue
(50.30.63–73)

District de l'Uele, Bas-Uele, Zone du Rubi et Zone de l'Uere-Bili (50.30.74–83): Correspondance générale expediée (50.30.84–139)
District de l'Uele, Bas-Uele, Zone du Rubi et Zone de l'Uere-Bili: Correspondance générale reçue (50.30.120–212)
Circulaires du Gouvernement à Boma et des Commissaires de Districts et Chefs de Zones (50.30.213–22)
Justice (50.30.292–317)
Démographie (50.30.318–33)
Service Médical (50.30.369–87)
Hygiène (50.30.388–9)
Affaires Indigènes – Main d'Oeuvre (50.30.517–53)
Dossier du personnel européen (50.30.615–45)

Emmanuel Muller, Commandant, Gurba-Dungu Zone. Papers

Copy letterbook, 13 August 1896–16 February 1897 and journal, December 1895–16 March 1897. Also enclosing Emile Christiaens copy letterbooks, 6 July 1893–4 December 1894 (54.95)

Adolphe de Calonne-Beaufaict

Correspondence, 1905–13

Repertoire Général de la Section d'Histoire (RG 1103)

André Landeghem papers, 1900–13 (RG 1010)
Expédition Lemaire, 1902–3
Felix Fuchs papers, Hygiène. Service Médical, 1901–14 (RG 765.114)
H. Orts papers, Hygiène et Médecine, 1906–7 (RG 167)
Dr A. Rodhain papers (58.20.47–73 and 58.20.45–6)

Musée Royal de l'Afrique Centrale, Section Ethnographique, Tervuren
Photographic collection

Archives Palais Royal. Brussels.

King's Cabinet Papers (1882–1912)

102 H. M. Stanley correspondence, 1884–97
370 Gouverneur-Général T. T. Wahis to Léopold II, 12 November 1905

Dominican House, Louvain

R. P. Van Mol, O.P., 'Herinneringen uit Mijn Missionarisleven in Uele-Kongo, 1921–1964', typescript, 477 pp., 1967.
C.-R. Lagae, 'Rapport extraordinaire sur le vicarat de Niangara (Congo Belge)

confié aux Dominicains de la Province Belge de Sainte Rose', 18 July 1927.

Le Propagateur du Rosaire, Louvain, 1875–1914, 1919–25

Les Missions Dominicaines, Hainaut, Belgium, 1922–

L'Année Dominicaine, Paris, 1899–

Tongerloo Abbey, Belgium, Prémontré Library Archives
Archives, 'Uele missie'. 2 boxes
P. N. Gevaerts' history of the mission, manuscript
Revue de l'Ordre Prémontré et ses Missions, Heverle, Belgium, 1898–

Primary sources: Sudan

Sudan Government Archives, Khartoum
Mongalla,, 19 January 1926, Governor, Bahr el-Ghazal to Civil Secretary (class 1, box 6, file 42)
19 June 1925. J. E. Philipps, District Commissioner, Tembura to Governor, Bahr-el Ghazal Province (class 1, box 6, file 42)
3 June 1926, Governor, Bahr el-Ghazal, enclosing H. Burges Watson, Tembura District, Intelligence Report (class 1, box 6, file 42)
28 November 1907, Cameron, Governor, Mongalla Province. 'Notes on the Lado Enclave and points in connection with its transfer from the Belgians' (class 1, box 8, file 51)
30 November 1919, 'Report by Principal Medical Officer, Egyptian Army, on sleeping sickness for the year ending 30 September 1919' (class 1, box 6, file 39)
5 January 1905, 'Notes from trader recently arrived from Congo Territory', enclosed in Wilson to Lansdowne (class 1, box 8, file 50)

Sudan National Archives, Khartoum
Historical Archives. Native Societies, Archive X. Subject: Native societies and cults, 17 October 1916, Dungu, TA T. Torissen to Inspector, Meridi District (Sudan).

Primary sources: United Kingdom
London School of Hygiene and Tropical Medicine. Ronald Ross Papers
Correspondence
Dutton to Ross. 13/076. 11 January 1902
Dutton to Ross. 13/070. 22 December 1901

J. L. Todd to Ross. 72/365. 10 July 1911
C. Christy to Ross. 50/271. 20 June 1901
Ross: draft letter to Editor of *British Medical Journal*. 13/163. 2 December 1902
Ross to Emile Van Campenhout. 20/123. 19 October 1909
Dr Leon E. Bertrand to Ross. 50/229–30. 13 March 1901; 51/059. 31 July 1903

Ross manuscripts. 13/159–63

Anon. 32/392. 'Sir Alfred Jones and the sleeping sickness'. 19 December 1905
Balfour, Andrew, 'Some tropical lacunae', Ms. lecture at Universities of Leiden, Utrecht and Amsterdam, March 1927 (Box 1 (12), Ms. FC: D1)
    'Medical science as a factor in imperial development, 1870–1921' (Box 2 (42), Ms. FC: D1)
    'Malaria as an enemy of the British Empire', address to the Guildhouse, Eccleston Square, 18 October 1925 (Box 1 (10), Ms. FC: D1)
Conférence International sur la Maladie du Sommeil. Rénuie à Londres en 1907–1908 (AD-P.17196)
Low, George Carmichael, ms. correspondence with Patrick Manson between June and October 1902. London School of Hygiene and Tropical Medicine Library, 2 packets

Liverpool School of Tropical Medicine, Liverpool University, Library Archives

TM/8/SX.1.1 Register of students 1899–1923
TM/14/TOJ 7.2 4 September 1904, Dr Thomas to Mrs Todd
TM/14/TOJ 7.6b 3 December 1920, J. L. Todd to MacPhail
TM/14/DUJ 7P n.d. Inge Heiberg/Todd/Christy/Dohet
TM/14/DUJ 10 1 February 1904, Dutton to Ross
TM/14/TOJ 10 November 1904, 'Life on the Congo: sleeping sickness ravages', *Standard*
TM/14/TOJ 6a 15 November 1920, Todd to MacPhail
TM/14/TOJ 6b 3 December 1920, Todd to MacPhail
TM/14/TOJ 3a, b 29 December 1969, Bridget Fialkowski to Dr Walker
TM/14/DUJ 11 22 November 1902, Dutton to 'Griff'

Wellcome Institute for the History of Medicine, London, Western Manuscripts Collection

A. Balfour Papers

Dutton, Joseph Everett

Ms. 2248 Gambia expedition. Diary, 1901
Ms. 2251 Diary of a journey with Dr Heiberg in Lowa region, 1904
Mss. 2255–61 Photograph albums of Liverpool Tenth and Twelfth Expeditions to Africa, vols. 1902–05

Ms. 2262 Congo expedition diary, vol. 1, 1903–4
Ms. 2263 Native examination book, 1903–4
Ms. 2267 Tse-tse fly book, 1904–5
Ms. 2268 Congo expedition diary, vol. 2, 2 July 1902–12 May 1905

Todd, John Lancelot

Ms. 4801 'Congo Free State as a political unit', 1908
Ms. 4802 Notes re: rick fever and sleeping sickness, 1910–12
Ms. 4795 Notebook, 1904–6
Ms 4794 Congo native and cattle examination notes, 1904–5
Ms. 4796 Congo expedition diary, vol. 3, 13 May 1905 to 29 August 1905
Ms. 4792 Congo expedition: casebook 1, 1903–8
Ms. 4793 Congo expedition: casebook 2, 1904–5

Todd, John L., 'Congo Free State as a political unit'.
Weatherhead, E. A., Ms. journal, 1902 (Church Missionary Society, Bugala, Sesse Islands).

Wellcome Institute for the History of Medicine, London, Autograph Letters

Dutton, Joseph Everett, Mss. 314522. Correspondence with family from Congo Free State, 1 April 1902–14 October 1904.

Wellcome Institute for the History of Medicine, London, Contemporary Medical Archives Centre

Hamerton, Lt-Col. Albert Ernest, Ms. notebook and photograph album while serving on Sleeping Sickness Commission, 1908–10, 2 vols. (Acc. no. 12, ref. GC/18)

Wellcome Tropical Institute, London

Carpenter, G. Hale, 'History of sleeping sickness in Uganda', 13 August 1924, manuscript.
A. J. Duggan Papers (papers concerning Cuthbert Christy) Report and three maps on sleeping sickness in Uganda, 31 October 1902.

Wellcome Foundation Archives, London

Autograph letter collection
Wellcome Foundation records
Henry Wellcome papers
A. W. Haggis, 'The life and work of Sir Henry Wellcome', 18 August 1941, typescript
Wellcome Bureau and Wellcome Research Institute papers

Royal Commonwealth Society, London

Cuthbert Christy Papers

(Thirty-nine notebooks, exercise books, etc.)
Notebooks 9–14. Diary of Royal Society Expedition to Uganda, 1902–3
Notebooks 15–16. Diary of Liverpool School Expedition to Congo Free State, September 1903–March 1904
Notebook 18. Zoological/rubber expedition to Belgian Congo, 1912
Notebook 19. Casenotes, 1904
Notebook 20. Casenotes of Liverpool School Expedition to Congo Free State, September 1903–March 1904
Notebooks, 23–28. Six letter books of Congo Free State expedition, February 1912–January 1916
Notebook 29. Diary of Nile–Congo Divide mapping expedition and inspection for Sudan Sleeping Sickness Commission, February–October 1916

Final report to the Sudan Sleeping Sickness Commission. 'General report on a tour through the Lado, Belgian Congo and southern Bahr el-Ghazal undertaken during 1916', typescript, 32 pp.
Mann, A. R. H., ms. diary, 15 July–9 August 1935, 2 vols.
Sanders, Alfred Harry, ms. 42, diary in Bahr el-Ghazal, 1902–3

The Royal Society, London

Sleeping Sickness Conference, correspondence, 1907–8
Lyndhurst Duke correspondence, 1911–12
C. Christy correspondence, 1910–11
Papers of the Tropical Diseases Committee including Muriel Robertson and W. F. Fiske

Rhodes House, Oxford

Boyd, Alexander, ms. diary, 1 April 1906–13 November 1906 (Mss. Afr. r.5).
Browne, Dr S. G., 'Links with the past as medical missionary, Yakusu' (Mss. Afr. S. 1227).
Foran, William Robert, Five undated mss. including 'Ivory poachers in the Lado Enclave (1902–1912)', 3 vols. (Mss. Afr. S. 771–5).
Gowers, Sir William Frederick, Governor of Uganda. Diary of a visit to the Belgian Congo, 18 April–3 May 1931 (Mss. Afr. S. 1150).
Harris, Sir John Hobbis, Mss. including 'Conditions in the Congo and proposed reforms', 1908 (Mss. Afr. r.69).
 Album of press cuttings on Congo Reform Movement, 1906–7 (Mss. Brit. Emp. S. 353).
McLaren, J. C. (Enclosed in Sir J. Hobbis Harris Papers, mss. Brit. Emp. S. 353), *Western Daily Mercury*, Report on trip through Congo Free State from Dufile to Boma via the Uele.

Sudan Intelligence Reports. Egypt (1892–9). Sudan (1899–1903)

Pitt-Rivers Museum, Balfour Library, Oxford

Pring, Samuel W., diary, 22 January 1919–12 July 1921, typescript, 230 pp. 'Belgian rule in the Congo', November 1919

The Royal Geographical Society, London

Schweinfurth, Georg, correspondence

Public Record Office, Kew, London

FO 367 (series) Re: 1908 Sleeping Sickness Conference, London
FO 367.259.2447 21 January 1911, J. P. Armstrong, Acting Consul, Leopoldville. Consular report on conditions of the natives in the Uele district
FO 367.323.31211 3 July 1913, A. C. Johnson to General Wilson
FO 367.69.24474 4 June 1907, G. B. Michell to C. F. Cromie
FO 367.69.27004 24 June 1907, Michell to Cromie
FO 367.69.29312 12 August 1907, Michell to Cromie
FO 367.363.56228 1 December 1916, Kitchener to Sir Edward Grey
FO 367.215.43829 25 November 1911, Acting Consul Campbell to Sir Edward Grey
FO 403.30493 5 March 1900, Captain Moreton F. Gage, Ft Berkeley, Equatoria. Memorandum on Belgian administration of the Upper Nile

Worldwide Evangelisation Crusade (Heart of Africa Mission), Bulstrode, Gerrard's Cross

In-house bulletins

Baptist Missionary Society, Didcot

'Yakusu Quarterly Notes', March 1912–July 1960
Sub-committee minute books, 1092–14
Chesterman, Dr Clement, Yakusu, Belgian Congo, correspondence, 1919–36
General Missionary Conference Reports, 1907, 1918, 1921, 1924, Belgian Congo
Bentley, William Holman, correspondence

Interviews

Belgium

Professor P. G. Janssens, formerly Medical Officer and Chief of Medical and Public Health Laboratories, Kilo-Moto Gold Mines (1936–50). Brussels, 10 April 1982; Antwerp, 20 July 1982; Brussels, 11 April 1984

Dr C. Calewaert, Kilo-Moto Gold Mines. Ghent, 31 July 1982
René Braibant, Engineer, Kilo-Moto Gold Mines. Liège, 24 July 1982
Dr Mokassa (Budu-speaker). Brussels, 23 August 1982
R. P. Mboli André (Azande-speaker). Tongerloo Abbey, 20–1 August 1982
R. P. Ngbato Gilbert (Babua-speaker). Tongerloo Abbey, 20–1 August 1982
R. P. Engelen, Tongerloo Abbey, 14 August 1982
R. P. Menu (Dominican). Louvain, 23 July 1982
R. P. Van der Crabbe (Dominican). Louvain, 23 July 1982
M. Houssiau, retired director of Cotonco (Congo, 1927–70). Brussels, 17 August 1982
Francis Busschots, Administrateur-Délégué, Cotoni. Brussels, 2 and 17 August 1982

United Kingdom

Professor George S. Nelson, parasitologist. Liverpool School of Tropical Medicine, 14 February 1985
Professor R. Mansell-Prothero, geographer. University of Liverpool, 14 February 1985
Dr R. A. Pullan, geographer. University of Liverpool, 14 February 1985
Dr Leonard S. Goodwin, Wellcome Museum for Medical Science, London, 15 October 1984
Dr Anthony J. Duggan, Wellcome Institute for the history of Medicine, London, 8–9 August 1983; 2 December 1983
Dr Stanley G. Browne (Baptist Missionary Society, Yakusu Hospital, Congo). Sutton, Surrey, 23 August 1983
André Singer, ethnographic film-maker, London, 29 February 1984

Theses

Bakonzi, Agayo, 'The gold mines of Kilo-Moto in northeastern Zaire: 1905–1960', Ph.D. dissertation, University of Wisconsin, 1982.
Bimanyu, Deogratis, K., 'The Waungwana of eastern Zaire', Ph.D. dissertation, University of London, 1977.
Dassas-Dewitte, Colette, 'La maladie du sommeil dans l'Etat Indépendant du Congo', Mémoire de Licence, Université Libre, Brussels, 1963.
Eyers, John E., 'A. D. P. Hodges and early scientific medicine in Uganda, 1898–1918: with a select bibliography on the early history of sleeping sickness in Uganda, 1900–1920', M.A. thesis, Loughborough University of Technology, 1982.
Headrick, Rita, 'The impact of colonialism on health in French Equatorial Africa, 1880–1934', Ph.D. thesis, University of Chicago, 1987.
Hodnebo, Kjell, 'Cattle and flies: a study of cattle-keeping in Equatoria Province, the southern Sudan, 1850–1950', Hovedoppgave i historie varen, Universitet i Bergen, Norway, 1981.
Keim, C. A., 'Precolonial Mangbetu rule: political and economic factors in

19th-century Mangbetu history (northeast Zaire)', Ph.D. dissertation, Indiana University, 1979.

Lloyd, David T., 'The precolonial economic history of the Avongara-Azande *c.* 1750–1916', Ph.D. dissertation, University of California, Los Angeles, 1978.

McMaster, M. A., 'Patterns of interaction: a comparative ethnographic perspective on the Uele region of Zaire, *ca.* 500 B.C., to 1900 A.D.', Ph.D. dissertation, University of California, Los Angeles, 1988.

Ndaye, Ladislas, 'La maladie du sommeil au Congo de 1900–1930', Mémoire de Licence, Université Libre, Brussels, 1970.

Shapiro, Martin Frederick, 'Medicine in the service of colonialism: medical care in Portuguese Africa, 1885–1974', Ph.D. dissertation, University of California, Los Angeles, 1983.

Soff, Harvey G., 'A history of sleeping sickness in Uganda: administrative response 1900–1970'. Ph.D. dissertation, Syracuse University, N.Y., 1971.

Worboys, Michael, 'Science and British colonial imperialism, 1895–1940', Ph.D. dissertation, University of Sussex, 1979.

Index

The Belgian Congo appears as such rather than as Zaire.

Sleeping sickness is abbreviated in sub-entries to s-s.